Practical Guide to the Evaluation of Clinical Competence

Eric S. Holmboe, MD, FACP
Senior Vice President for Quality Research and Academic Affairs
American Board of Internal Medicine
Philadelphia, Pennsylvania
Adjunct Professor of Medicine
Yale University School of Medicine
New Haven, Connecticut

Richard E. Hawkins, MD, FACP
Vice President, Assessment Programs
National Board of Medical Examiners
Philadelphia, Pennsylvania

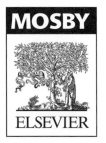

MOSBY

ELSEVIER

1600 John F. Kennedy Blvd.
Suite 1800
Philadelphia, PA 19103-2899

Library of Congress Cataloging-in-Publication Data

Practical guide to the evaluation of clinical competence / [edited by]
Eric S. Holmboe, Richard E. Hawkins.—1st ed.
    p. ; cm.
Includes bibliographical references and index.
   ISBN 978-0-323-04709-8
1. Clinical competence—Evaluation. 2. Clinical medicine—Ability testing. I. Holmboe, Eric S. II.
Hawkins, Richard E.
   [DNLM: 1. Clinical Competence. 2. Internship and Residency. 3. Education, Medical,
Graduate—standards. 4. Educational Measurement—methods. 5. Fellowships and Scholarships.
W 20 P895 2008]
R837.A2P73 2008
616—dc22   2007018058

Acquisitions Editor: James Merritt
Developmental Editor: Nicole DiCicco
Electronic Developmental Editor: Carol Emery
Project Manager: Bryan Hayward
Design Direction: Gene Harris
Cover Photo: Gene Frassetto

Printed in the United States of America.

Last digit is the print number: 9   8   7   6   5

Preface

Evaluation of medical trainees is hard but invaluable work. Evaluation of clinical competence is a core element of professionalism and underlies effective self-regulation; it is essential to fulfilling our professional obligation to assure the public that the graduates of medical training programs are competent to enter the next stage of education and/or practice. As medical educators, it is also important that we develop and use high-quality evaluation methods and systems in order to fulfill a primary obligation to our students, residents, and fellows. Here, effective evaluation provides the feedback and guidance to support their professional growth and development.

We have spent much of the last 15 years of our professional lives thinking, learning, and then teaching, about evaluation. We have had the good fortune to participate in developing or refining evaluation methods and systems across the spectrum of education and practice. Like many of you, much of our initial learning was largely through trial and error, occurring as a result of being assigned positions of responsibility in determining the competence of students and residents. Subsequently, we adopted a more deliberative approach to developing and implementing evaluation methods, and the slope of our learning curves began to increase. Our efforts to appraise the impact and effectiveness of new or enhanced evaluation methods helped us gain additional knowledge and understanding of evaluation, more so than did review of the relatively limited amount of medical literature on resident evaluation available at the time.

The impression that our knowledge and understanding about evaluation was advanced more significantly through "on-the-ground" development and measurement of evaluation approaches than through reading the literature led us to believe that sharing our experiences and knowledge might be valuable to others in the community. We started by giving faculty development workshops at various professional conferences and began to write about our experience. The organization of this book, including most of the chapters, reflects the evolving structure and content of the materials developed for our faculty development workshops.

Although originating from, and built on, previous faculty development work, this book also reflects our own professional growth and enhanced understanding of evaluation. Our discussions and collaboration with experts in the medical education and evaluation community helped us become more comfortable in applying knowledge and the "science of evaluation" principles to the day-to-day challenges confronting clerkship and program directors.

The primary purpose of this book is to provide a *practical* guide to developing evaluation systems. However, we hope that it also serves as a useful resource through inclusion of the underlying evidence base to support recommendations and facilitate understanding. The book has been organized around the various evaluation tools and how individuals with responsibilities for evaluation can apply these tools in their own setting. Each chapter provides information on the strengths and weaknesses of the evaluation method, along with information about specific tools. However, no single tool can do the whole job; effective evaluation requires a multifaceted approach.

Effective evaluation also depends upon collaboration among a *team* of faculty and other educators; thus any change to an evaluation system must include not only buy-in from others, but also the investment to train educators to use evaluation tools effectively. Evaluation tools are only as good as the individual using them. If done well, evaluation can have a profoundly positive effect on patients, trainees, and faculty. Nothing can be more satisfying than knowing each and every one of your graduates is truly ready to move to the next career level. The public expects no less, and we should expect no less from ourselves. In that spirit, we welcome comments from you the reader on how we can improve upon this book.

Eric S. Holmboe
Richard E. Hawkins

Contributors

Robert McL. Boote, BS, JD
Ballard, Spahr, Andrews & Ingersoll, LLP
Philadelphia, Pennsylvania

John R. Boulet, PhD
Assistant Vice President
Research and Evaluation
Educational Commission for Foreign
    Medical Graduates
Philadelphia, Pennsylvania

Carol Carraccio, MD, MA
Associate Chair for Education
Department of Pediatrics
University of Maryland School of Medicine
Baltimore, Maryland

Brian E. Clauser, EdD
Associate Vice President
Measurement Consulting Services
National Board of Medical Examiners
Philadelphia, Pennsylvania

Stephen G. Clyman, MD
Executive Director
Center for Innovation
National Board of Medical Examiners
Philadelphia, Pennsylvania

Margery H. Davis, MD
Professor of Medical Education
Director of the Centre for Medical
    Education
University of Dundee
Dundee, Scotland

F. Daniel Duffy, MD, MACP
Professor of Medicine
University of Oklahoma
Norman, Oklahoma
Former Executive Vice President
American Board of Internal Medicine
Philadelphia, Pennsylvania

Michael L. Green, MD, MSc
Associate Professor of Medicine
Yale University School of Medicine
Associate Program Director for Ambulatory
    Education
Yale Primary Care Internal Medicine
    Program
New Haven, Connecticut

Richard E. Hawkins, MD, FACP
Vice President
Assessment Programs
National Board of Medical Examiners
Philadelphia, Pennsylvania

Eric S. Holmboe, MD, FACP
Senior Vice President for Quality Research
    and Acadamic Affairs
American Board of Internal Medicine
Philadelphia, Pennsylvania
Adjunct Professor of Medicine
Yale University School of Medicine
New Haven, Connecticut

S. Barry Issenberg, MD, FACP
Associate Professor of Medicine
University of Miami Miller School of
    Medicine
Gordon Center for Research in Medical
    Education
Miami, Florida

Jocelyn M. Lockyer, MHA, PhD
Professor
Department of Community Health Sciences
Associate Dean
Continuing Medical Education and
    Professional Development
University of Calgary
Calgary, Canada

Catherine R. Lucey, MD, FACP
Professor of Medicine
Vice Dean for Education
College of Medicine
Ohio State University
Columbus, Ohio

Melissa J. Margolis, MS
Measurement Scientist
Measurement Associates
National Board of Medical
   Examiners
Philadelphia, Pennsylvania

John J. Norcini, PhD
President and CEO
Foundation for Advancement of
   International Medical Education and
   Research
Philadelphia, Pennsylvania

Louis Pangaro, MD
Professor and Vice Chair
Depatment of Medicine
Uniformed Services University of the
   Health Sciences
Bethesda, Maryland

Ross J. Scalese, MD
Assistant Professor of Medicine
University of Miami Miller School of
   Medicine
Gordon Center for Research in Medical
   Education
Miami, Florida

David B. Swanson
Deputy Vice President
Professional Services
National Board of Medical Examiners
Philadelphia, Pennsylvania

Acknowledgments

Much love to my wife of 25 years, Eileen Holmboe, and for supporting me through many career turns and moves.

Gratitude and love to my children, Ken and Lauren, who have to put up with their all too often "part-time" dad.

Thanks and love for Mom, Dad, Kristi, and Kevin.

Eric Holmboe

Much love and gratitude to my wife, Marguerite Hawkins, and my mother, Jacqueline Hawkins, for their support over many years.

Richard Hawkins

We both would like to sincerely thank the many trainees with whom we worked over the years. More than any other group, we learned the most working with you. Your dedication and cooperation were much appreciated.

Eric Holmboe
Richard Hawkins

Faculty Guidelines to Training DVD

This DVD provides a set of video recorded trainee–patient encounters intended to facilitate faculty development programs focusing on improving direct observation and feedback skills. These tapes can be used in conjunction with the training methods discussed in Chapter 9.

This DVD provides brief descriptions of training scenarios. The scenarios are scripted to depict varying levels of trainee proficiency. Trainee deficiencies are demonstrated in each level—none are scripted to be "perfect." There are three scenarios for each clinical skill of medical interviewing, physical examination, and counseling; each successive scenario displays progressively better performance. Following a brief introduction regarding the context of the trainee-patient encounter, the deficiencies, or "errors," for each clinical encounter scenario are outlined. It is important to note that the deficiencies range from minor to more severe; the judgment of the faculty is an important component of the training exercises. You can use this guide to help you discuss and calibrate your own faculty in workshops. We recommend you review the scenarios carefully on your own with the guidelines to become comfortable with the clinical encounters before using them in workshops with your own faculty.

How Faculty Should Conduct an Effective Observation

A separate video is provided to illustrate important concepts in direct observation. The focus of this scenario is on the faculty physician performing the observation of a resident or student. This scenario provides multiple examples of what *not* to do as a faculty member in performing an observation. A number of points should be noted about this direct observation by the faculty attending:

1. The faculty member is late, disrupting the flow of the trainee–patient encounter.
2. He does a poor job of explaining to the patient what his role will be during the observation, and was not explicit with the trainee about what he will do during the physical examination.
3. His positioning to observe the physical examination is poor; he is seated behind the patient and in front of the trainee. This makes it very difficult for him to see if the physical examination maneuvers were done correctly, and having the observer right in front of her may be distracting to the trainee.
4. He disrupts the blood pressure measurement by trying to wash his hands during the measurement.
5. He disrupts the eye examination by moving around and inserting himself into the examination process. One reason this may have distracted the trainee was the lack of explanation by the faculty physician on what he would do during the examination (see item 2 above).
6. He further disrupts the examination by asking the patient questions during the trainee's examination of the lungs. This could have been avoided had the faculty physician reviewed the patient's history and presenting complaint with the trainee before observing the physical examination. The medical history presentation could have been done at the bedside. This then cues the faculty physician on what he should be looking for during the physical examination.
7. The faculty physician is distracted by a knock at the door. This distraction causes him to miss a critical component of the examination; the cardiac examination in a patient with a presenting complaint of syncope.

These are the major take-home points from this direct observation encounter. Some basic principles for effective direct observation are as follows:

- Prepare for the observation.
  - Faculty: Know what you are looking for.
  - Resident: Let him/her know what to expect.
  - Patient: Let him/her know why you are there.
- Minimize intrusiveness—correct positioning using "triangulation," when possible.
- Minimize interference with the trainee–patient interaction.
- Avoid distractions.

Medical Interviewing Tapes (Scenarios 1–3)

Context

The patient presents with chest discomfort that started early in the morning. The setting is an emergency department and the resident is performing the history to decide whether the patient requires admission. This patient has several "key features" in his history: exertional nature of the pain and relief with rest; prior symptoms consistent with angina; and positive risk factors. These findings, along with past history, strongly suggest coronary artery disease.

Facilitator Notes

The videos show progressively better information collection (1 = poor, 3 = best of the three, but still with deficiencies), what may be referred to as the "doctor-centered" portion of the medical history. Suboptimal in all of the videos are the "patient-centered" aspects of the medical interview such as responding to concerns, body language, and so on. Video 3 is a little better in that the trainee starts with an open-ended question, asks for patient's questions, and so forth.

Physical Examinations (Scenarios 4–6)

Context

A new patient presents to an urgent care clinic with a 2-day history of productive cough and mild shortness of breath. He states he has felt warm at home. He has difficulty performing activities of daily living without dyspnea on exertion. He has an 80 pack-year smoking history and still smokes 1 pack of cigarettes per day. He was told he had a "heart murmur" some years ago, but that no further evaluation was needed. He denies a history of heart attack or angina. He also denies chest pain or paroxysmal nocturnal dyspnea. This patient has not received regular medical care since moving to a retirement apartment complex 4 years ago. His only surgical history was an appendectomy as a child. He denies any change in his stools or bowel habits, but has noted a 5-pound weight loss in the last 6 months. He notes a little swelling in his ankles that usually goes down overnight. His only medication is a multivitamin and a daily aspirin when he "remembers to take them." BP taken by nurse is 110/72 mm Hg and temperature is 101.5°F.

Physical Examination

1. Components of examination
   a. Blood pressure measurement
   b. HEENT examination
      Should examine the throat and ears
      Should examine the mucosa for pallor (eyes, mouth at minimum)—assessment for signs of anemia
   c. Neck examination—should assess for adenopathy (assessment of nodes should cover all important lymphatic areas to include supraclavicular area)
   d. Pulmonary exam—should assess for pneumonia and pleural effusion; should at minimum percuss and auscultate

e. Cardiac examination including assessment of jugular venous pressure
f. Assessment of extremities

Facilitator Notes

This patient has a right middle lobe pneumonia. Look particularly for proper examination by the trainee of the right middle lobe.

Counseling (Scenarios 7–9)

Context

This female patient has hyperlipidemia and has failed a trial of weight loss and dietary modification with no change in cholesterol level. Recent laboratory test results follow: total cholesterol is 285 mg/dL; High-density lipoprotein level is 45 mg/dL; triglyceride level is 170 mg/dL; and low-density lipoprotein level is 206 mg/dL. She returns to office today to start statin therapy. Other cardiovascular risk factors are age (>45 years); hypertension; father had heart attack at age 53; currently smoking.

Important issues for counseling are as follows:

a. Discussion of patient's role in decision making
b. Discussion of the clinical issue or nature of the decision
c. Discussion of the alternatives
d. Discussion of pros and cons of the choices
e. Discussion of the uncertainties with the decision
f. Assessment of patient's understanding
g. Exploration of patient preference

Facilitator Notes

These videos can be used to highlight important components of informed decision making for a very common scenario. They could be useful as a way to incorporate the new Adult Treatment Panel (ATP) cholesterol guidelines to discuss how the feedback to the resident on these tapes could incorporate evidenced-based medicine principles. The video also demonstrates emotion from the patient—How should one respond? The video could be used to facilitate discussion of the NURS model (**N**ame the emotion/reflect **U**nderstanding/show **R**espect/give **S**upport) of responding to emotions from patients.

The Core Elements of Informed Decision Making

Level of Decision Making Required	Component
Basic (e.g., ordering a lab test)	1, 2, 7
Intermediate (e.g., prescribing new medication)	1, 2, 3, 4, 6,. 7
Complex (e.g., invasive procedure)	All 7

Braddock Core Informed Decision-Making Components

Rate each required component performed by the trainee.

1. Discussion of patient's role in decision making
   Rationale: Many patients are not aware that they can and should participate in decision making.
   Example: "I'd like us to make to make this decision together."

2. Discussion of the clinical issue or nature of the decision
   Rationale: A clear statement of what is at issue helps to clarify what is being decided and allows the physician to share some of her/his thinking about it.
   Example: "This is a medication that would help with . . . ."

3. Discussion of alternatives
   Rationale: A decision is always a choice among certain options, including doing nothing at all.
   Example: "You could try the new medication or continue the one you are taking now."

4. Discussion of the pros (benefits) and cons (risks) of the options
   Rationale: MDs frequently discuss the pros of one option and the cons of another option without fully exploring the pros and cons of each.
   Example: "The new medication is more expensive, but you need to take it only once a day."

5. Discussion of the uncertainties associated with the decision
   Rationale: While often difficult, a discussion of the uncertainties is crucial for a patient's comprehensive understanding of the options.
   Example: "Most patients with your condition will respond to this medication, but not all."

6. Assessment of the patient's understanding
   Rationale: Once the core disclosures are made, the physician must check with the patient to know if what the doctor said so far makes sense: This is a central goal of informed decision making.
   Example: "Does that make sense to you?" "Do you have any questions so far?"

7. Exploration of patient preference
   Rationale: Physicians may assume that patients will speak up if they disagree with a decision, but patients often need to be asked for their opinion.
   Example: "Does that sound reasonable?"

Facilitator Key to the Clinical Scenarios

As noted previously, videos were scripted to illustrate varying levels of trainee proficiency; each contains some deficiencies. The scenarios were developed iteratively for use in a research study on direct observation. Provided on the following pages are the deficiencies for each encounter. You may not agree with all of them; this could be a rich source for dialogue with your workshop group. Some deficiencies are more blatant than others; the key simply denotes presence or absence of the deficiency, not degree. All of these videos can be used for direct observation of competence training described in Chapter 9.

The facilitator key is provided in the format of an abstraction instrument. The key can be used to assess faculty performance in direct observation, and to provide feedback to the faculty. The criteria are based on an absolute (criterion-based) scale, not a relative (normative-based) scale for optimal patient care. Your faculty may have different points of view depending on the level of trainee you choose for your direct observation exercises.

Scenario 1: Level 1 History Taking

Clearly Unsatisfactory. On the 9-point mini-CEX instrument, this trainee should receive a rating of 3 or lower.

Description of Deficiency

Primary

1. Failed to introduce himself
2. No open-ended questions; all questions closed-ended
3. Question about quality of pain leading ("pressure or squeezing")
4. Failed to ask if patient is having chest pain now
5. Did not ask what made pain better (alleviating)
6. Did not ask duration of discomfort
7. Failed to ask about any prior episodes of chest discomfort
8. Failed to ask about diaphoresis
9. Did not ask how severe the pain was
10. Did not ask about past medical history (except cholesterol)

Secondary

11. Lacked patient centeredness
12. Failed to ask if the patient had ever smoked
13. Failed to ask about occupation
14. Did not ask age of father at time of his heart attack
15. Family history closed-ended
16. Failed to ask patient if patient had any questions
17. Failed to recognize patientconcern atend of interview/offer empathetic or reassuring comment

Scenario 2: Level 2 History Taking

Marginal to low satisfactory. On a 9-point scale, this performance received an average rating of 4 among a group of communication experts. Research has shown that a 4 on a 9-point scale equates to a marginal, or barely satisfactory, performance.

Description of Deficiency

Primary

1. Failed to ask if patient is having chest pain now
2. Did not ask about duration of chest discomfort
3. Did not ask what made pain better

4. Did not ask about any prior episodes of chest discomfort

Secondary

5. Did not ask age of father at time of heart attack
6. Failed to ask about occupation
7. Lacked patient centeredness
8. Did not ask explicitly about heart disease in other family members
9. Failed to ask patient if patient had any questions

Scenario 3: Level 3 History Taking

High satisfactory (from a data-gathering perspective). Some experts viewed this scenario as poor in patient-centeredness.

Description of Deficiency

Secondary

1. Could be more patient centered (subjective)
2. Failed to ask patient if patient had any questions
3. Failed to ask about leg edema

Scenario 4: Level 1 Physical Examination

Clearly unsatisfactory. On the 9-point mini-CEX instrument, this trainee should receive a rating of 3 or lower.

Description of Deficiency

Primary

1. Failed to take blood pressure
2. No respiratory rate taken
3. No pulse taken
4. Cursory examination of oral cavity, no light or tongue blade
5. No examination of ears in patient with fever
6. No examination of nasal cavity
7. Did not examine sinuses
8. Lymph node examination incomplete and cursory (e.g., does not examine posterior nodes or supraclavicular)
9. Lung examination incomplete—no anterior or right middle lobe (RML) auscultation
10. Lung examination technique incorrect—does not compare from side to side (subtle to detect)
11. Lung examination—no percussion
12. Cardiac examination—no assessment of point of maximal impulse (PMI)
13. Cardiac examination—no use of bell to assess S3 or S4
14. Cardiac examination—does not listen to heart in recumbent position
15. Cardiac examination—no assessment of jugular venous distension (JVD)

Secondary

16. Abdominal examination not performed

17. Carotid examination not performed
18. Thyroid examination not performed

Scenario 5: Level 2 Physical Examination

Marginal performance. This performance was rated a 4 on a 9-point scale by two experts in physical diagnosis.

Description of Deficiency

Primary

1. Pulse not taken
2. Respiratory rate not taken
3. Did not examine ears
4. Did not examine nasal passages
5. Lymph node examination too rapid and cursory (did not examine posterior, supraclavicular nodes completely)
6. Lung examination incomplete—no anterior or RML auscultation
7. Cardiac examination—no assessment of JVD

Secondary

8. Took blood pressure in incorrect position
9. Did not ask if sinuses tender when palpated
10. Thyroid examination not performed
11. Carotid examination not performed
12. Abdominal examination not performed

Scenario 6: Level 3 Physical Examination

High satisfactory to low superior. This trainee should receive a score of 6 or 7 on a 9-point mini-CEX scale.

Description of Deficiency

Primary

1. Respiratory rate not taken
2. Did not examine nasal passages
3. Pulmonary—did not listen anteriorly with stethoscope
4. Cardiac—did not assess PMI

Secondary

5. Did not listen to complete respiratory cycle before moving stethoscope
6. Thyroid examination not performed
7. Posterior lymph node examination not completed
8. Abdominal examination not performed

Scenario 7: Level 1 Counseling

Clearly unsatisfactory. On the 9-point mini-CEX instrument, this trainee should receive a rating of 3 or lower.

Description of Deficiency

Primary

1. No discussion of patient role in decision making
2. No discussion of the risks (side effects)

3. No discussion of alternatives
4. No mention of dose
5. No assessment of patient's understanding (Do you have any questions?)
6. No discussion of the uncertainties of starting the medicine
7. No exploration of patient preference
8. Failed to address patient reluctance to take medicine

Secondary

9. No discussion of the degree/magnitude of benefit for stroke or acute myocardial infarction (AMI) prevention
10. Did not respond to nonverbal cues
11. Follow-up interval too long
12. Never told patient her cholesterol level
13. Never told patient her goal cholesterol level

Scenario 8: Level 2 Counseling

Marginal performance. Although the resident is pleasant, a number of key items necessary for informed decision making are lacking. Two experts in informed decision making rated this performance a 4 on a 9-point scale.

Description of Deficiency

Primary

1. No discussion of patient role in decision making
2. No discussion of alternatives
3. No discussion of other side effects (e.g., myopathy)
4. No mention of dose
5. No exploration of patient preference

6. No discussion of the uncertainties of starting the medicine
7. No response to patient reluctance to take medicine

Secondary

8. No discussion of the degree/magnitude of benefit for stroke or AMI prevention
9. Follow-up interval too long
10. Failed to counsel on need for blood test at 6 weeks
11. Never told patient her goal low-density lipoprotein level
12. Missed opportunity to counsel on tobacco use

Scenario 9: Level 3 Counseling

High satisfactory to low superior. This trainee should receive a score of 6 or 7 on a 9-point mini-CEX scale. The trainee may have provided *too* much information for patient, and was not sufficiently patient-centered.

Description of Deficiency

Primary

1. No discussion of the uncertainties of starting the medicine

Secondary

2. No mention of dose
3. Did not completely respond to patient fear
4. Frames other medications negatively

Contents

1

Evaluation Challenges in the Era of Outcomes-Based Education

John J. Norcini, PhD, Eric S. Holmboe, MD,
and Richard E. Hawkins, MD

DRIVERS OF CHANGE IN ASSESSMENT
Outcomes-Based Education
Accountability and Quality Assurance
Technology
Psychometrics

FRAMEWORK FOR ASSESSMENT
Dimension 1: Competencies
  Medical Knowledge
  Interpersonal and Communication Skills
  Patient Care
  Professionalism
  Practice-Based Learning and Improvement
  Systems-Based Practice
Dimension 2: Levels of Assessment
  Miller's Pyramid
  The Cambridge Model
Dimension 3: Assessment of Progression

CRITERIA FOR CHOOSING A METHOD

ELEMENTS OF EFFECTIVE FACULTY DEVELOPMENT

FUTURE CHALLENGES
Methods of Assessment
  Traditional Measures
  Methods Based on Observation
  Simulation
  Work
New Competencies: Teamwork and
  Systems-Based Practice
Systems of Assessment

CONCLUSION

REFERENCES

Through the early 1950s, physicians were assessed in limited ways.[1] Medical knowledge was evaluated with essays and other open-ended question formats that were graded by an instructor. Clinical skill and judgment were tested using an oral examination that often required the student to go to the bedside, gather patient information, and present it along with a diagnostic list and treatment plan to one or more examiners who asked questions. Because these were the only generally accepted methods available, they were applied to most assessment problems even if they were not completely suitable to the task.

From that point to the present, there have been extensive changes in the way assessment is conducted. Methods have proliferated, as has the sophistication of their use. Much progress has been made in the assessment of medical knowledge with a variety of written and computer-based techniques offering reliable and valid results. In the last few decades, considerable

gains have been made in defining and enhancing the psychometric qualities of objective structured clinical examinations (OSCEs), particularly related to their use in high-stakes examinations. However, assessment in the context of clinical education has lagged to some degree, especially in the areas of clinical skills and performance. Equally important, the methods that have been developed to support clinical education often rely on faculty who are inexperienced in their use, do not share common standards, and have not been trained to apply them in a consistent fashion. Faculty development has failed to keep pace with the application of these new educational methods.

This chapter will present an overview of the drivers of change in the assessments used during clinical education, a framework for such assessment, criteria for choosing methods, elements of an effective faculty development effort, and the nature of future challenges.

Drivers of Change in Assessment

The increase in the number of methods and the enhanced sophistication of assessment overall has been motivated by public pressure for accountability and quality improvement. This has been accompanied by curricular changes in the form of outcomes-based education and supported by improvements in technology and psychometrics.

Outcomes-Based Education

Consistent with trends in all of education, the past two decades have seen an evolution in the thinking about how physicians should be trained.[2,3] A focus on the educational process has given way to an emphasis on what a physician should look like at the end of training and at important junctures during the training process. Outcomes-based education starts with a specification of the competencies expected of a physician, and these requirements drive the content and structure of the curriculum, the selection and deployment of teaching and learning methods, the site of training, and the nature of the teachers. Assessment plays a central role in determining whether students and residents have actually achieved the competencies that have been specified and whether the educational program has been efficacious.

This change in thinking and the need to assess the diverse competencies of the physician has been an important factor in the development of new methods of assessment. Pressure for additional developments will persist as more schools and programs implement changes to attain the goals of an outcomes-based education.

Accountability and Quality Assurance

The movement to outcomes-based education has been accompanied by significant efforts to enhance the accountability of physicians.[4] Motivated in part by high-profile cases such as those involving Michael Swango in the United States and Howard Shipman in the United Kingdom, the public has pressured medicine to increase its level of oversight and eliminate the "bad apples."[5,6] Medical educators are also more keenly aware that too many trainees graduate with substantial deficiencies in knowledge and clinical skills.[7,8] Promoting trainees who lack competence erodes the trust between the medical profession and the public.

At the same time, there has been a variety of efforts to improve the quality of health care.[9–11] These efforts have relied on methods devised by workers in the field of quality management science and, in some cases, used successfully in industry for over 50 years. Central to both accountability and quality assurance is assessment. It offers a means of identifying those whose overall performance is well below standards and identifying areas of weakness, helping to drive the continuous quality improvement process. These developments have helped to fuel the creation of several new methods of assessment and to increase the use of those already available.

Technology

Over the past 50 years, the availability of more sophisticated technology has changed the testing of medical knowledge and judgment in fundamental ways.[12,13] The introduction of the computer heralded an era of large-scale testing by encouraging the use of multiple-choice questions (MCQs) that could be scanned by machine, turned into scores, and then reported in an efficient and objective fashion.

More recently, the intelligence of the computer has improved assessment in two ways:

1. On the one hand, it has enabled the application of significant psychometric advances to the assessment of medical knowledge. Specifically, the computer's intelligence has improved efficiency by allowing the selection of questions that are targeted to the ability of particular examinees. Sequential testing and adaptive testing permit gains in efficiency and precision.
2. On the other hand, it has improved the assessment of clinical decision making by permitting the use of interactive item formats that more closely simulate the types of judgments physicians need to make in practice.

The impact of technology on assessment of clinical skills has been slower to develop but there are now a number of tools that recreate aspects of the clinical encounter with considerable fidelity. These methods have a growing impact on assessment, especially in the area of procedural skills.

Psychometrics

At the same time that the technology has improved, there have been significant advances in psychometrics, the basic science of assessment. Classical test theory, prominent from the turn of the 20th century, has gradually given way to measurement models based on strong assumptions about test items and examinees. The family of item response theory models now makes it possible to produce equivalent scores even when examinees take tests made up of different questions.[14] They also support the computer-based administration of examinations that are tailored to the ability level of individual test-takers; this allows tests to be shortened by as much as 40%.[15] The ability to shorten tests has cost and validity implications; less test material exposure decreases the likelihood that future examinees are familiar with examination content.

Generalizability theory, another major development, makes it possible to identify how much error is associated with different facets of measurement (e.g., raters, patients).[16] Based on this information, assessments can be prospectively designed to make the best use of resources, such as faculty time, while maintaining the reliability of the results.

In addition to these major developments, there have been a number of other advances. For example, there is a variety of systematic methods available for setting standards on tests and for identifying when test questions are biased against particular groups of examinees.[17,18] Test development methods have gotten better, as have the means for judging whether particular items are working properly. Overall, these advances have improved both the quality and efficiency of assessment.

Framework for Assessment

As methods of assessment have proliferated, so has the need to use them efficiently and to combine them into a system of evaluation. Developing, implementing, and sustaining effective systems for the evaluation of clinical competence in medical school, residency, and fellowship programs require consideration of what competencies need to be assessed, how to best assess them, and the level of the trainee being assessed. Consequently, a three-dimensional framework for structuring an assessment system is needed. Along the first dimension are the competencies that need to be assessed, along the second is the level of assessment required, and along the third is the trainees' stage of development.

Dimension 1: Competencies

As shown in Table 1-1, there are several schemes for describing the knowledge, skills, and attributes of the physician.[4,19–21] The Canadian Medical Education Directions for Specialists (CanMEDS) model, which was developed by the Royal College of Physicians and Surgeons in Canada, describes the competencies in terms of the roles of a physician. Good Medical Practice, which was created by the General Medical Council in the United Kingdom, describes the elements of good practice.

In the United States, two influential groups developed a set of core competencies. The Accreditation Council for Graduate Medical Education (ACGME) and the American Board of Medical Specialties (ABMS) adopted six general competencies. These competencies are the outcomes framework for residency and fellowship training as well as maintenance of certification programs throughout a physician's career in the United States. The Institute of Medicine (IOM) has recommended five core skills, or competencies, that create a framework for evaluating performance and stimulating the reform of education. They are intended to improve professional education and practice with a goal of enhancing the safety and quality of health care. Although there are some differences among the schemes, there is also significant overlap in these descriptions of a physician.

For purposes of this chapter, we will focus on the six ACGME/ABMS competencies: medical knowledge, interpersonal and communication skills, patient care, professionalism, practice-based learning and improvement, and system-based practice. Definitions for each of these follow with more emphasis on the last two, which are relatively new.

These competencies are intended as the first step in identifying the learning objectives of graduate training programs, and it is anticipated that they will be adapted to the content, education, and practice of the particular specialty/subspecialty. The data produced by the assessment of these competencies serve as a basis for judging the quality of the trainees and their training, as well as supporting the continuous improvement of both.

Medical Knowledge

Students, residents, and practicing physicians must possess knowledge of the basic and clinical sciences and be able to apply them to patient care. Moreover, they are expected to demonstrate an appropriate approach to reasoning about clinical problems.

Table 1-1 **The Competencies of Physicians as Described by Four Organizations**

CANMEDs	GMC	ACGME/ABMS	IOM
Medical expert	Good clinical care	Medical knowledge	Employ evidence-based practice
Communicator	Maintaining good medical practice	Interpersonal and communication skills	Work in interdisciplinary teams
Collaborator	Teaching and training appraising and assessing	Patient care	Provide patient-centered care
Manager	Relationships with patients	Professionalism	—
Health advocate	Working with colleagues	Practice-based learning and improvement	Apply quality improvement
Scholar	Probity	Systems-based practice	Utilize informatics
Professional	Health	—	—

ABMS, American Board of Medical Specialists; ACGME, Accreditation Council for Graduate Medical Education; CanMEDS, Canadian Medical Education Directions for Specialists; GMC, General Medical Council (UK); IOM, Institute of Medicine.

Interpersonal and Communication Skills

Students, residents, and practicing physicians must possess the interpersonal and communication skills that produce effective information exchange and relationships among members of the health care team. With patients, this competence supports the development and maintenance of a therapeutic and ethical relationship.

Patient Care

Good patient care requires that physicians are both compassionate and effective. They must be able to communicate well and demonstrate caring while gathering the data they need. This competence necessitates informed decisions based on medical knowledge and patient preferences, management plans that are carried out fully, and counseling of both patients and their families. Essential procedures must be carried out safely and effectively.

Professionalism

Students, residents, and practicing physicians must be committed to carrying out their professional responsibilities, adhering to ethical principles, and being sensitive to patients. Professionalism is ingrained in overall clinical competence and includes the aspirations to excellence, humanism, accountability, and altruism.

Practice-Based Learning and Improvement

Trainees and practicing physicians are expected to apply scientific evidence and use methods to investigate, evaluate, and continuously improve the quality of care for patients. This requires trainees to identify areas of opportunity for improvement, identify and correct medical errors, and use information technology at the point of care for the benefit of patients. The appropriate knowledge, skills, and attitudes in quality improvement and evidence-based medicine are needed for this competency.[22]

Systems-Based Practice

Trainees and practicing physicians require a deep understanding of both the micro- and macro-systems in which health care is provided. Trainees must learn to apply this knowledge to utilize efficiently and effectively the resources, health care providers, and technology to optimize the care delivered not only to individual patients, but to populations of patients as well. Knowledge, skills, and attitudes in effective teamwork are crucial to this general competency.[22,23]

Dimension 2: Levels of Assessment

The multifaceted nature of the competencies makes it apparent that no single method could provide a sufficient basis for making judgments about students or residents. In an organized approach to this problem, Miller proposed a classification scheme that stratifies assessment methods based on what they require of the trainee. Often referred to as Miller's pyramid, it is composed of four levels: knows, knows how, shows how, and does.[24]

Miller's Pyramid

Knows. This is the lowest level of the pyramid and it contains methods that assess what a trainee "knows" in an area of competence. Forming the base of the pyramid, knowledge represents the foundation upon which clinical competence is built. An MCQ-based examination composed of questions focused on ethics and principles of patient confidentiality would provide an assessment of what a trainee "knows" about professionalism.

Knows how. To function as a physician, a good knowledge base is necessary but insufficient. It is important to know how to use this knowledge in the acquisition of data, the analysis and interpretation of findings, and the development of management plans. For example, a method that poses a moral dilemma, asks trainees to reason through it, and evaluates the sophistication of their moral thinking would provide a "knows how" assessment of professionalism.

Shows how. Although trainees may know and know how, they may not be able to integrate these skills into a successful performance with patients. Consequently, certain assessment methods require the trainee to show how they perform with patients. For example, a standardized patient presenting with an ethical challenge would offer the trainee an opportunity to "show how" he or she would respond to a professionalism challenge.

Does. No matter how good traditional assessment methods become, there remains the concern that what happens in a controlled testing environment does not generalize directly to what happens in practice. The highest level of Miller's pyramid, therefore, focuses on methods that provide an assessment of routine performance. For example, the development and use of a critical incident system, such as the one currently used in some medical schools, offers an assessment of what students actually do in terms of professionalism.

Miller's pyramid is a useful framework for considering differences and similarities among assessment methods. However, the fact that it is a pyramid might imply to some that methods addressing the higher levels are better. Instead, superior methods are those best aligned with the purpose of the test. For example, if an assessment of medical knowledge is needed, a method associated with that level (e.g., multiple-choice questions) is better than a method associated with another level (e.g., standardized patients).

The Cambridge Model

As physicians near the end of training and enter practice, external forces come to play a very large role in performance. The Cambridge Model, a variation on Miller's pyramid, proposes that performance in practice (the highest level of the pyramid) is influenced by two large forces beyond competence.[25] Systems-related factors, such as government programs, patient expectations, and guidelines, strongly influence what physicians do. Similarly, factors related to the individual physician such as state of mind, physical and mental health, and relationships with peers and family have a significant effect. Consequently, assessment becomes more difficult because it is harder to disentangle the effects of the context of care from the competence of the individual physician. Here, a focus on health care processes and outcomes as a measure of what a physician "does" may provide a more valid assessment of a physician's ability to integrate multiple competencies within a complex social context.

Dimension 3: Assessment of Progression

Acquiring competence is not an overnight process. Trainees progress through a series of stages that begin in undergraduate medical education and continue throughout their careers. Educators must be able to recognize when a trainee has attained sufficient knowledge, skills, and attitudes to enter the next stage and this requires appropriate standards and benchmarks for the transition. Hubert and Stuart Dreyfus have created a developmental model of learning applicable to the health professions that proposes five stages of educational development (Table 1-2).[26]

The Dreyfus model proposes that each stage of learning requires a different method of teaching. The novice needs instructor-driven teaching, but the expert needs

Table 1-2 The Stages of Learning as Proposed by Dreyfus

Stage of Learning	Method of Learning (Teaching Style)	Learning Steps	Learner Characteristics
1. Novice	Instruction (instructor) Breaks skill into context-free, discrete tasks, concepts, rules	Recognizes the context-free features Knows rules for determining actions based on these features	Learning occurs in a detached analytic frame of mind
2. Advanced beginner	Practice (coach) Experiences coping with real situations Points out new aspects of material Teaches rules and reasoning techniques for action	Recognizes relevant aspects based on experience that makes sense of the material Learns maxims about actions based on new material	Learning occurs in a detached, analytic frame of mind
3. Competence	Apprenticeship (facilitator) Develops a plan or chooses perspective that separates "important" from "ignored" elements Demonstrates that rules and reasoning techniques for choosing are difficult to come by Role models are also emotionally involved in making decisions	Volume of aspects is overwhelming Performance is exhausting Sense of what's important is lacking Stands alone making correct and incorrect choices Coping becomes frightening, discouraging, elating	Learner is emotionally involved in the task and its outcome Too many subtle differences for rules; student must decide in each case Makes a mistake, then feels remorse Succeeds, then feels elated Emotional learning builds competence
4. Proficiency	Apprenticeship (supervisor) Gains more specific experience with outcomes of one's decisions Applies rules and maxims to decide what to do	Rules and principles are replaced by situational discrimination Emotional responses to success or failure build intuitive responses that replace reasoned ones	Learner immediately sees the goal and salient features Learner reasons how to get to the goal by applying rules and principles
5. Expertise	Independence (mentor) Experiences multiple, small random variations Observes other experts or experiences nonrandom simulations Working through the cases must emotionally matter	Gains experience with increasingly subtle variations in situations Automatically distinguishes situations requiring one response from those requiring another	Immediately sees the goal and what must be done to achieve it Builds on previous learning experiences

From Dreyfus HL: On the Internet. Thinking in Action Series. New York, Routledge, 2001.

independence. Likewise, the characteristics of learners and the steps they must go through to acquire competence will change over the five stages of development. Necessarily, the methods of assessment applied at each developmental level must also evolve. For example, at the level of the novice, an MCQ-based knowledge test might be most appropriate, but a standardized patient–based examination might be better suited to trainees who are in the competence or proficiency stages. Educators need to recognize this developmental sequence when designing an assessment system and it will be critical to ensure that the chosen method is suitable to the task.

Criteria for Choosing a Method

Decisions about which method of assessment to use in a particular circumstance have traditionally rested on validity and reliability. Validity is the degree to which the inferences based on the scores of an assessment are correct. Reliability, a closely related concept, is a measure of the repeatability or consistency of scores, akin to the 95% confidence intervals often provided with medical tests. Valid inferences regarding a particular test score or assessment result are to a large extent dependent upon the reliability of these outcomes. These are certainly critical characteristics of educational tests and they have the further advantage of being quantifiable.

For purposes of assessment in medical education, van der Vleuten and Schuwirth have recently added educational effect, feasibility, and acceptability as factors to be considered in choosing a method of assessment. In terms of educational effect, they argue that trainees will work hard in preparation for an assessment.[27] Consequently, the method should direct them to study in the most relevant way. For example, if an educational objective is for trainees to know the differential diagnoses for a particular chief complaint, then assessment using extended matching questions will induce better learning than assessment based on standardized patients.

Feasibility is the extent to which an assessment method is affordable and efficient. Although high-fidelity simulations might be a good way to assess procedural competence, the use of a method such as direct observation of procedural skills (DOPs), which is based on faculty observation, is likely to be more feasible in most graduate training settings.[28]

Acceptability is the degree to which the trainees and faculty believe that the method produces valid results. This factor will influence motivation of faculty to use the method and reduce the trainees' distrust of the results. It is important that educational leaders not underestimate trainee knowledge and understanding of assessment and their ability to participate in decisions regarding assessment practices.

In addition to these five factors, it is important to consider how a particular method fits into the overall system for assessment. The same method can be used to assess more than one competence. For example, peer assessment can provide a measure of both professionalism and interpersonal skills. Likewise, two different methods can be used to capture information on the same competence, thereby increasing confidence in the results. For example, patient care can be assessed using both the mini-CEX (clinical evaluation exercise) and monthly ratings by attending physicians.

Educational effect, feasibility, and acceptability are not easily quantifiable, nor is the relationship among methods of assessment in a system. However, these factors plus reliability and validity should be weighed when considering selection of a particular method.

Elements of Effective Faculty Development

Although faculty members are important to evaluation regardless of method, they play a particularly critical role in assessment in the clinical setting because it is often based on observation. Recall that Miller placed "performance," meaning the care of actual patients, at the tip of the pyramid. Envision the pyramid as a spear and at the tip of that spear are patients. Using this metaphor helps faculty appreciate the central role of observation in both assuring trainee competence and guaranteeing that patients receive high-quality, safe care in the context of training.

In many respects, assessment methods based on observation are only as good as the individuals using them. Although there has been substantial progress in creating these new methods, significantly less attention has been paid to the development of approaches to training faculty in how to use them most effectively. This omission continues to occur despite repeated studies demonstrating significant problems with the quality of faculty assessments.[29–31]

There are three significant reasons why faculty training is urgently needed. First, in order to perform quality assessment, faculty members must possess sufficient knowledge, skill, and attitudes in that competency. For example, the decline of clinical skills teaching in the 1980s and 1990s resulted in many of today's educators failing to acquire a high level of clinical skills themselves. This limits the degree to which they can validly assess clinical performance.

Second, the competencies will evolve and change over time. Witness the birth of the "new" competencies of practice-based learning and improvement and systems-based practice. The majority of faculty today never received any formal instruction in these competencies during their own training and thus they are often learning new knowledge and skills alongside their trainees.

Finally, assessment is a core tenet of professionalism for medical educators. Too often, faculty members view it as someone else's job, especially when a negative performance appraisal is involved. Faculty development reinforces the importance of assessment and provides medical educators the opportunity to develop common standards for performance.

To make effective use of the methods of assessment based on observation, educational institutions must commit the necessary resources for faculty development. However, too often faculty development translates into a project or a brief workshop. If faculty development is to be truly successful, medical educators need to embrace new strategies that embed faculty development in real-time teaching and clinical activities. Faculty development, like quality improvement and maintenance of competence, must become a continuous process and appropriately rewarded. As noted earlier, the quality and safety of patient care depend on it.

Medical educators must also end their quest for the holy grail of evaluation, the perfect rating form imbued with special powers to solve all evaluation needs. Evaluation is hard work and it requires a multifaceted approach. Landry and Farr, in a landmark article in the performance appraisal field nearly 25 years ago, pleaded with researchers to redirect development efforts from a search for the perfect rating form to training the assessors.[32] Researchers in this field subsequently developed a number of validated approaches that can lead to better evaluations. Table 1-3 provides a summary of several approaches with applicability for medical educators. Most, if not all, of these approaches can be used in small, repeated aliquots of time longitudinally, and there is some evidence that they work in the medical education setting.[33,34] Chapter 9 provides detail on how these training approaches

were modified to create a faculty training program to improve observation skills.

Future Challenges

Although considerable strides have been made in assessment, much work remains to be done. Specifically, effort is needed to continue to (1) refine the different methods of assessment, (2) expand their application to new competencies such as teamwork and systems-based practice, and (3) develop systems that integrate them in support of ongoing quality improvement.

Methods of Assessment

Traditional Measures

Traditional measures will continue to play an important role in the assessment of clinical proficiency. Specifically, written methods such as MCQs and standardized patients will be mainstays of all assessment programs for the near future. All of these methods can be improved and work on each must continue.

Methods Based on Observation

Even though assessment has been woven through the basic science curriculum, historically it has not been as

Table 1-3 **Methods to Train Faculty in the General Competencies**

Training Method	Description	Example
Performance dimension training (PDT)	Familiarize faculty with appropriate performance dimensions or standards for use in evaluation by reviewing the dimensions of a performance or competency. Faculty members work in small groups to improve their understanding of these definitions with review of actual trainee performance or clinical evaluation vignettes. PDT should focus on optimal performance.	Faculty members discuss the elements of what constitutes a safe and efficient discharge of a patient who needs home assistance and follow-up (systems-based practice).
Frame-of-reference training	Using the results of the PDT exercise, faculty members define what would constitute "satisfactory" performance (the anchor point). Faculty members then practice evaluating trainees performing at various levels of competence using the evaluation instrument of choice. The group discusses reasons for the differences between faculty ratings.	Faculty members are given several vignettes along with examples of the medical record, etc., regarding a discharge performed by a resident. For each vignette, the faculty members rate the level of performance (unsatisfactory, marginal, satisfactory, superior). The vignettes provide examples of different levels of competence in systems-based practice. After each rating, group members discuss their ratings with each other. This exercise helps to "calibrate" faculty to be able to discriminate between different levels of competence.
Rater error training	Faculty members discuss the common errors (such as halo effect or compensation fallacy) in ratings. Each error is described and defined.	Examples of each error are provided for discussion and review. Actual examples from the program could be used.

well integrated with clinical education. Nonetheless, assessment methods based on the observation of routine encounters in the clinical setting offer a rich and feasible target for assessment. Continued refinement of the methods themselves is needed, as is faculty development, which is a key to their successful use. Furthermore, the opportunity for educational feedback as part of these methods is probably as important as their assessment potential.

Simulation

Improvements in technology have spurred the development of a series of simulators that recreate reality with high fidelity. The use of simulation in assessment is in its infancy, the technology remains expensive, and several developments are needed before widespread adoption and use. Researchers will need to continue to focus on identifying appropriate scoring methods, optimizing the generalizability of scores, and ensuring their relevance to performance in practice.[35] Particularly in the area of procedural skills, however, these methods will offer the ability to test under a variety of conditions without concern for harm to patients. Educators will confront difficult decisions requiring them to balance the cost, variable fidelity of individual simulation methods, and potential risks to patients (and trainees) in making decisions regarding how best to assess procedural skills.[36]

Work

The assessment of physicians' performance at work (the "does" level of Miller's pyramid) is a relatively recent development. Despite the need for significant research, the day-to-day performance of physicians is being used increasingly in the settings of continuous quality improvement and physician accountability. Assessment in this context is a matter of identifying the basis for the judgments (e.g., outcomes, process of care), deciding how the data will be gathered, and avoiding threats to validity and reliability (e.g., patient mix, patient complexity, attribution, and numbers of patients).[37] Given the pressure to increase quality and decrease costs, it is important that improvements in this form of assessment happen quickly.

New Competencies: Teamwork and Systems-Based Practice

The concepts of systems-based practice and interdisciplinary team education are only now taking shape in clinical practice and medical education. Educators are struggling to determine how to incorporate these new competencies into their curricula, so it is not surprising that the current science around evaluating competencies is in its infancy. However, several groups are defining the specific knowledge, skills, and attitudes required for competent interdisciplinary teamwork and interaction with health care systems.[23,38] Chapter 11

provides a framework for integrating systems-based thinking and practice into the educational environment and a starter set of evaluation measures and methods.

Systems of Assessment

The movement toward outcomes-based education and assessment presents many challenges for medical educators. Educational leaders will need to integrate traditional and new assessment methods into their educational programs to ensure that individual trainees meet important educational and professional objectives and to inform continued quality improvement of their programs. Assessment approaches must be clearly aligned with educational objectives and congruent with teaching and learning methods. Assessment should be closely intertwined with instructional activities in order to optimize efficient use of resources and to consolidate learning. The assessment system will need to include multiple methods to capture each of the general competencies and ideally to provide for the assessment of different aspects of each competency by different methods. Program and clerkship directors will need to prepare the assessors, through the implementation of robust faculty development programs, and inform and engage trainees in order for the assessment system to succeed.

Beyond the performance of individual trainees, the assessment system will need to support the continuous collection and analysis of aggregate data to provide feedback regarding the quality of the educational program. This includes information from more traditional assessment methods, such as program-level subscores on MCQ examinations or aggregate case-level data from clinical skills examinations, as well as composite scores or ratings from newer methods such as multisource feedback and computer simulation–based exercises. It also involves collection and analysis of clinical information, such as compliance with evidence-based health care processes or patient health outcomes that can provide the impetus for curricular change or feedback on the quality of educational interventions. Establishing such a connection, at least at the institutional level, will facilitate conduct of needed research to elucidate the relationships between educational activities and health care practices and outcomes.

In addition to compiling aggregate data within programs to inform quality improvement initiatives, assessment systems will need to enable information gathering regarding the performance of program graduates. As with concurrent measures, educational leaders will need to access and incorporate into their assessment systems information about future competence and performance of program graduates in order to guide quality improvement efforts. Some information, such as licensure actions, in-training or board certification examination scores, or program director ratings may not be difficult to obtain. Obtaining other sources of information, such as specific performance measures or clinical data, to provide additional feedback regarding educational program quality will require more effort. The formation of collaborative projects and networks linking professional and clinical outcomes across the spectrum of education and practice will facilitate understanding and incorporation of information critical to the continuous quality improvement of educational programs.

Conclusion

Public and professional pressure to increase accountability and quality improvement in clinical care has resulted in important changes in medical education and assessment. Delineation of essential physician competencies and a move toward outcomes-based medical education has led to a critical review of the quality and methods used in the assessment of competence and performance. Advances in technology and psychometrics have supported continued refinement of traditional assessment modalities and the development of new approaches. Educational leaders now face difficult challenges in developing and integrating assessment systems into their educational programs. They must understand the psychometric properties of various assessment tools, consider their relevance to trainee level, as well as to instructional methods and educational objectives, and then balance these factors against program culture and resource availability in deciding what methods to use in their assessment system. The chapters that follow are intended to help guide educational leaders in designing their assessment systems to support evaluation of individual trainees and continuous quality improvement of their educational programs.

REFERENCES

1. Norman GR: Research in medical education: Three decades of progress. BMJ 2002;324:1560–1562.
2. Harden RM, Crosby JR, Davis M: An introduction to outcome-based education. Med Teacher 1999;21(1):7–14.
3. Association of Medical Education in Europe: Education Guide No 14: Outcome-based Education. Dundee, AMEE, 1999.
4. Institute of Medicine: Crossing the Quality Chasm: A New Health System for the 21st Century. Washington, DC, National Academy Press, 2001.
5. Stewart JB: Blind Eye: How the Medical Establishment Let a Doctor Get Away with Murder. New York, Simon & Shuster, 1999.
6. The Final Report of the Shipman Inquiry. Accessed at http://www.the-shipman-inquiry.org.uk/backgroundinfo.asp, July 26, 2007.
7. Mangione S, Nieman LZ: Cardiac auscultatory skills of internal medicine and family practice trainees. A comparison of diagnostic proficiency. JAMA 1997;278(9):717–722.
8. Reilly BM: Physical examination in the care of medical inpatients: An observational study. Lancet 2003;362(9390):1100–1105.
9. Berwick DM, Godfrey AB, Rossener J: Curing Health Care: New Strategies for Quality Improvement. San Francisco, Jossey-Bass, 1990.
10. Laffel G, Blumenthal D: The case for using industrial quality management science in health care organizations. JAMA 1989;262:2869–2873.
11. Plsek PE: Quality improvement methods in clinical medicine. Pediatrics 1999;103(Suppl):203–214.
12. Bunderson CV, Inouye DK, Olsen JB: The four generations of computerized educational measurement. In Linn RL (ed):
Educational Measurement. Washington, DC, American Council on Education, 1989.
13. Norcini JJ: Computers in physician licensure and certification: New methods of assessment. J Educ Computing Res 1994;10:161–171.
14. Hambleton RK, Swaminathan H: Item response theory: Principles and applications. Dordrecht, Kluwer, 1985.
15. Green BF: Adaptive testing by computer. In Ekstrom RB (ed): Principles of Modern Psychological Measurement. San Francisco, Jossey-Bass, 1983, pp 5–12.
16. Brennan RL: Generalizability Theory. New York, Springer-Verlag, 2001.
17. Norcini JJ: Standard setting. In Dent JA, Harden RM (eds): A Practical Guide for Medical Teachers. Churchill Livingstone, 2005, pp 293–301.
18. Ekstrom RA (ed): Handbook of Methods for Detecting Test Bias. Baltimore, Johns Hopkins Press, 1982.
19. Frank JR, Jabbour M, Tugwell P, et al: Skills for the new millennium: Report of the societal needs working group, CanMEDS 2000 Project. Ann R Coll Phys Surg Can 1996;29:206–216.
20. General Medical Council: Good Medical Practice. London, General Medical Council, 2001.
21. Leach DC: A model for GME: Shifting from process to outcomes. A progress report from the Accreditation Council for Graduate Medical Education. Med Educ 2004;38(1):12–14.
22. American Board of Internal Medicine (ABIM): Portfolio for Internal Medicine Residency Programs. Philadelphia, ABIM, 2004.
23. Baker GR, Gelmon S, Headrick L, et al: Collaborating for improvement in health professions education. Qual Manag Health Care 1998;6(2):1–11.
24. Miller G: The assessment of clinical skills/competence/performance. Acad Med 1990;65(Suppl):S63–S67.
25. Rethans JJ, Norcini JJ, Barón-Maldonado M, et al: The relationship between competence and performance: Implications for assessing practice performance. Med Educ 2002;36:901–909.
26. Dreyfus HL: On the Internet. Thinking in Action Series. New York, Routledge, 2001.
27. Van der Vleuten CP, Schuwirth LW: Assessing professional competence: From methods to programmes. Med Educ 2005;39(3):309–317.
28. National Health Service: Modernising Medical Careers: The Foundation Programmes. Accessed at http://www.mmc.nhs.uk/pages/foundation, Nov. 17, 2006.
29. Herbers JE Jr, Noel GL, Cooper GS, et al: How accurate are faculty evaluations of clinical competence? J Gen Intern Med 1989;4:202–208.
30. Noel GL, Herbers JE Jr, Caplow MP, et al: How well do internal faculty members evaluate the clinical skills of residents? Ann Intern Med 1992;117:757–765.
31. Kroboth FJ, Hanusa BH, Parker S, et al: The inter-rater reliability and internal consistency of a clinical evaluation exercise. J Gen Intern Med. 1992;7:174–179.
32. Landy FJ, Farr JL: The Measurement of Work Performance: Methods, Theory and Applications. Orlando, FL, Academic Press, 1983.
33. Holmboe ES, Hawkins RE, Huot SJ: Effects of training in direct observation of medical residents' clinical competence: A randomized trial. Ann Intern Med. 2004;140(11):874–881.
34. Berbano EP, Browning R, Pangaro L, Jackson JL: The impact of the Stanford Faculty Development Program on ambulatory teaching behavior. J Gen Intern Med 2006;21(5):430–434.
35. Boulet JR, Swanson DB: Psychometric challenges of using simulations for high-stakes assessment. In Dunn D (ed): Simulators in Critical Care Education and Beyond. Philadelphia, Lippincott, Williams & Wilkins, 2004, pp 119–130.
36. Ziv A, Wolpe RP, Small SD, Click S: Simulation-Based Medical Education: An Ethical Imperative. Acad Med. 2003;78: 783–788.
37. Norcini JJ: Current perspectives in assessment: The assessment of performance at work. Med Educ 2005;39:880–889.
38. Ogrinc G, Headrick LA, Foster T: Teaching and assessing resident competence in practice-based learning and improvement. J Gen Intern Med 2004;19(5 Pt 2):496–500.

2

Issues of Validity and Reliability for Assessments in Medical Education

Brian E. Clauser, EdD, Melissa J. Margolis, MS, and David B. Swanson, PhD

The purpose of this chapter is to provide an overview of the concepts of validity and reliability as they apply to assessment in medical education. The discussion begins with a brief history of validity theory and a description of how the conceptualization of validity has changed. Michael Kane's approach to validity, in which the validation process has come to be viewed as a structured argument in support of the intended interpretations made based on test scores, will be the main structural focus of the chapter. Kane's approach is important because the view that the validation process is one of collecting evidence to construct a coherent argument in support of the intended interpretations leads to a notable conclusion: there is no such thing as a *valid test*! The score from any given test could be used to make a variety of decisions in different contexts and with different examinee populations; evidence to support the validity of one type of interpretation in one context with one population may or may not support the validity of a different interpretation in a different context with a different population. This point will be discussed in greater detail later; it is introduced here because it is central to the understanding of the argument to be made throughout this chapter.

Within the components of Kane's validity framework, various medical education assessment contexts will provide a structure for examples of the types of evidence that might be collected to create a validity argument. The discussion of reliability will be presented within the context of generalizability theory, and the generalizability of scores will be considered in the context of the overall validity argument. It is hoped that this chapter will provide the reader with a greater understanding of issues that are central to validity and reliability as these concepts pertain to assessment in medical education.

Historical Context

Practically speaking, the history of test theory as we know it begins with Charles Spearman around the turn of the 20th century. Spearman's interest was not in assessment but in the psychological study of intelligence. Most of the basic equations from classical test theory were developed by Spearman to aid his research on the presence of a common (g) factor shared by most if not all tests of mental proficiency.[1–4] These equations are all dependent on Karl Pearson's mathematical formulation of the correlation coefficient.[5]

This groundwork laid the foundation for a science of testing that expanded explosively during the First World War. The U.S. Army had a monumental personnel problem: tens of thousands of recruits had to be placed in jobs. Testing provided a potentially effective and efficient means of determining appropriate job placements.[6] This effort established psychological testing in the United States, and not surprisingly the science of testing was used in an effort to boost industrial efficiency after the war. In both the military and industrial contexts, the question of interest was, "How well do these tests predict performance on the job?" Evidence to justify the use of the test naturally conformed to the approach established by Spearman and took the form of a correlation between the test scores and an independent assessment of job performance.

The explosion in placement testing did much to define the view of validity during the period from 1920 through 1950. Correlational evidence, referred to as criterion validity, was the standard during this period; in his 1951 chapter in the first edition of *Educational Measurement*, Edward Cureton defined validity "in terms of the correlation between the actual test scores and the 'true' criterion score."[7]

As a practical matter, criterion validity has obvious utility. In placement testing, it has clear relevance to the interpretation of the score and it provides an objective basis for comparing multiple assessments available for a given purpose. However, the strength of this approach is less apparent for applications outside placement testing. One problem is that an obvious and practical criterion may not be available. No clear and objective external criterion is likely to exist for an achievement test. If such a criterion is identified, the test developer would need to provide validity evidence to support the use of the criterion. This has the potential to lead to a kind of infinite regression.[8]

Questions about the appropriateness of criterion validity as a primary evaluation of assessments of academic achievement led to the development of procedures for assessing content validity. The purpose of such evidence is to establish that the content of the test reasonably represents the domain of interest. This type of evidence clearly is necessary but not sufficient to establish the validity of interpretations for an achievement test. As Messick pointed out, evidence that the test is domain relevant provides no direct support for inferences based on the test scores.[9]

During the period after the Second World War, interest in personality testing pushed researchers to continue to consider the types of evidence required to support the use of these new instruments. Neither criterion nor content validity models provided a particularly good fit to these tests. It was in this context that Cronbach and Meehl introduced the idea of construct validity.[10] In describing the issues that led to their formulation of construct validity, Cronbach commented in the second edition of *Educational Measurement*[11]:

> The rationale for construct validation (Cronbach and Meehl, 1955) developed out of personality testing. For a measure of, for example, ego strength, there is no uniquely pertinent criterion to predict, nor is there a domain of content to sample. Rather, there is a theory that sketches out the presumed nature of the trait. If the test score is a valid manifestation of ego strength, so conceived, its relations to other variables conform to the theoretical expectations.

This approach to validation greatly expanded the types of evidence that could be considered in evaluating an assessment. For example, in the context of achievement testing, construct validation might argue for collecting evidence to demonstrate that examinees with advanced training in the topic area outperform those with less training.

The 1950s brought two other important changes in the conceptualization of validity. First, Campbell and Fiske introduced the multitrait-multimethod matrix.[12] The matrix provided correlational evidence about the relative strength of relationship between different traits measured by a single method and measures of the same trait using different methods. In the context of personality testing, examples of traits included extroversion and aggression; methods may have included individual examiner-administered assessments and group-administered paper-and-pencil assessments. Campbell and Fiske's matrix provided an empirical means of assessing the impact of what was later to become known as construct-irrelevant variance (signaled by relatively higher correlations between different traits measured by the same method compared with the same trait measured by different methods). The second important change in the conceptualization of validity came when Loevinger focused attention on the proposed interpretation of test scores.[13] This represented an important shift in perspective from consideration of the relationship between the construct the test was designed to measure and the test score to consideration of the correspondence between what is measured by the test and the proposed interpretations.

By the publication of the third edition of *Educational Measurement*, Messick was able to present a unified theory of validity.[9] Rather than being defined as "the correlation between the actual test scores and the 'true' criterion score,"[7] validity now was viewed as the "... degree to which empirical evidence and theoretical rationales support the adequacy and appropriateness of interpretations and actions based on test scores."[9] Messick's model built on the contributions of his predecessors; following Cronbach and Meehl[10] and Loevinger,[13] he emphasized the need to specify the intended meaning and use of the test score before validation. Consistent with Cronbach and Meehl and Campbell and Fiske,[12] Messick emphasized the importance of considering alternative hypotheses such as the impact of construct-irrelevant variance. Additionally, like these predecessors, Messick argued that the process of validation would involve an extended program of research.

Much of Messick's formulation of validity can be seen as completely consistent with Cronbach and Meehl's conceptualization. In one important respect, however, Messick diverged from that earlier perspective: he viewed evidence relating to the consequences of testing to be equally important in evaluating an assessment. Messick believed that both the actual and potential social consequences of a test must be evaluated. Considering as an example a test for medical licensure, at a minimum this requirement leads to examination of consequences such as the test's impact on what teachers choose to teach and learners choose to learn. More broadly, consequential validity would require consideration of the test's impact on the availability of medical practitioners to the community at large and perhaps specifically for underserved communities. Messick's view of consequential validity went beyond these considerations; his views additionally required consideration of the impact that such an examination might have on the entrance of minority candidates into the profession. This broad definition of consequential validity emphasizes the importance of test developers and administrators accepting responsibility for their actions. The definition takes the validation process beyond the scientific evaluation of the assessment into the arena of social and political values.

The history of validity theory should make it clear that the definition of validity has expanded over time. The emphasis also has changed as the focus of testing has changed. Criterion validity has not been replaced; this type of evidence remains essential in evaluating admissions and employment tests. Similarly, content validity represents an important source of evidence in support of tests of achievement. The history of validity is a history of both an expansion in meaning and a shift in emphasis. Recently, Kane has introduced an additional shift in perspective by representing validity as an argument in support of the proposed interpretations of a test score.[8,14] As with previous stages in the evolution of validity theory, Kane's view does not deny the importance of the evidence and perspectives that have been discussed during the last half century; those readers familiar with Messick's writing on validity will find that Kane provides more of a shift in perspective than a rejection of the basic arguments. That shift in perspective does have one important characteristic: it highlights the fact that the collection of evidence in support of the interpretations of test scores must form a structured and coherent argument that leads from the test administration to the interpretation. That structured argument is only as strong as its weakest component.

Kane's View of Validity

Implicit in the interpretation of a test score is a series of assertions and assumptions that support that interpretation. The interpretation of a passing score on a licensing examination requires the assumption that the test was administered under standardized conditions and that the examinee did not have prior access to the test material. If the examinee cheated, no interpretation can be made about the score regardless of other characteristics of the test. Interpretation of the test score requires assumptions about the precision of the score; if the test score is not reproducible, there is no basis for making an interpretation. Interpretation of the score assumes that the test measures some relevant aspect of the overall set of knowledge, skills, and abilities

required for the practice of medicine. It also assumes that the cut-score has been established in a way that supports the interpretation. If any one of these assumptions is unfounded, the strength of the others is of little relevance.

Kane provides a structure for this validity argument that outlines four links in the inferential chain from the test administration to the final decision or interpretation.[8,14] He labels these four components *scoring, generalization, extrapolation*, and *interpretation/decision*. Support for the *scoring* component of the overall argument includes evidence that the test was administered properly, examinee behavior was captured correctly, and scoring rules were appropriate and applied accurately and consistently. The *generalization* component of the argument requires evidence that the observations were appropriately sampled from the universe of test items, clinical encounter, and the like. Generalization also requires evidence that the sample of observations was large enough to produce scores with an acceptable level of precision. Broadly speaking, this stage in the argument asks the question: Is the test reliable? The *extrapolation* component of the argument requires evidence that the observations represented by the test score were relevant to the target proficiency or construct measured by the test. This requires a demonstration that the observations were relevant to the interpretation and that the scores were not unduly influenced by sources of variance that are irrelevant to the intended interpretation. The *decision/interpretation* component of the argument requires evidence in support of any theoretical framework required for score interpretation or evidence in support of decision rules. For tests with an established cut-score, this evidence would include support for the procedure used to establish that cut-score. Again, the score user can have confidence in an interpretation only if there is evidence for each component of the overall argument. The types of evidence required will vary with the purpose and characteristics of the assessment. Table 2-1 provides examples of some of the kinds of questions that arise at each stage of the argument. The questions are provided as examples and are not intended as an exhaustive list. The next sections will describe these four aspects of the validity argument in some detail. Within each section, details will be provided for three types of assessments as examples: (1) a high-stakes test of clinical knowledge; (2) a standardized patient–based (SP-based) examination of clinical skills required for progress in medical school; and (3) an assessment of residents' clinical skills based on direct observation by faculty.

Scoring

The *scoring* component of the validity argument must provide evidence that test data have been collected appropriately and scored accurately. This will include consideration of a variety of types of evidence such as the extent to which the stated conditions of standardization have been implemented, the accuracy of the

Table 2-1 **Questions Associated with Each of the Four Components of Kane's Argument-Based Approach to Validity**

Component	Questions
Scoring	1. Were the observations made or stimulus materials administered under standardized conditions? 2. Were the scores recorded accurately? 3. Were the scoring algorithms applied correctly? 4. Were appropriate security procedures implemented?
Generalization	1. What are the sources of measurement error that contribute to the observed scores on the assessment? 2. How similar would scores be across replications of the measurement procedure? 3. How similar would classification decisions be across replications of the measurement procedure? 4. To what extent are test forms constructed using a systematic process?
Extrapolation	1. To what extent do the scores correspond to real-world proficiencies of interest? 2. Are there factors that interfere with assessment of the proficiencies of interest? 3. Do scores predict real-world outcomes of interest? 4. Are there artificial aspects of the testing conditions that impact the scores?
Decision	1. Was the standard established through implementation of a defensible and properly implemented procedure? 2. Do examinees identified for remediation improve to meet the standard or benefit more from a remediation program than would those who were not identified?

scoring process, and the choice and implementation of scaling procedures. As with each of the four components of the validity argument, the specifics of the evidence that will be relevant to the scoring aspect of the argument will vary with the characteristics of the test.

Example I: A High-Stakes Standardized Assessment

Standardized tests have been developed to provide the strongest possible evidence for the *scoring* and *generalization* components of the validity argument. Adherence to the conditions of standardization ensures that the data are collected in the same manner for all examinees. Factors such as the time allowed for the examination, seating, lighting, screen size, or print quality are controlled. To the extent that administration procedures require documentation of violation of these conditions and annotation of score reports, the score user will have confidence in the conditions under which the test responses have been collected. Similarly, professionally administered and scored tests routinely will have quality control steps built into the scoring process. If responses are recorded on paper and scanned, the accuracy of the scanner must be verified. ''Key validation''—statistical analyses of examinee responses designed to verify that the keyed answer is correct—also provides evidence that the scoring rules have been applied accurately. This step includes analyzing responses to examine the proportion of examinees receiving credit for each item and comparing the probability of a correct score on the item for examinees at different proficiency levels.

One important consideration for scores from high-stakes tests is security. Examinees with low proficiency may be motivated to cheat. When items are reused from one administration to another, the possibility

exists that examinees will memorize items and make them available to individuals testing on a later date. When tests are computer administered on a continuous basis, this threat to validity may be increased. Evidence about the size of the item pool and the frequency with which items are reused will support the user's confidence that prior exposure has not threatened the integrity of the score. When printed test books are used, the possibility of theft also threatens the integrity of the scores. When tests are computer-based, encryption of test items at all times except when they are displayed on screen may provide additional confidence in the security of the test material. For both paper-and-pencil and computer delivery, carefully documented and monitored security procedures are necessary to ensure that all test materials remain secure until the test is administered.

Evidence that the identity of the examinee is verified and that the examinee has no electronic (or other) means of obtaining assistance during the examination will be important. Score interpretations will be useless if the examinee whose name is shown on the score report is not the one who completed the examination. Similarly, if an examinee was able to use a mobile phone to receive assistance, the meaning of the score will be in doubt. Again, evidence that appropriate security procedures exist is not necessarily compelling; it also is necessary to verify that these procedures are implemented consistently.

Example II: A Standardized Patient–Based Assessment

The reproducibility of the stimulus material and scoring procedures is, as previously noted, a strength of standardized tests comprising multiple-choice items. Relatively little effort is required to be satisfied that two examinees assigned to the same test form but sitting at different computer terminals are seeing the same items and that those items are being scored in the same way. The same is not necessarily true for a test using standardized patients. Adding the human element creates the possibility that two standardized patients trained to portray the same scenario may perform in a less-than-perfectly-standardized manner; the same standardized patient may not portray the same scenario in the same way on two different occasions. The scoring phase of the validity argument will need to include evidence that standardized patients are trained to an acceptable standard, and it also will require evidence that standardized patients are monitored over time to ensure both inter- and intrapatient consistency. Similar issues arise with scoring for these tests; whether the scores are produced by the standardized patients or observers, it will be necessary to assess the accuracy of the process. Again, this aspect of testing must be verified before testing begins and must continue to be monitored over time. It also is important to remember that collecting evidence of a high level of rater agreement during a small-scale pilot administration should not replace collecting the same evidence once the test is being administered operationally.

In addition to verifying that the overall error rate is low both in standardized patient portrayal and in the scoring process, it will be important to provide evidence that there are not significant interactions between examinee characteristics and standardized patients' performance or scoring. For example, the examinee's gender or ethnicity should have no impact on the way the scenario is portrayed and scored. If significant interactions are found suggesting that examinees of otherwise equal proficiency are likely to receive better scores if they are male rather than female, this would be a serious threat to the valid interpretation of scores. This type of effect is more serious than random error in portrayal or scoring because random errors tend to average out across encounters; systematic effects do not.

Security issues also may be important with SP–based tests. If the test is used to make important decisions, examinees may attempt to improve their scores by gaining prior access to test information. In most circumstances, SP-based tests are administered on multiple occasions. This creates the opportunity for examinees who have completed the examination to share information with others who will test in the future; in most situations, prior knowledge about the patient presentations that will appear on a test should be expected to influence examinee scores. This threat to validity is analogous to the problem associated with the reuse of material on tests comprising multiple-choice items, but in the case of SP-based examinations it is much more difficult to produce large banks of test ''items.'' When tests are administered during a relatively short period, sequestering examinees to prevent the sharing of information may provide evidence that this threat to validity has been controlled. With SP-based tests, an additional threat to security exists in that standardized patients themselves may share information with

examinees before the test administration. This threat to security will be even more dangerous when the standardized patient scores the examination; in this situation, the patient could give the examinee an inappropriate advantage by misrepresenting the examinee's score.

Compelling evidence for score interpretation for SP-based assessments will require support for the assertion that security risks have been controlled. For administrations at medical schools, partial support for this assertion may be based on procedures that sequester examinees or provide for different test forms to be delivered on different days. For large-scale administrations, development of large case banks may limit the potential impact of an examinee obtaining prior access to information about a small number of cases. Although the evidence has been inconsistent, some authors have argued that prior access to information has no appreciable impact on scores (see Swanson and associates[15] for a more complete discussion). The methodological difficulties associated with demonstrating the absence of an effect are sufficiently complex as to make this a problematic form of evidence, but conceptually it does provide an example that highlights the varied types of evidence that may be called into the construction of the validity argument.

Example III: An Assessment Based on Direct Observation

Evaluation of a trainee's clinical skills through direct observation involves taking another step away from the completely standardized stimulus material of the written examination and the partially standardized conditions that exist in SP-based assessment to the relatively uncontrolled conditions of observation on the ward or clinic. In order to support the interpretations of scores produced in this setting, it will be necessary to produce evidence that different evaluators working in different settings are, in fact, assessing the same construct in the same way. One means of providing such evidence would be to carefully define the characteristics of performance to be rated. A combination of careful definition and thorough training of evaluators may provide reasonable support for the assertion that individuals are being assessed on the same construct. The disadvantage of carefully defining the characteristics to be assessed is that it may lead to a restriction in assessment to those aspects of the construct that can be defined easily; this will have an impact on the potential to extrapolate from the scores to the construct of interest. The alternative may be that each evaluator defines the construct in his or her own way, but this approach clearly leaves the scoring aspect of the validity argument seriously weakened.

Even with careful definition and training of the evaluators, it will be important to collect evidence that demonstrates that evaluators are assessing the same constructs; think-aloud or other interview-based procedures may provide evidence regarding the specific attributes the evaluators are considering.

Presumably, the nature of direct observation reduces problematic issues related to security. However, depending on the relationship between the observer and the observee, verification of identity may be an issue; a faculty member may mistakenly rate the wrong trainee. Similarly, the conditions of observation must be equitable in the sense that everyone being observed has similar knowledge (or ignorance) about when they will be observed and what behaviors will be assessed.

Generalization

This stage of the argument focuses on the relationship between the observed scores and the associated universe scores or true scores. Both universe scores and true scores are conceptualizations; the universe score represents the score that an examinee would receive if it were possible for that examinee to respond to all items representing the universe of acceptable observations (that is, if the examinee responded to all items in the domain). The true score is a closely related concept representing the mean score that the examinee would receive if she or he completed an unlimited number of randomly equivalent forms of the test. (The observed score is the score that is actually recorded when an examinee completes a specific test form.) The details of these definitions and the related theories are beyond the scope of this chapter; the interested reader is referred to Gulliksen[1] and Lord and Novick[16] for a detailed discussion of classical test theory and to Cronbach and associates[17] and Brennan[18] for discussions of generalizability theory.

Two kinds of evidence are required for this stage of the argument. First, it is necessary to show that the sample of items presented or observations made of the examinee are representative of the domain to which the score is to be generalized. Second, it is necessary to demonstrate that the sampling is sufficiently extensive to prevent the observed scores from being unduly influenced by sampling error. The extent to which the sample is representative will depend on the procedures used for test construction (or data collection); the adequacy of the sampling can be examined directly through a well-developed set of theory-based statistical procedures.

The samples will be representative to the extent that data collection follows specified rules. In some cases, random selection from a specified domain will be appropriate, while in other cases stratified sampling will be preferred. In some contexts, rules for the range of conditions under which observations may (or must) be made will replace the sampling of stimulus material.

Far and away, the most developed aspect of test theory relates to evaluation of reliability; conceptually this methodology is designed to assess the relationship between observed scores and true scores or universe scores. The most common index of this relationship is the reliability coefficient; this coefficient represents the correlation between the observed test scores from two equivalent forms of the test. The square root of this value represents the correlation between observed scores and true scores on the test. In the classical test theory framework, the reliability coefficient is also directly related to the standard error of measurement, which represents the distribution of observed scores around a given true score.

A wide variety of approaches have been developed to estimate the relationship between observed scores and true scores. The usefulness of these procedures will depend on how one conceptualizes the meaning of "a replication of the measurement procedure."[19] Because the specific set of items and the specific time and date on which the test was administered are rarely central to how the scores are to be interpreted, it is generally desirable to view "replication" as including measurements with different test forms on different occasions. This common condition makes correspondence between scores achieved on two forms of a test on different occasions as one standard for assessing replicability. The value of this standard rests on the assumption that the characteristic to be measured has not changed between administrations. This includes change in the narrow sense of learning as well as change in relevant conditions of observation such as motivation and familiarity with the test format.

When it is unlikely that *relevant* conditions of testing remain constant across occasions, it may be more appropriate to conceptualize a replication so that occasion is held constant. In the practical sense in which the test is administered twice on the same day, replication on the same occasion is open not only to the effects of fatigue but also to the effects of practice leading to increased familiarity with the format. In the literal sense of replication on the same occasion (in which two forms are administered simultaneously), these effects are absent but actual replication is not possible; only a conceptual or theoretical replication can exist.

For a test based on multiple-choice items, the definition of replication must include consideration of occasion and the selection of items. For more complex testing formats, the definition of replication similarly will be more complex. Consider, for example, an essay examination. In this instance, the stimulus will be standardized but a replication reasonably may involve a different set of essay prompts to which an examinee will respond on a different occasion. Additionally, the responses may be scored by a different set of judges and the judges may evaluate the material on different occasions. The definition of a replication therefore will depend on which features are considered fixed and which are considered random. In this context, the definition of fixed and random variables is guided by the desired interpretation of scores. In the event that score interpretation assumes that judgments were made by a specific group of experts and that all examinees were judged by the same experts, judges will be a fixed facet in the design. If it is sensible to view the specific judges as sampled from a larger group of similarly acceptable judges, the judges should be viewed as a random facet. Similarly, if the score interpretations assume a specific set of test items or other stimulus materials, then this facet is fixed; otherwise, if the stimuli may be viewed as sampled from a larger domain, items must be viewed as a random facet. Random facets will vary from one replication to the next; fixed facets will not vary.

The appropriate methodology for examining the relationship between observed scores and true scores or estimating the standard error of measurement will depend on the complexity of the data collection design. When practicality allows, actually repeating the measurement procedure will provide a sound basis for assessing the relationship of interest. The correlation between scores produced across replications will provide an appropriate estimate of the reliability of the test. Again, the square root of this value will represent the correlation between observed and true scores, and the well-known formula

$$\sigma_e = \sigma_x \sqrt{1 - r_{xx'}}$$

provides an estimate of the standard error of measurement. (In this formula, σ represents the standard deviation of the observed scores and $r_{xx'}$ represents the reliability of the test.)

In many circumstances, replication will not be practical; for example, candidates for licensure cannot be called upon to retest under the same high-stakes conditions after they have completed and passed an examination. Numerous procedures are available to evaluate test scores based on a single administration of an examination. Nearly a century ago, Spearman and Brown introduced the first of these procedures based on the correlation between split halves (e.g., even- and odd-numbered items) of an examination.[4,20] KR20[21] and coefficient alpha[22] estimate a value equal to the average of all possible split halves. These procedures provide estimates of reliability based on the strength of relationship between items in a single test form. They work on the assumption that the strength of relationship (covariance) between item n and item m (n ≠ m) on a single test form will provide a good approximation of the strength of relationship between item ''n'' on test form 1 and item ''m'' on test form 2.

Coefficient alpha and the Kuder-Richardson formulas are useful tools for collecting evidence about the generalization of test scores. Unfortunately, they have become a kind of knee-jerk response to the question of score reliability. Too often, researchers seem to view estimating reliability as a requirement that allows them to report a coefficient that a journal editor will demand rather than as an opportunity to better understand the characteristics of their assessment. When applying these procedures, two important considerations arise. First and foremost, the evaluator must again ask the question about what is meant by a replication of the measurement procedure. These procedures are appropriate when generalization is viewed in terms of replication across items (or test forms) with all other conditions of measurement held constant. In the relatively simple context of tests based on multiple-choice items, this approach generally will underestimate the standard error of measurement that would be observed for replications across both test forms and testing occasions. For more complex testing formats, interpretation of the results of applying these procedures will be more difficult and often much more problematic.

A second important consideration in applying these procedures is related to the assumptions used in their derivation. The central assumption in interpreting coefficient alpha (or KR20) is that, on average, the strength of relationship between any two items on a single test form is equal to that between any two items on different forms of the test. When this assumption is violated, the results may misrepresent the actual reliability of the assessment substantially. Typically, this violation will result in an overestimate of reliability. Consider, for example, the case in which a passage describing a clinical scenario is followed by several questions. It is common that the strength of relationship between questions associated with the same passage will be greater than the strength of relationship between items from different passages. Because the scenarios typically will be different from one test form to the next, the average relationship between items across test forms will be best approximated by the relationship between items from different scenarios on a single test.

Another example of a situation in which these procedures may be misapplied occurs in assessments in which multiple judges assess an examinee's performance on the same task. For example, consider the circumstance in which judges work in pairs to evaluate an examinee's interaction with a real patient. The assessment requires that each examinee interact with five patients, and each interaction is evaluated by a different pair of judges. If the judges score separately, the examinee will receive ten scores. If all examinees have interacted with the same five patients and been scored by the single set of judges assigned to that patient, the evaluator may be tempted to calculate coefficient alpha based on this set of ten scores. Again, however, because the strength of relationship between scores from judges evaluating performance with the same patient will be greater than that between pairs evaluating performance with different patients, this approach will not appropriately approximate the strength of relationship between scores from different tests. In this instance, the error in estimation may be substantial (e.g., the estimated standard error may be 50% of the correct value) and may grossly overestimate score precision.

Another common error in application of coefficient alpha is calculation of the coefficient based on the combination of data from multiple administrations of a test in which the mean difficulty of the test varies across administrations. Consider a test based on standardized patients in which (a) the same cases are administered at three different schools, and (b) each school recruits and trains a separate group of standardized patients. If all examinees complete the same set of cases, the evaluator may be tempted to combine the data sets for estimating the reliability of the test. However, differences due to variation in mean difficulty (stringency) across patients at different schools will in this analysis be indistinguishable from differences in examinee proficiency. The result may be a substantially inflated estimate of reliability.

The assumption that the covariance between items on a single test form approximates the covariance between items across forms is central to the interpretation of coefficient alpha as an estimate of the correlation between scores from two forms of a test. There are, however, instances in which this may not provide an appropriate estimate of the correlation between scores across forms of a test even when this assumption is met. Much of classical test theory is built on the assumption that multiple forms of a test will be classically parallel. If different examinees take different forms (of varying difficulty) on occasions one and two, the correlation between scores will be influenced by the difficulty of the forms. In this situation, an additional source of error has been introduced and classical test theory models will be insufficient; it is in response to this type of complexity that Cronbach and colleagues developed generalizability theory.

Generalizability Theory

Classical test theory divides observed scores into two components: true score and error. Because an examinee's true score is defined as uncorrelated with error, it follows that observed-score variance is composed of true-score variance and error variance. Generalizability theory expands this framework to divide the overall variance into multiple components. Consider as an example the simple testing situation in which examinees respond to essay prompts that are evaluated by raters. To study the generalizability of the results, a researcher collected data for a group of examinees; all examinees responded to the same prompts, and all responses were evaluated by the same raters. In the framework of generalizability theory, essay prompts and raters become distinguishable sources of error variance. As in the classical test theory framework, it is possible to take data from a single administration, estimate the reliability (or generalizability) of the test, and project the expected reliability of the test with differing numbers of essay prompts. However, because generalizability theory provides a means of making explicit the error contributed by variability both in essay prompts and raters, this framework makes it possible to further project how the reliability of the test would change if the number of raters evaluating performance on each prompt also was varied.

The estimates made in a generalizability analysis are based on analysis-of-variance procedures. However, Cronbach emphasized that the central feature of generalizability theory was the focus on an explicit description of the aspects of the measurement procedure that were considered fixed and those that potentially contributed to measurement error. He viewed analysis of variance as one of a number of potential approaches to estimation.

Example I: A High-Stakes Standardized Assessment

The focus of the *generalization* stage of the validity argument is on the extent to which scores will be comparable across replications of the assessment procedure. In the context of high-stakes standardized assessments, the interpretation of scores typically will require that they are comparable across multiple test forms. For example, a licensing or certifying examination would lose credibility if examinees could expect widely varying scores based on which test form they were assigned on a given day.

Viewed from a generalizability theory framework, this part of the argument will require several types of evidence. First, it will be necessary to demonstrate that the sampling procedure used for test construction supports the creation of comparable test forms. The simplest case of the construction of multiple forms would be based on random selection of items from an available pool of acceptable items. This is conceptually simple, but it is unusual for standardized tests. A more common approach would be to select items to meet the constraints of a table of specifications or test "blueprint." In this case, items may be randomly selected from each of a number of content categories (see Table 2-2 for a hypothetical 200-item multiple-choice test in internal medicine). When different item formats are included on the test, the table of specifications may specify the number of items from each combination of format and category. A common variation on this theme is to write items for a new form of the test to meet the specifications of the previous form. When systematic differences exist in the test construction procedure across forms, estimation of the correlation between scores on multiple forms based on generalizability analysis of a single form will be inappropriate.

When systematic test construction procedures are used, standardized tests typically will have a reasonably simple data collection design, examinees will typically be the object of measurement, and the sampling of items will represent a potential source of measurement error. With the simple design, three sources of variance can be estimated: a person variance component, which is conceptually equivalent to true-score variance in classical test theory; an item variance component, which represents the variability in item difficulty; and a person-by-item variance component, which represents residual variance not explained by the other two effects. The person-by-item variance component divided by the number of items will represent the error variance when comparisons are being made between examinees who have completed the same test form; when comparisons

Table 2-2 **Sample Blueprint for a 200-Item Multiple-Choice Test in Internal Medicine**

Disease Category/Organ System*	Number of Questions per Clinical Task				
	Making a Diagnosis	Making Therapeutic Decisions	Preventing Disease	Using Diagnostic Studies	Total
Cardiovascular disorders	10	9	5	6	30
Dermatologic disorders	4	2	2	2	10
Endocrine and metabolic disorders	7	6	3	4	20
Gynecologic disorders	3	3	2	2	10
Hematologic disorders	3	3	1	3	10
Immunologic disorders	3	3	2	2	10
Mental disorders	4	3	1	2	10
Musculoskeletal disorders	8	6	2	4	20
Neurologic disorders	6	4	2	3	15
Nutritional and digistive disorders	8	9	4	4	25
Renal, urinary, male reproductive disorders	6	3	2	4	15
Respiratory disorders	8	9	4	4	25
Total	**70**	**60**	**30**	**40**	**200**

*Items related to infectious and neoplastic diseases are included in the affected organ system.

are being made between examinees who have completed different test forms, a clear definition of error variance is more complicated. If the test forms are constructed through a process that approximates random sampling from an undifferentiated item pool and there is no formal equating procedure, the appropriate error variance will be the sum of the item variance component and the person-by-item variance component divided by the number of items. When statistical equating procedures are used, the impact of the item variance component may be reduced; because equating is not likely to be error free, the error variance estimate based on the person-by-item variance component alone will represent a lower bound of the error variance when forms are equated.

When items are sampled from fixed content categories, generalizability analysis becomes more complicated. In this situation, there are variance components for: persons (p); content categories (c); items nested in content categories ($i{:}c$); persons by content categories ($p \times c$); and persons by items nested in content categories ($p \times i{:}c$). In this case, the c component will not contribute measurement error because this structure is fixed across test forms. Similarly, because the categories are fixed, the $p \times c$ variance component will contribute to universe or true score variance. The $p \times i{:}c$ component will contribute to error, and when comparisons are made across forms the $i{:}c$ will contribute to measurement error. The impact of this latter component again will be mitigated to the extent that test forms are constructed or equated to be statistically equivalent. This stratification process typically will yield a smaller standard error and larger generalizability coefficient than analysis without stratification; this is the reason

that coefficient alpha is referred to as a lower bound estimate of reliability. It should be noted, however, that in practice the improvement typically is modest.

The error variance estimates produced using generalizability theory provide a basis for estimating the standard error of measurement for the test; these are useful for providing confidence intervals around scores. Generalizability coefficients also may be produced as the ratio of the universe score variance divided by the sum of the universe score variance and the error variance. Although these indices are commonly reported, caution is required because they will be sensitive to the specific sample of examinees used in the estimation. Consider, for example, estimation of such an index for one of the Steps of the United States Medical Licensing Examination; if the coefficient is estimated based on the relatively homogeneous group of U.S. graduates taking the test for the first time, it may be several points lower than if it is estimated based on all examinees completing the test. In contrast, the standard error of measurement tends to be more stable across groups, making it a more interpretable and useful index of precision.

Example II: A Standardized Patient–Based Assessment

The logic of the argument described in the previous example holds in the context of SP-based assessment. In order to draw conclusions from analyses based on a single administration of the assessment, the rules employed in test construction must guarantee that there will not be systematic differences in test forms.

The logistic realities of test delivery may make this more difficult when the items are people, but clearly generalization across test forms will be threatened if the patients on one form are systematically different than those on another. Important differences could include changes in the types of problems portrayed as well as changes in the level of experience and training of the patients; demographic characteristics such as age and gender also could impact the credibility of generalization across forms.

The generalizability of standardized tests composed of multiple-choice items is relatively easy to evaluate, and even the simpler classical test theory models provide adequate tools. The complexity of performance assessments, however, makes evaluation of the generalizability of scores a more difficult matter. Consider a test in which examinees rotate through a set of stations and at each station they interact with a patient and complete a patient note. The notes then are scored by a group of raters. When examinees complete the same set of stations and notes are rated by the same set of raters, variance components can be estimated for persons, stations, raters, persons by stations, persons by raters, stations by raters, and persons by stations by raters. The evaluator will need to determine which of these components contributes to measurement error in the specific context. Interaction terms that include the person and station effect almost always will contribute to measurement error, regardless of the intended score interpretation, because the *generalization* argument is about the extent to which the score from this test form is comparable to the score from a similarly constructed test form. By contrast, generalization over raters may or may not be important. If the test is administered in a context in which the same group of raters rates all examinees, and if there is no intention to draw inferences about how the examinees may have performed with other raters, then raters are considered a fixed facet in the design. In this case, the rater and station-by-rater variance components will not contribute to measurement error and the person-by-rater component will contribute to universe score variance. However, in most circumstances users of test scores will wish to draw inferences that extend beyond the group of raters scoring an examinee's performance, and these variance components are best viewed as contributing to measurement error (often substantially if the typical examinee is scored by a small number of raters).

Up to this point, it should be clear that when a facet in the design is considered fixed, the scores will have a smaller error variance and a higher level of generalizability. The evaluator may be tempted to try to increase the generalizability of scores by considering facets fixed. This strategy is without merit; it gives a promising, encouraging answer to the wrong question.

Example III: An Assessment Based on Direct Observation

When examinees are observed in a practice setting, the *generalization* portion of the validity argument may be problematic. Although there may be explicit rules controlling the sampling of observations, the logistics of practice-based assessment could make it likely that the environmental factors and patient characteristics are more similar from one observation to another within versus between examinees. This may lead to an overly optimistic report on the generalizability of scores. In this setting, the scores will be influenced by the rater effect as well as an effect for the specific patient. Depending on the design used to assign raters, it may be difficult to accurately estimate a rater effect. It also may be difficult or even impossible to fully differentiate between variance associated with the difficulty of the patient's presentation and the residual variance.

It usually is the case that the generalizability of scores will decrease as the type of assessment changes from a highly structured format, such as a professionally developed multiple-choice test, to a standardized patient or direct observation format. There are two reasons for this. First, it is possible to sample from the domain of interest more widely and efficiently with multiple-choice items because it takes relatively little time to respond to them and they are inexpensive to score. Second, both the sampling of content and the scoring can be more highly standardized with multiple-choice assessments so that the contribution of these factors to measurement error can be markedly reduced.

The potential to sample more widely reduces the impact of the examinee-by-item interaction as well as the effect of any higher-order interaction terms (including residual variance). There is a widely held view that the examinee-by-item interaction term in the typical person-by-item design represents "content specificity," or the tendency for physician knowledge to be highly problem-specific. The pervasive nature of the effect is well documented: the examinee-by-item (or case) interaction term is routinely the largest single source of error variance. It is, however, less clear whether this term represents content specificity or other sources of uncontrolled variability in the design. There is relatively little research investigating how consistently examinees respond to the same items or cases on different occasions. To the extent that the effect of interest actually is content specificity, examinees completing the same multiple-choice items or interacting with the same standardized patients on multiple occasions would receive highly consistent scores. There is some evidence from outside the domain of medical assessment to suggest that scores may not be highly reproducible across occasions. Similarly, there is evidence that the generalizability of test scores can be increased by building test forms to consistently sample from fixed content categories; however, the absolute magnitude of this increase generally is not large.

As noted previously, a second reason for the lower generalizability of scores based on assessments utilizing standardized patients or direct observation is that the conditions of observation and the scoring are more difficult to standardize. This argues for enhancing the structure of the assessment, but this process requires careful thought. The decision to implement a less structured assessment instead of one that is more highly structured (e.g., a clinical rather than a multiple-choice examination) is based on the perceived need to more directly assess the construct of interest. The problem lies in the fact that changing the scoring procedure may increase the standardization of the assessment by altering what is being assessed; the focus of the assessment therefore may shift in the direction of proficiencies that are more easily quantified and away from its original intent. This is not to argue against making every effort to structure the assessment; the key is to structure the assessment with a careful eye on the intended interpretation of the scores. Inevitably, it will be necessary to strike a balance between the generalizability of scores and the extent to which one can extrapolate from those scores to the actual proficiencies of interest. The next section will examine the *extrapolation* phase of the argument.

Extrapolation

Evaluators rarely are interested in knowing about an examinee's ability to answer multiple-choice items, or for that matter, the examinee's ability to interact with standardized patients. Instead, evaluators are interested in factors such as an examinee's knowledge base, problem-solving skills, clinical judgment, and ability to communicate effectively. Scores from assessments provide indirect evidence about the proficiencies of interest; the *extrapolation* phase of the validity argument is concerned with how indirect that evidence is.

This is the most difficult stage of the validity argument because the evidence is by nature inferential and the analytic framework is less well developed than that for the generalizability argument. The *extrapolation* stage of the argument is every bit as vital as the *generalization* phase. A highly reliable score that measures the wrong characteristic is of no value. However, it is equally important to remember that the *appearance* that an examination measures the proficiency of interest is not a substitute for actual evidence. Such "face validity" may support the political acceptability and perhaps the legal viability of an assessment,[23] but it does not contribute to the validity argument.

As noted in the introduction to this chapter, test validity cannot be reduced to a correlation with a criterion measure because completely valid criteria are rarely (if ever) available. Nonetheless, information about the relationship between test scores and other relevant measures will contribute to the argument. Similarly, evidence about the content of the examination will be of interest. Beyond these two types of supportive evidence, the *extrapolation* argument must be guided by the quote from Cronbach that began this chapter, "A proposition deserves some degree of trust only when it has survived serious attempts to falsify it."[24] The evaluator will be called upon to assess both

the extent to which scores are influenced by sources of variability that are not related to the proficiency of interest and the extent to which scores fail to reflect aspects of the proficiency of interest; these two threats to validity are referred to as construct-irrelevant variance and construct under-representation.

Evidence regarding the presence of construct-irrelevant variance and construct under-representation may be in the form of convergence or divergence of scores with other measures. One potential source of construct-irrelevant variance is the assessment format. When tests are delivered via computer, for example, it is reasonable to be concerned about the extent to which scores may be influenced by computer skills. Consider an assessment in which an examinee is called upon to interview and examine a patient and then to describe the critical features of the case. If examinees are required to respond using a computer keyboard, performance may be influenced by typing skills; if responses are time-limited, the impact of these skills may not be trivial. Presuming that typing is not part of the construct of interest, the impact of typing skills on test scores would be considered construct-irrelevant variance. The multitrait-multimethod matrix could provide a means of examining the presence of such an effect. For a sample of examinees, the ability to interview and examine a patient and to describe the critical features of the case could be evaluated based on the typed responses and oral presentation by the examinee. These same two response formats could be used to evaluate an apparently distinct proficiency such as the examinee's knowledge of mechanisms of disease. If the scores across proficiencies within response format are more highly correlated than the scores across formats within proficiencies, this could be a matter of concern. (Note that it is possible for such correlations to systematically vary in magnitude for different examinee groups, suggesting that validity varies by group.)

Example I: A High-Stakes Standardized Assessment

Tests of this sort typically assess a defined domain of interest. Extrapolation of test scores to performance in practice (or readiness for advancement in training) requires that the content of the test is matched appropriately to the demands of practice. Evidence for the content validity of the test will follow from the procedures used to define the domain and sample from it in assembling test forms. A job (or practice) analysis may be used to collect information about the requirements of practice, and additional studies may include collecting expert judgments about the relevance of items on actual test forms.[25]

Criterion-related evidence is conceptually central to the *extrapolation* stage of the validity argument. While some researchers have been successful in collecting this type of evidence,[26] it has generally been elusive. Studies based on limited or biased samples using flawed criteria are of questionable value, and the evaluator should be aware that well-constructed studies providing indirect evidence about the relationship between test scores and the proficiency of interest may be much more compelling than correlational evidence based on flawed criteria.

As noted previously, an important part of the argument will require evaluation of potential sources of construct-irrelevant variance. Because logistic constraints necessitate administering high-stakes multiple-choice examinations within structured time limits, one potentially important source of construct-irrelevant variance with such tests is the impact of speededness. It may be the case that the ability to respond quickly is not a part of the construct of interest and is not consistent with the intended score interpretations. The effects of speededness are an example of a potential source of construct-irrelevant variance, and the validity argument will be weakened to the extent that this issue is left unaddressed.

Differential item functioning is a topic that has been given considerable attention in the educational measurement literature (see references 27 and 28 for a review of relevant literature), and numerous statistical procedures have been developed to identify test items that perform differentially for examinees in different groups (after matching the examinees on the proficiency that the test is intended to measure). These procedures provide a useful means of identifying items that are sensitive to construct-irrelevant variance, and their use can bolster the validity argument. The classic case of differential item function occurs when an item requires knowledge of content that is not germane to the construct of interest. For example, if a reading comprehension test includes a passage about the American Civil War, it may differentially favor examinees raised in the United States over those who were not. These procedures may be used equally well to compare examinees who saw the item at the beginning of the test to those who saw it at the end (potentially testing for the presence of the effect of time constraints or examinee fatigue). Comparisons similarly could be made between examinees viewing images on a high- as opposed to low-resolution monitor or examinees responding to an item that has been exposed on previous test forms as opposed to those responding to the same item when it was initially administered. Each of these comparisons could provide evidence about the presence of construct-irrelevant variance, and the presence of such effects clearly would threaten the argument that scores can be extrapolated appropriately.

Example II: A Standardized Patient–Based Assessment

The primary attraction of performance-based assessment formats is that they have the potential to more directly measure constructs of interest; weakening the *generalization* argument is considered acceptable because the *extrapolation* argument is strengthened. However,

even though simulations may be of high fidelity, there always are aspects of them that are artificial. There has been relatively little research into the degree to which interactions with standardized patients differ from interactions with real patients, but it is inevitable that differences will exist. Even when standardized patients appear to be indistinguishable from actual patients, the choice of scoring algorithms may impact the extent to which the scores can be extrapolated to the performance of interest in practice. Checklists may fail to capture more subtle interviewing skills that would facilitate information gathering. Similarly, knowledge that the interaction is being scored based on a checklist may alter an examinee's approach to interviewing in order to maximize score points.

The previous comments are intended to highlight the fact that the appearance of similarity between the assessment setting and the practice setting is not in itself validity evidence. Using an assessment task that closely approximates the practice setting has the potential to limit the effects of construct-irrelevant variance and construct under-representation, but this similarity does not ensure that the score appropriately represents the proficiency of interest.

Example III: An Assessment Based on Direct Observation

As with performance-based assessment formats, such as those using standardized patients, direct observation with real patients is attractive because it has the potential to strengthen the *extrapolation* stage of the validity argument. Because observations are done in the practice setting, differences between the features of the assessment and those of practice may be minimized or eliminated. This characteristic may facilitate construction of an assessment that directly relates to real-world performance, but again it does not in itself make the argument for extrapolation. The act of observing may alter the environment. More important, the scoring algorithm will shape what is observed and how that observation is transformed into a score. It is the score and not the setting that is of interest, so collecting observations in the practice setting does not ensure against the effects of construct-irrelevant variance or construct under-representation. Assessments based on direct observation are particularly susceptible to halo effects.[29] In an effort to more clearly define the behaviors to be assessed and to avoid such effects, evaluators may shift from the construct of interest to a set of easily defined behaviors. In an effort to avoid the effect of construct-irrelevant variance, the scores may suffer from construct under-representation. For example, the complex concept of physician-patient communication may be reduced to a set of descriptions, such as "asks open-ended questions" and "makes eye contact." To support the *extrapolation* stage of the validity argument, evidence will be required to demonstrate the link between the scores and the intended interpretation, regardless of whether the data resulted from direct observation or from gridding answers with a number 2 pencil.

Decision/Interpretation

The *decision/interpretation* stage of the validity argument provides support for the decision rules and theory-based interpretations that are applied to test scores. The most common decision rules will be simple pass/fail classifications based on a single cut-score, but conjunctive or partially compensatory rules are not uncommon. Arguments supporting the reasonableness of these rules will be needed if the score interpretations associated with the resulting classification decisions are to be credible.

Similarly, score interpretations based on psychological theories about cognition, judgment, or decision making will only be as credible as the theories themselves. For example, if a score is used to classify practitioners as experts or novices based on their patterns of data collection in reaching a diagnosis, the theory of expert judgment supporting scoring would be critical; if the theory were shown to be flawed, score interpretations would be suspect.

Example I: A High-Stakes Standardized Assessment

When performance on multiple-choice tests is used to make a decision about eligibility for licensure or certification, the appropriateness of the cut-score will be a critical part of any validity argument supporting the interpretation that passing candidates are capable of performing in a safe and effective manner. This said, it must be remembered that standard setting decisions are policy judgments; they are not scientifically verifiable. Given this reality, Kane has argued that appropriate evidence to support the use of a cut-score will demonstrate that the procedure used to establish the standard was sensible.[30] Information about the choice of procedure, selection of judges, and implementation of the procedure will be central.

The credibility of the decision rule is central to score interpretation for high-stakes standardized tests, but this does not reduce the potential importance of theory-based assumptions. For example, the use of multiple-choice items may be based on the theoretical assumption that the knowledge and judgment required to respond to such items form a necessary prerequisite for decision making in practice.

Example II: A Standardized Patient–Based Assessment

Standardized patient–based examinations are sometimes used to make classification decisions in medical schools or postgraduate education, and in these situations failing examinees may be required to complete remedial training. When this is done, the assessment takes on the characteristics of a placement test. Evidence to support the decision rule used in this setting might include results demonstrating that examinees classified as requiring remediation will show differential improvement when exposed to the remediation program. Alternatively, evidence could be collected to demonstrate that examinees so identified have a significantly greater chance of succeeding in future training if they complete the remediation program.

Scoring procedures for SP-based examinations also may be based, implicitly or explicitly, on theoretical assumptions about how information is to be aggregated in drawing conclusions about an examinee's proficiency. Decisions will need to be made about the relative value of thoroughness and efficiency. Similarly, decisions must be made about the importance of physical examination maneuvers. If the practitioner will confirm both negative and positive results with a diagnostic test, the theoretical basis for drawing conclusions about the diagnostic ability of an examinee based on his or her use of a nondiscriminating physical examination maneuver would be suspect. These comments are not intended to advocate for or against specific approaches to scoring such examinations; they are intended to highlight the fact that the structure of the scoring procedure ultimately rests on a theoretical view of the diagnostic process, and the strength of that model limits the extent to which scores can be interpreted with respect to the examinee's diagnostic proficiency.

Example III: An Assessment Based on Direct Observation

As with the formats discussed previously, assessments based on direct observation will depend on theoretical assumptions. Assumptions about the nature of the construct being assessed will dictate the choice of process as opposed to product or outcome measures. Similarly, theories relating to expert-novice differences or cognitive theories about the nature of the medical diagnosis process—and, more broadly, medical decision making—may influence the data that are collected and the way that those data are aggregated and the resulting scores interpreted.

Conclusion

One perspective on validity theory that has not received much attention in this chapter is consequential validity.[9] If the impact of a test is evaluated from a policy perspective, the consequential argument may be the only argument of significance. In this chapter, the validity argument is seen as the accumulation of scientific evidence in support of intended score interpretations. Judgments of value and social policy may motivate an evaluator to administer an examination. Tests may be used to motivate curricular change or to draw trainees' attention to aspects of the curriculum that may have been underemphasized. Such motivations may be appropriate, but they do not reflect on the interpretation of scores and therefore are not viewed as part of the validity argument. That said, it is important to remember that testing programs—whether implemented within the classroom or on a national or international level—have consequences, and programmatic review of the positive and negative consequences is an important responsibility of the program administrator.

This chapter has presented an overview of validity and reliability. Validity has been conceptualized within Kane's framework as a systematic argument in support of score interpretation. Reliability has been viewed as a component of the overall validity argument. The details of the specific examples should be viewed as unimportant, and whether a specific piece of evidence is seen as part of the *extrapolation* stage or the *interpretation* stage of the argument is secondary. The central issue is that the overall argument must be complete and coherent. There is no such thing as a valid test; the validity argument must focus on intended interpretations of test scores. To construct such an argument, researchers must self-critically and systematically collect a wide array of evidence relevant to the credibility of those interpretations.

REFERENCES

1. Gulliksen H: Theory of Mental Tests. New York, John Wiley & Sons, 1950.
2. Spearman C: Proof of the measurement of association between two things. Am J Psychol 1904;15:72–101.
3. Spearman C: "General intelligence" objectively determined and measured. Am J Psychol 1904;15:201–292.
4. Spearman C: Correlation calculated with faulty data. Br J Psychol 1910;3:271–295.
5. Pearson K: Mathematical contributions to the theory of evolution: III. Regression, heredity, panmixia. Phil Trans R Soc Lond [Series A] 1896;187:253–318.
6. Yoakum CS, Yerkes RM: Mental Tests in the American Army. London, Sidgwick & Jackson, 1920.
7. Cureton EE: Validity. In Lindquist EF (ed): Educational Measurement. Washington, DC, American Council on Education, 1951, pp 621–694.
8. Kane M: Validation. In Brennan RL (ed): Educational Measurement, 4th ed. Westport, CT, American Council on Education/Praeger, 2006, pp 17–64.
9. Messick S: Validity. In Linn RL (ed): Educational Measurement, 3rd ed. New York, American Council on Education/Macmillan, 1989, pp 13–103.
10. Cronbach LJ, Meehl PE: Construct validity in psychological tests. Psych Bull 1955;52:281–302.
11. Cronbach LJ: Test validation. In Thorndike RL (ed): Educational Measurement, 2nd ed. Washington, DC, American Council on Education, 1971, pp 443–507.
12. Campbell DT, Fiske DW: Convergent and divergent validation by the multitrait-multimethod matrix. Psych Bull 1959;56:81–105.
13. Loevinger J: Objective tests as instruments of psychological theory. Psych Rep 1957;3:635–694.
14. Kane M: An argument-based approach to validation. Psych Bull 1992;112:527–535.
15. Swanson DB, Clauser BE, Case SM: Clinical skills assessment with standardized patients in high-stakes tests: A framework for thinking about score precision, equating, and security. Adv Health Sci Educ 1999;4:67–106.
16. Lord FM, Novick MR: Statistical Theories of Mental Test Scores. Reading, MA, Addison-Wesley, 1968.
17. Cronbach LJ, Gleser GC, Nanda H, Rajaratnam N: The dependability of behavioral measurements: Theory of generalizability for scores and profiles. New York, John Wiley & Sons, 1972.
18. Brennan RL: Generalizability Theory. New York, Springer-Verlag, 2001.
19. Brennan RL: An essay on the history and future of reliability from the perspective of replications. J Educ Meas 2001;38:295–317.
20. Brown W: Some experimental results in the correlation of mental abilities. Br J Psych 1910;3:296–322.
21. Kuder GF, Richardson MW: The theory of estimation of test reliability. Psychometrika 1937;2:151–160.
22. Cronbach LJ: Coefficient Alpha and the internal structure of tests. Psychometrika 1951;16:297–334.
23. Clauser BE, Margolis MJ, Case SM: Testing for licensure and certification in the professions. In R.L. Brennan RL (ed): Educational Measurement, 4th ed. Westport, CT, American Council on Education/Praeger, 2006, pp 701–731.
24. Cronbach LJ: Validity on parole: How can we go straight? New directions for testing and measurement. Proceedings of the 1979 ETS Invitational Conference. San Francisco, Jossey-Bass, 1980, pp 99–108.
25. Cuddy MM, Dillon GF, Clauser BE, et al: Assessing the validity of the USMLE Step 2 Clinical Knowledge Examination through an evaluation of its clinical relevance. Acad Med 2004;79(10):S43–S45.
26. Tamblyn R, Abrahamowicz M, Dauphinee WD, et al: Association between licensure examination scores and practice in primary care. JAMA 2002;288(23):3019–3026.
27. Holland PW, Wainer H: Differential Item Functioning. Hillsdale, NJ, Lawrence Erlbaum Associates, 1993.
28. Clauser BE, Mazor KM: Using statistical procedures to identify differentially functioning test items (ITEMS Module). Educ Meas Issues Pract 1998;17(1):31–44.
29. Margolis MJ, Clauser BE, Cuddy MM, et al: Use of the Mini-CEX to rate examinee performance on a multiple-station clinical skills examination: A validity study. Acad Med 2006;81(10):S56–S60.
30. Kane M: Validating the performance standards associated with passing scores. Rev Educ Res 1994;64:425–461.

Evaluation Forms and Global Rating Scales

Louis Pangaro, MD, and Eric S. Holmboe, MD

As noted in earlier chapters, assessing trainee competence in the actual practice setting is critical to effective evaluation. Educators often label this activity as in-training assessment.[1] Effective in-training assessment requires a multifaceted approach including input from both faculty and nonphysician observers.[1,2] The most common evaluation method used by faculty is the global rating scale included as part of an evaluation form, in which the term "global" means all-inclusive, or overall; "scale" describes a linear analog (usually numeric) for distinguishing levels or steps of performance; and "rating" refers to the act of locating a person's performance on the continuum or at a specific level.[3,4] The rating scale is one component of an evaluation form; the form should include some space for descriptive, written comments.[5] Thus, the evaluation documented on the form should equal the sum of the scale rating(s) on specific competencies plus descriptive, written evaluation:

$$\text{Evaluation Form} = \text{Scale Rating(s)} + \text{Written Evaluation}$$

Where do evaluation forms fit into the evaluation system (Fig. 3-1)? Comprehensive evaluation of a trainee is a multidimensional composite, authored by a program director or clerkship director, and typically includes both summary evaluations of learners by one or more teachers and a series of quantified measurements. Evaluations by individual teachers, in turn, may be their own synthesis of multiple observations over days or weeks, with or without single direct observations of competence at individual tasks.

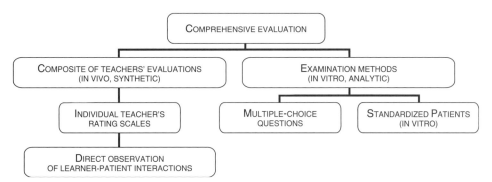

Figure 3-1 Placing evaluation forms into a comprehensive system.

It is the role of academic managers, such as program or clerkship directors, to achieve consistently credible evaluations of trainees, both for the sake of society and future patients (summative evaluation) and to enhance the improvement of trainees through feedback (formative evaluation). The creation of evaluation forms, with or without rating scales, is one strategy academic managers can use to create credible evaluations that are valid (not arbitrary), are reliable across observations by teachers (not capricious), and in formative stages can be relied upon by learners as anticipations of summative grading.[6] Faculty development, in general, and training of teachers in the use of evaluation forms and scales, specifically, are intended to minimize variation between observers, and eliminate unacceptable variation, in which ratings would depend more upon teacher characteristics (or teacher preferences) than upon attributes of the trainee.

Evaluation forms are in themselves, implicitly or explicitly, frameworks to guide teachers' observations and documentation of learners' performance. Therefore, they usually include an explicit statement of goals for the learners, or at least, the criteria by which learners are to be judged. As an official and legal document of a program or institution they publicly express curricular goals and are intended to avoid variance that is "arbitrary," due to having inconsistent goals and standards across teachers. However, they are not guarantees that teachers will not be "capricious" (inconsistent or idiosyncratic) in applying them to individual learners. Experienced program directors will recognize these terms—arbitrary and capricious—as legal terms derived from cases designed to protect learners' Fourteenth Amendment due process rights.[7]

We will begin this chapter by discussing the importance of evaluation frameworks to guide the effective use of evaluation forms. Next, we provide an outline of the advantages and disadvantages of rating scales and evaluation forms, including some important psychometric rating error issues that limit the effectiveness of evaluation forms. The chapter will close with practical suggestions on how to prepare faculty to more effectively use evaluation forms.

Evaluation Forms and Frameworks

In any evaluation form that is to be used by a teacher in evaluating a trainee, there is an underlying set of assumptions about what we expect of the trainee (the educational goals) and about the tasks that a trainee must complete successfully in order to demonstrate that the goals have been achieved (curricular objectives). This set of assumptions can be considered to be the underlying "framework" that encompasses ("frames") everything that is necessary to decide whether the trainee is progressing. Teachers commonly divide the educational goals into three familiar categories (knowledge, skills, and attitudes), but this is simply one useful framework (described in the next section) among several other alternatives.

Analytic Framework

In the traditional framework used in education, including elementary and secondary school, there are three domains: knowledge, skills, and attitudes (KSA). It is straightforward to place learning objectives for learners, especially in preclinical rotations, into the three KSA domains: for instance, *knowledge* of the structures within the chest cavity, *skill* in the physical examination of heart and lungs, and a proper *attitude* of respect for the patient's physical comfort and privacy.

The analytic approach to formulating educational goals provides a generic set of terms that can be applied to any curricular task in any field of education. The analytic approach is particularly useful when trying to measure discrete aspects, and course and program directors are quite familiar with using a single multiple-choice test as a measure of knowledge, and perhaps with using a checklist to rate skill in examining a patient's knee, or in giving informed consent. By isolating one particular aspect of performance, for instance, the ability to interview the patient about an alcohol use history, or the ability to place a central venous catheter, the analytic method allows us to create a fairly detailed set of performance tasks that can be compiled into a checklist, which can in turn be placed on a rating form. Such a checklist can be as detailed as necessary to help the teacher document whether each aspect of a particular task can be performed separately, then combined into a single (global) rating. Together, all these items (checklist and overall global rating) constitute the criterion description of what ultimate proficiency (or competency) looks like for this task. The analytic method requires an evaluation form to have at least three scales (Fig. 3-2).

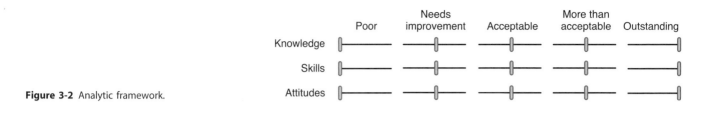

Figure 3-2 Analytic framework.

Developmental Framework

The growth of human beings has often been used as a metaphor for the growth of students in an educational process. The pedigree of this approach is ancient, and Plato describes the growth of the individual from a pre-occupation with superficial, concrete details toward a perception of the true meaning and form underlying them. In the well-known *Taxonomy of Educational Objectives in the Cognitive Domain*, Bloom provides a vocabulary for describing the progressively higher mental skills acquired by students in primary education: knowledge, comprehension, application, analysis, synthesis, and evaluation.[8] Dreyfus and Dreyfus provided a generic vocabulary of educational progress for adult learners from novice, to advanced beginner, competent performance, proficient performance, intuitive expert, and master.[9] Developmental models are very useful for medical school faculty because they reflect the fact that students grow, and that not all learners are at the same level of performance. The models of Bloom and Dreyfus focus on cognitive aspects of development, and personal and attitudinal characteristics are not evident. Bloom, and to some extent Dreyfus, choose to treat the attitudinal ("affective") domain separately from the cognitive; however, their advantage over analytic models, which lack an explicit terminology to capture change, is that the recognition of growth and progress is explicit, and does not have to be inferred by the teacher or the student. To this extent, any curriculum that has learners at different stages, such as medical school, requires some explicitly developmental aspect. Using the Dreyfus model, a linear rating scale similar to a Likert scale could be constructed in which the word "novice" was at the left and "master" was at the extreme right (Fig. 3-3).

The Dreyfus terms used as "anchors" on the linear scale shown in Figure 3-3 are global, and such a developmental scale could be developed for a specific domain within the analytic framework.

This scale can be made less vague, although still abstract, using Bloom's taxonomy for the growth of clinical reasoning. For example, Figure 3-4 demonstrates how you might judge a resident's case presentation.

In this example, the "criterion" against which the resident is to be rated is clinical reasoning, and the

program director has to decide what level of performance is acceptable (the "standard") for a PGY-1, PGY-2, PGY-n.

Given the ACGME framework of six competencies in each of which a *finishing* resident is judged to be successful (or not), such static, or pass/fail, dichotomous ratings of competence must be modified for those earlier in their training. The faculty or program director then must determine what is the "standard" to be met within the criterion for each level. In other words, it is the responsibility of the program director to reframe each of the specific ACGME competencies into a developmental model which can describe what the acceptable/passing "standard of performance" is for student, intern, resident, or fellow.

A Synthetic Model

As students and residents progress toward independence, we expect that they themselves will spontaneously and consistently bring whatever skills, knowledge, and attitudes are necessary to help a patient, today; the learner is himself/herself responsible for deciding (whether or not consciously) what this patient needs. This leads to a "synthetic" definition of competence as "the ability to bring to each patient seen in one's practice everything that that patient needs, and nothing else." In other words, competence at the point of independent practice requires that the resident make the decisions about what the task is, right at this moment, and summon whatever skill, knowledge, or attitude is needed.[10,11] In rating performance we might comment individually on a resident's fund of knowledge, or "attitude," but in the end, we have to judge whether residents have been able to master all the necessary attributes and, on their own, combine them successfully. A synthetic framework[6] "puts things together" in a vocabulary that emphasizes progressively higher expectations as a student progresses through the clinical years and through residency. The underlying premise is that the purpose of medical education is growing independence. Interns are in supervised practice, but their level of responsibility is clearly higher than that of students. More important, when residents graduate and move into practice, their ability

Figure 3-3 Developmental framework—Dreyfus.

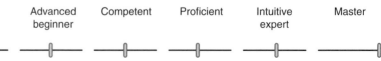
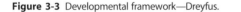

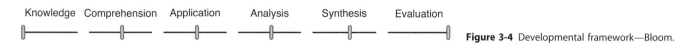

Knowledge   Comprehension   Application   Analysis   Synthesis   Evaluation

Figure 3-4 Developmental framework—Bloom.

to function without supervision must be documented. These concepts of "responsibility" and "function" are both synthetic, in which a combination of knowledge, skills, and attitudes is required.

Independence does not mean a lack of accountability, or freedom to function outside the medical care system; in fact, the opposite is now taught in training programs under the "system-based practice" competency of the ACGME. However, growing independence is the underlying premise of the synthetic model, and it has this in common with developmental models (differences will be discussed later).

RIME Framework

Box 3-1 presents a useful framework for evaluating students and residents. Its name uses a descriptive, developmental vocabulary: reporter, interpreter, manager/educator (RIME).

The RIME framework is explicitly developmental and distinguishes basic and advanced expectations of performance. Each RIME step is a final, "common pathway" of professional competencies that synthesizes skills, knowledge, and attitude and can be used for setting minimal expectations for learners in each year of training.[6] The RIME framework does not set the upper bound of what a student or resident is allowed to do, but rather the minimal standard of acceptable performance for the learner's level of training. In this respect RIME is a "razor," helping teachers to set a clear "cutpoint" below which the learner is classified as not yet ready for higher responsibility.

The RIME framework is different from other developmental models in that it is not necessarily sequential. Progress toward higher learning is usually apparent in the basic tasks; for instance, residents typically gather and interpret patients' findings together, and prepare

for management discussions at the same time. Even residents might function at a "reporter" level for something uncommon, like Cushing syndrome, but be at "manager" level for community-acquired pneumonia. In other words, the RIME synthetic framework has an explicit developmental aspect, but is not, strictly speaking, developmental. It focuses on visualizing what success looks like for learners at each level, and in this sense it is behavioral. In rating an individual learner-patient encounter, the RIME method can be applied directly to the level of performance just observed. On the other hand, for an end of rotation evaluation form, it is up to the teacher to be sure that the overall rating reflects the level that the learner has achieved consistently, and considers the common, core medical issues that are likely to be encountered at the next level of training or practice. The RIME vocabulary (Box 3-2) is an attempt to provide a portable vocabulary that teachers can use to observe and categorize a learner's performance with a specific patient, or overall for a rotation.

Although it appears that the terms of the RIME scheme describe developmental stages through which a student progresses systematically, this is not strictly true. Learners may be quite proficient at interpreting chest pain in a hospitalized patient, but complete novices in dealing with nodular goiter. This content-based expertise is true for both students and residents. The RIME framework describes how a learner interacts with a particular patient, and it is up to a teacher to make a judgment about the overall level of performance with common, core problems that are expected to be seen within each educational experience. As noted in the section Developmental Frameworks, advanced learners do not typically separate the tasks of reporting and interpreting, or reporting and managing. For an expert, the fundamentals of differential diagnosis underlie the way patients are interviewed and examined; in other words, the task of interpretation is contained within the gathering of data, and a good oral case presentation typically contains an implicit interpretation.

Likewise, the "manager/educator" relationship with patients is established during the act of interviewing them, and so is also present within what appears to be merely the reporter function. The RIME scheme guides teachers' observations in looking for the signs of interpretation or management within the student's act of reporting. Perhaps more important, the apparent stages of the RIME scheme can be used to establish a minimally acceptable level of performance for learners at each level. A clinical clerk must always be an acceptable reporter, even though interpreting is not yet proficient. A resident, on the other hand, must always be successful as reporter, interpreter, and manager. In other words, the RIME is a "razor" and can be used to set pass/fail thresholds.

In the global rating scale, we can infer that interpreter is a higher level of performance than the reporter role, and that manager is higher than interpreter (Fig. 3-5).

BOX 3-1	**The RIME Scheme: A Synthetic Framework for Progress of Clinical Trainees**

Reporter: fulfills the promise of reliably, respectfully, and honestly gathering information from patients and communicating with faculty; gets the basic work done; answers the "what" questions.

Interpreter: reporting shows selectivity and prioritization and implies analysis; takes ownership for thinking through patient problems, and of acquiring the knowledge to offer a reasonable differential diagnosis; answers the "why" questions.

Manager: takes ownership for working with patients on diagnostic and therapeutic decisions, and fulfills a promise of developing the expertise to do so; consistently answers "how" to resolve problems.

Educator: personal planning and reflection fulfill a commitment to deeper expertise for self, colleagues, and patients; takes ownership for self-correction and self-improvement.

Reporter	Interpreter	Manager/Educator

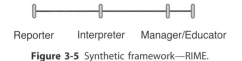

Figure 3-5 Synthetic framework—RIME.

BOX 3-2   RIME Vocabulary

Reporter: A learner must be reliable in working with patients, must accurately gather and communicate the clinical findings on his/her own patients, and can answer the "what" questions (What is the patient's blood pressure? What medications is the patient on?). Proficiency as a reporter requires the skill to do an accurate history and physical examination and the basic knowledge of what to look for. Like a newspaper journalist, the learner must independently gather the information, and communicate it in a variety of formats of different lengths.

Interpreter: A successful interpreter accepts ownership for thinking independently, and consistently offers an explicit differential diagnosis, explicitly supported by findings learned in basic science courses, for problems that are common in medical practice. Interpreters can answer the "why" questions (Why does my patient have abdominal pain? Why is this liver enlarged?) Overall, interpreting requires a higher level of knowledge and more skill in stating the clinical findings that support possible diagnoses and in applying test results to specific patients. A student has to make the transition, emotionally, from "bystander" to become an active participant in patient care.

Manager: Managing patient care takes even more knowledge, more confidence, and more judgment in deciding when action needs to be taken and to propose and select among options; the learner accepts ownership for answering the "how" questions for getting things done. An essential element is the ability to work with each particular patient's circumstances and preferences, that is, to be patient-centered, which depends upon interpersonal skills and the ability to educate patients.

Educator: This is part of the strategy of management, focused on a learning plan for the physician and for bringing the patients to the point at which they (and their families) can participate in decisions. Defining important questions to learn about in more depth takes insight. Having the drive and time-management skills to look for the evidence on which clinical practice can be based and knowing whether current evidence will stand up to scrutiny are qualities of an advanced trainee; to share leadership in educating the team (and even the faculty) takes maturity and confidence. Residents and fellows are generally expected to systematically learn from their own practice experience and be educators. We would also argue that those ready for independent practice should be able to explain the essence of their management to their interns and to their patients.

Adapted from Pangaro, LN: Evaluating professional growth: A new vocabulary and other innovations for improving the descriptive evaluation of students. Acad Med 1999;74:1203–1207.

Are the distances between the three equal? There is no empirical data to support this, and because being an educator is part of the action phase of the process, it is difficult to assign a visual distance between them.

Descriptive Terminology for Evaluation

Why is it necessary to have a vocabulary of descriptive evaluation for use by teachers in the clinical setting? Such evaluations are often felt to be "subjective" and susceptible to biases of the individual teacher,[12] to student-teacher interactions, and to halo effects (in which the

student's strengths prevent adequate recognition of limitations). "Objective" assessment tools, such as multiple-choice tests or an objective structured clinical examination (OSCE) using stan-dardized patients, have been considered to be more reliable.[12,13] However, such highly structured examinations are resource intensive, under the control of program and clerkship directors rather than everyday teachers, and are difficult to arrange frequently enough to provide ongoing feedback. Moreover, clinical teachers spend so much time with students that some descriptive vocabulary and framework are essential if their observations are to be used for formative evaluation (feedback) or summative evaluation (grading). We hope to persuade teachers that their descriptions of a student's behavior are not inevitably inferior to computerized tests and high-fidelity simulations using mannequins; in fact, because of its feasibility and easy application, we feel that "low-tech" can be "good tech."

The RIME scheme is an attempt to help teachers make their observations more structured and more consistent, by providing a useful description of what success looks like for each trainee. In fact, using the RIME scheme it is possible to achieve the level of reliability that is sufficient for pass/fail decisions,[14] that has predictive validity for identifying poor performance during internship,[15] and that helps achieve a high degree of intersite consistency in a multisite curriculum.[16] In other words, evaluations using words can be both reliable and valid, if they are part of a system of regular *frame of reference* training for teachers.[17,18] It may be more appropriate to refer to such evaluations by teachers as "descriptive," avoiding the term "subjective," which carries a pejorative connotation for those trained in the sciences.[10] Teachers are more reluctant to offer comments on personal behaviors, which they or students might consider hard to measure ("subjective"); yet these aspects are exactly what we must capture if we are to give feedback on professional growth.[11,19] The RIME descriptive vocabulary has been reported to be feasible and fair by students and faculty at multiple institutions.[20–22] Perhaps more important, several studies by Hemmer and associates have shown what would probably seem intuitive: teachers will tell you what they will not write down on evaluation forms, and that this information is more sensitive in detecting students who have deficiencies of general knowledge on multiple-choice final examination scores and in detecting students with professionalism problems.[19,23] In other words, the "low-tech" method of asking teachers what they think about students can be helpful in providing students with interim information about their progress that can help them anticipate summative evaluations.

The synthetic RIME framework provides a way for teachers and trainees to visualize what success looks like. Its terms are more concrete, more behavioral

Table 3-1 **The Analogous Rhythm of the Scientific, Clinical, and RIME Processes**

Classical Scientific Method	Clinical Process	RIME Scheme
Observation	History and physical examination	Reporter
Reflection	Diagnosis	Interpreter
Action	Therapy	Manager
Reflection/further observation	Follow-up	Educator

than the generic terms of the analytic models (knowledge, skills, and attitudes) or the developmental Dreyfus model (novice, beginner, expert, etc.). Because its rhythm (observation-reflection-action) parallels the day-to-day activities of clinicians and scientists, it has an intuitive value and acceptance by teachers (Table 3-1).

There is probably not an intern in the United States who has not written a "SOAP" note in which that classic rhythm of observation-reflection-action is reproduced, with observations recorded as "Subjective, Objective" and reflection-action as "Assessment and Plan"). In other words, the rhythm within the RIME scheme captures what physicians and scientists do every day. It is simple, without being simplistic.

Complementary Frameworks—ACGME General Competencies and RIME

It is helpful to explain how frameworks can be complementary and not mutually exclusive. The first three items of the ACGME competencies framework are the traditional knowledge, skills, and attitudes of the analytic approach and are implicit, not explicit, in the RIME framework. In other words, if after a night on call the resident can successfully propose an evidence-based management plan that incorporates patient preferences, it follows that he/she has the needed medical knowledge and reasoning skills, as well as interpersonal and communication skills, and has accepted professional ownership of the need to do so. The ACGME term of "patient care" is essentially a synthetic term that embraces the four terms of the RIME scheme. System-based practice is contained in the term "manager," and practice-based learning and improvement is an advanced form of being an educator.

Frameworks: Concluding Thoughts

Frameworks are not inherently right or wrong. They are methods that can help teachers clarify and students learn. Frameworks are useful in their different ways to help teachers assess trainees' progress toward independence. Synthetic models are strongest in structuring observations made of learners in their actual care of patients (in vivo), because these acts involve complex

tasks that require multiple attributes. Analytic models are best at looking at discrete tasks whether in the care of patients (in vivo) and under testing conditions (in vitro).

We wish to stress two principles of assessment in the clinical setting. One is that the framework must be accepted by the teacher rating the learner; that is, it must not appear arbitrary, or the teachers will instead feel free to use their own intuitive, and potentially less effective, frameworks. Second, the framework has to be applied consistently across teachers and across students; otherwise, the process is capricious. We should not assume that any form or framework is so intuitively valid and easy to use that a teacher will apply it with consistency. Therefore, there must be ongoing training and feedback about the framework and the use of rating scale (see later section in this chapter on faculty development).

To some extent the integrity of the assessment process for trainees depends on teachers using it, and using it consistently. This in turn may depend on its ease of use, its portability from one trainee or location to another, and its ability to be remembered. Our strategy is that simplicity leads to acceptance; acceptance leads to use; use leads to consistency, and consistency is an important element of fairness.

Rating Scales

Rating scales arose from a need to evaluate areas of performance not captured by standard knowledge-based instruments. Impetus for the development of rating scales came from two sources in the early 1900s: (1) psychologists looking to measure human attitudes and (2) military branches that wanted to better evaluate trainees who were using new technologies.[3,4] Thurstone and Likert were two influential individuals in the development of rating scales. In the late 1920s Thurstone developed a cumbersome process for developing scales but advanced the important notion of using "equal-appearing intervals" when devising scales. In 1932 Likert developed the well-recognized scale employing not only equal intervals but adding descriptors at each point along the scale (i.e., strongly agree, agree, undecided, disagree, strongly disagree). Over the past 60 years many scales have been developed with better psychometric properties, including specific rating scales and evaluation forms for medical education. These forms were developed with the goal of evaluating such important competencies as clinical skills, clinical judgment and decision making, interpersonal and communication skills, and professionalism.

Although the Likert scale approach is still commonly used in surveys and survey research, most evaluation forms in medicine training use a *behaviorally anchored rating scale (BARS)*. A BARS form provides descriptors of performance at various points along the scale. An example of a behaviorally anchored rating scale is the American Board of Internal Medicine (ABIM) evaluation form for residents and fellows (Fig. 3-6).

INTERNAL MEDICINE RESIDENT EVALUATION FORM

Resident's Name

Attending's Name

Rotation Name

Rotation Period

Evaluation Date

In evaluating the resident's performance, use as your standard the level of knowledge, skills and attitudes expected from the clearly satisfactory resident at this stage of training. **For any component that needs attention or is rated a 4 or less, please provide specific comments and recommendations on the back of the form.** Be as specific as possible, including reports of critical incidents and/or outstanding performance. Global adjectives or remarks, such as "good resident," do not provide meaningful feedback to the resident.

	Unsatisfactory		Satisfactory			Superior		
	1	2	3	4	5	6	7	8	9

1. Patient Care
Incomplete, inaccurate medical interviews, physical examinations, and review of other data; incompetent performance of essential procedures; fails to analyze clinical data and consider patient preferences when making medical decisions

❏ Insufficient contact to judge

1 2 3 4 5 6 7 8 9

❏ Performance needs attention

Superb, accurate, comprehensive medical interviews, physical examinations, review of other data, and procedural skills; always makes diagnostic and therapeutic decisions based on available evidence, sound judgment, and patient preferences

2. Medical Knowledge
Limited knowledge of basic and clinical sciences; minimal interest in learning; does not understand complex relations, mechanisms of disease

❏ Insufficient contact to judge

1 2 3 4 5 6 7 8 9

❏ Performance needs attention

Exceptional knowledge of basic and clinical sciences; highly resourceful development of knowledge; comprehensive understanding of complex relationships, mechanisms of disease

3. Practice-Based Learning Improvement
Fails to perform self-evaluation; lacks insight, initiative; resists or ignores feedback; fails to use information technology to enhance patient care or pursue self-improvement

❏ Insufficient contact to judge

1 2 3 4 5 6 7 8 9

❏ Performance needs attention

Constantly evaluates own performance, incorporates feedback into improvement activities; effectively uses technology to manage information for patient care and self-improvement

4. Interpersonal and Communication Skills
Does not establish even minimally effective therapeutic relationships with patients and families; does not demonstrate ability to build relationships through listening, narrative or nonverbal skills; does not provide education or counseling to patients, families, or colleagues

❏ Insufficient contact to judge

1 2 3 4 5 6 7 8 9

❏ Performance needs attention

Establishes a highly effective therapeutic relationship with patients and families; demonstrates excellent relationship building through listening, narrative and nonverbal skills; excellent education and counseling of patients, families, and colleagues; always "interpersonally" engaged

30

	Unsatisfactory			Satisfactory			Superior		
	1	2	3	4	5	6	7	8	9	

5. Professionalism
Lacks respect, compassion, integrity, honesty; disregards need for self-assessment; fails to acknowledge errors; does not consider needs of patients, families, colleagues; does not display responsible behavior

☐ Performance needs attention

Always demonstrates respect, compassion, integrity, honesty; teaches/role models responsible behavior; total commitment to self-assessment; willingly acknowledges errors; always considers needs of patients, families, colleagues

☐ Insufficient contact to judge

6. System-Based Learning
Unable to access/mobilize outside resources; actively resists efforts to improve systems of care; does not use systematic approaches to reduce error and improve patient care

☐ Performance needs attention

Effectively accesses/utilizes outside resources; effectively uses systematic approaches to reduce errors and improve patient care; enthusiastically assists in developing systems' improvement

☐ Insufficient contact to judge

Resident's Overall Clinical Competence in Internal Medicine on Rotation

☐ Performance needs attention

Attending's Comments

_____

_____

_____

_____

_____

_____

Signatures: Resident's _____ **Attending's** _____

Figure 3-6 Internal medicine resident evaluation form.

31

MEDICINE CLERKSHIP EVALUATION FORM

Student Name: _____   Dates: From _____ TO: _____

Site: _____

For each area of evaluation, please check the appropriate level of ability. Qualities should be <u>cumulative</u> as rating increases, e.g. an outstanding rating for physical exam skills assumes that major findings are identified in an organized, focused manner AND that subtle findings are elicited. Indicate the level at which the student is <u>consistent</u>.

OUTSTANDING	*ABOVE AVERAGE*	*ACCEPTABLE*	*NEEDS IMPROVEMENT*	*UNACCEPTABLE*
DATA GATHERING				
Initial History/Interviewing Skill			If Not Observed, Check Here O	
O Resourceful, efficient, appreciates subtleties, prepares for management.	O Precise, detailed, appropriate to setting (ward or clinic), focused/selective.	O Obtains basic history. Identifies new problems. Accurate data gathering.	O Inconsistent reporter. Incomplete or unfocused. Inconsistent data gathering.	O Unreliable reporter. Inaccurate, major omissions, inappropriate.
Physical Examination Skill			If Not Observed, Check Here O	
O Elicits subtle findings	O Organized, focused, relevant	O Major findings identified	O Incomplete, or insensitive to patient comfort	O Unreliable PE, unable to gather findings; major gaps
DATA RECORDING				
Written Histories & Physicals			If Not Observed, Check Here O	
O Concise, reflects thorough understanding of disease process & patient situation	O Documents key information, focused, comprehensive, reporting implies interpretation	O Accurate, complete, timely reporting. Fulfills Reporter role.	O Often late; poor flow in HPI, lacks supporting detail, labs, or incomplete problem lists. Gaps in reporting.	O Inaccurate data or major omissions. Unreliable reporting, recording.
Progress Notes/Clinic Notes			If Not Observed, Check Here O	
O Analytical in assessment and plan	O Precise, concise, organized	O Identify on-going problems & documents plan	O Needs organization, omits relevant data	O Not core or inaccurate data
Oral Presentations			If Not Observed, Check Here O	
O Tailored to situation (type of rounds); emphasis and selection of facts teaches others key points	O Fluent reporting; focused; good eye contact; selection of facts implies interpretation	O Maintains format, includes all basic information; minimal use of notes	O Major omissions, often includes irrelevant facts, rambling	O Consistently ill-prepared, does not know facts about patient, reports inaccurate information
KNOWLEDGE				
In General			If Not Observed, Check Here O	
O Understands therapeutic interventions, broad-based	O Thorough understanding of diagnostic approach, can move to interpreter	O Demonstrates understanding of basic pathophysiology	O Marginal understanding of basics, struggles to interpret data for others'	O Major deficiencies in knowledge base
Relating To Own Patients			If Not Observed, Check Here O	
(check as applicable) O Broad textbook mastery O Directed literature search O Educator of others	O Expanded differential diagnoses, can discuss minor problems; sufficient to suggest management	O Knows basic differential diagnoses of active problems in own patients; fills promise of growing knowledge	O Inconsistent understanding, insufficient to interpret consistently on own patients	O Lacks knowledge to understand own patients' problems; rarely sufficient to interpret
DATA INTERPRETATION				
Analysis				
O Understands complex issues, interrelates patient problems	O Consistently offers reasonable interpretation of data	O Constructs problem list, applies basic, reasonable differential diagnosis	O Frequently reports data without analysis; problem lists need improvement	O Cannot interpret basic data; problem lists inaccurate/not updated
Judgment/Management				
O Insightful approach to management plans	O Diagnostic decisions are consistently reasonable	O Appropriate patient care, aware of own limitations	O Inconsistent prioritization of clinical issues	O Poor judgment, actions affect patient adversely
MANAGEMENT SKILLS				
Patient Care Activities			If Not Observed, Check Here O	
O Functions at senior level, negotiates with patients, coordinates health care team	O Efficient & effective, often takes initiative in follow-up (clinic or ward)	O Monitors active problems, maintains patient records, fulfills duty toward patient	O Needs prodding to complete tasks; follow-up is inconsistent	O Unwilling to do expected patient care activities; unreliable
Procedures			If Not Observed, Check Here	
O Unusually proficient and skillful	O Careful, confident, compassionate	O Shows reasonable skill in preparing for and doing procedures	O Awkward, reluctant to try even basic procedures	O No improvement even with coaching, insensitive

June 2006

Figure 3-7 Medicine clerkship evaluation form.

PROFESSIONAL ATTITUDES

Reliability/Commitment

O Accepts full personal ownership in education & patient care	O Seeking responsibility as manager; views self as active participant in patient care	O Fulfills responsibility, accepts ownership of essential roles in care	O Often unprepared, not consistently present and not reporting accurately	O Unexplained absences, unreliable. Makes no promise of duty.

Response to Instruction/Feedback

O Continued self-assessment leads to further growth; insightful reflection	O Seeks and consistently improves with feedback; self-reflective	O Generally improves with feedback	O Inconsistent, does not sustain improvement;	O Lack of improvement; defensive/argumentative; avoids responsibility

Self-Directed Learning (knowledge and skills)

O Outstanding initiative, consistently educates others	O Sets own goals; reads, prepares in advance when possible	O Reads appropriately, and accepts ownership for self-education.	O Needs prompting, not meeting promise of growing expertise.	O Unwilling, lack of introspection. Makes no promise of expertise.

PROFESSIONAL DEMEANOR

Patient Interactions

O Preferred provider; seen as care manager by patient/teachers	O Gains confidence & trust, duty is evident to patient/healthcare team	O Sympathetic, respectful, develops rapport, gains trust	O Occasionally insensitive, inattentive	O Avoids personal contact, tactless, rude, disrespectful.

Response to Stress

O Outstanding poise, constructive solutions	O Flexible, supportive	O Appropriate adjustment	O Inflexible or loses composure easily	O Inappropriate coping

Working Relationships

O Establishes tone of mutual respect & dignity	O Good rapport with other hospital staff	O Cooperative, productive member of own team	O Lack of consideration for others	O Antagonistic or disruptive

COMMENTS: (Written comments are also required. **What's the "next step" for this student?** Thanks.)
Please check <u>each</u> step the student has <u>consistently</u> reached: o Reporter   o Interpreter   o Manager   o Educator

Recommended Grade: _____   Have you discussed this report with the student? ____

			Intern	Resident	Attending	Preceptor
_____	_____	_____	_____	_____	_____	_____
Printed Name	Signature	Date				

Our System is Based on Performance Criteria Rather Than Percentages. Please Use These to Describe Current Level of Student Work

PASS:
(Reporter)   Satisfactory performance. Obtains and reports basic information completely, accurately, reliably; is beginning to interpret; professional qualities are solid. Distinctive personal qualities should be recognized in descriptive comments.

HIGH PASS:
(Interpreter)   Clearly more than typical work in most areas of evaluation. Proceeds consistently to interpreting data; good working fund of knowledge; an active participant in care. Consistent preparation for clinics. Promises of duty/expertise evident.

HONORS:
(Manager/
Educator)   Outstanding ratings in most major areas of evaluation. Fourth-year level of patient care, actively suggesting management options; excellent general fund of knowledge, outstanding (broad/deep) knowledge on own patients. Strong qualities of leadership and excellence in interpersonal relationships, and able to the lead with patients/families/professionals on solutions. Promises of duty and growing expertise clearly evident and exceptional.

LOW PASS: Overall Marginal performance—performs acceptably in some areas but clearly needs improvement in others. Has shown evidence of progress and may be able to perform acceptably as a physician with additional experience in Medicine during Fourth Year without having to repeat the entire third year clerkship.

FAIL: Overall inadequate performance or unacceptable performance in any major area of evaluation. Little improvement with guidance. A grade of Fail will require repeating the clerkship.

June 2006

Figure 3-7, cont'd Medicine clerkship evaluation form.

This form contains the ACGME competencies of patient care, medical knowledge, professionalism, interpersonal skills and communication, practice-based learning and improvement, and systems-based practice graded on a 9-point scale (1 to 3 denoting unsatisfactory, 4 to 6 satisfactory, and 7 to 9 superior performance). Figure 3-7 shows an example of a BARS form for medical students from the Uniformed Services University of the Health Sciences containing detailed descriptors (incorporating RIME terms) at each level of performance on a 5-point scale.

The optimal range of a numeric scale is debated, but most experts recommend a scale contain between 4 and 9 gradations. A 9-point scale is helpful when comparing a large population of trainees, and for this reason organizations like the certification boards use a 9-point scale on tracking forms for residents and subspecialty fellows. Many programs have adopted 4- or 5-point scales on the belief that when rating an individual trainee, it is difficult to distinguish more than 4 or 5 levels of performance. For example, some residency program forms target only four categories of performance: unsatisfactory, marginal, satisfactory, and superior/outstanding. The logic of this approach is that varying "degrees" within categories of unsatisfactory, satisfactory, or superior performance are not terribly useful from an educational and formative assessment standpoint.

Purposes and Advantages of Evaluation Forms

Relative to other evaluation tools, evaluation forms can be relatively time efficient and flexible. Programs can modify or develop evaluation forms to suit specific needs. However, several caveats should be noted if you choose to develop a new evaluation form with a rating scale. First, the training program should assess, at a minimum, the reliability if not also the validity of the forms. Second, development of "new" forms, independent of efforts to teach faculty how to effectively use the new forms, does not necessarily lead to more reliable or valid assessments of the resident.[24] In fact, attention has shifted away from developing "better" forms because most performance appraisal experts believe that more focus is needed on how to train raters to use the form more effectively.[25,26] This is where the importance of evaluation frameworks comes in, and we will provide suggestions for faculty training later in the chapter. We should emphasize that reliability can be increased by increasing the number of observers and the number of observations in a composite evaluation (see Chapter 2).

Evaluation forms, if used effectively, can provide a longitudinal "composite" assessment. Other tools, such as standardized patients, although very valuable, usually only provide a cross-sectional assessment at a single point in time. Evaluation forms have the potential to capture judgments of individual faculty based on multiple observations conducted over time. The

first task of rating forms should be to structure the observations of faculty so that their "findings" (analogous to a patient's symptoms or vital signs) are focused to the goals of the program and are not idiosyncratic to the observer. Observations must then be interpreted, and placed in the framework of the program, and a conclusion reached as to whether this learner is meeting the expectations or values of the program; this interpretation of the observations is called evaluation. The evaluation may be used to provide feedback to the learner about his/her progress. Finally, there may be a conversion of the evaluation into a grade. In this respect grading is an administrative action rather than simply an educational one.

The evaluation form, as stated by Streiner,[3] is "far less intrusive than other grading techniques." Evaluation forms are intended to minimize the potential bias of the "Hawthorne effect," that is, when the process of measurement itself affects what is being measured. Evaluation forms should serve as an important template for feedback. Since evaluation forms usually contain the competencies of interest, reviewing the form with the trainee will help her or him gain knowledge about the content and characteristics of the clinical competencies, and understand the framework used for evaluation. In the United States, the six ACGME competencies not only apply to all residency and fellowship programs, regardless of specialty, but also will be the same competencies certification boards use to assess practicing physicians in maintenance of certification programs. Therefore, consistently reviewing an evaluation form containing these six competencies will help to prepare the trainee for lifelong assessment.

The trainee should be able to review completed evaluation forms as part of a comprehensive evaluation program, ideally as part of a portfolio approach to comprehensive assessment (see Chapter 7). It is important to remember that one of the evaluation form's major purposes is to document the professional development of the trainee dependent on his/her stage of training. Ideally, the evaluation record, whether paper or electronic, should provide space for the trainee to react and respond to the evaluation. And the trainee should be strongly encouraged to provide in writing their reactions and subsequent plans for personal development based on the evaluation. In this respect, a portfolio may be more than a tool for documentation or assessment, and may move into a curricular device for stimulating reflection (see Chapter 7). However, to be most effective, faculty must take responsibility for completing and returning evaluation forms in a timely fashion and review the evaluation form with the trainee prior to the end of an educational or training experience.

Written Assessment

Little attention has been given to the written comments often provided on the rating forms, and, as noted in the section Descriptive Terminology for Evaluation, descriptive evaluation is a crucial aspect of trainee evaluation. However, educators have often found the quality of written comments to be poor. Most comments tend to be brief and cryptic, such as "works hard" or "should read more." Obviously, such comments would not be sufficiently helpful for the trainee if the goal is to guide improvement by specific direction. One study involving two internal medicine residency programs investigated the effectiveness of a brief, multifaceted educational intervention with faculty to improve their written evaluation of residents on inpatient ward rotations.[27] The intervention was quite simple: a brief 15-minute review of evaluation and feedback prior to the start of the rotation and a folded 5-inch by 7-inch card that contained educational reminders and space to record observations (e.g., an "aide-de-memoir" card). The main goals of that study were (1) to improve the specificity of the comments with regard to the areas of competence being evaluated (e.g., medical knowledge versus clinical judgment), and (2) to encourage faculty to provide behavioral examples in support of any rating between 1 and 3 (poor performance) or 7 and 9 (superior performance).

Ninety-one faculty members were randomized among four teaching hospitals; a total of 273 resident evaluation forms were analyzed. The investigators found a modest increase in the number of category-specific written comments and the comments related to clinical skills (e.g., history taking, physical examination) categories in the intervention group compared to the control group. However, residents in the intervention group also reported two important effects: residents were more likely to change their medical management based on feedback from the attending, and they rated the feedback from the attending significantly higher than residents in the control group. The study suggests that a fairly simple, brief faculty intervention may lead to changes in faculty written evaluations. Given the increasingly busy nature of academic clinical practice, training programs truly need educational interventions that are both brief and effective. More work is needed to see if repeated interventions would produce sustained or greater improvement in written evaluations.

Evaluation Sessions

Unfortunately, many forms do not provide enough space for written comments because they are meant to provide a summative, rather than formative, evaluation. Perhaps more important, any descriptive comments written down by teachers are often classified with the pejorative term "subjective" because they are neither quantified nor consistently anchored in specific behaviors observed by all teachers. It is possible that research into the use of descriptive terminology has been inappropriately retarded by the "subjective–objective" terminology, and we should refer to numerical methods (such as multiple-choice examinations) more appropriately as "quantified" or "objectified" rather than "objective."[9–11,28] Given the limitations of written comments on evaluation forms, what else can

educators do to enhance the value of evaluation forms used for longitudinal educational experiences?

Evaluation sessions can be a powerful adjunct to evaluation forms. After the introduction of formal evaluation sessions—regularly scheduled meetings of clerkship directors with teachers[17]—studies documented the intuitive expectation that teachers would report verbally what they had not initially written down on their forms.[18,23] All programs should consider using in-person evaluation meetings with faculty. These sessions do not need to be long; 10 to 15 minutes is sufficient to explore professionalism issues and additional detail about the trainee's performance during the educational rotation.

Psychometric Issues

Global rating scales must possess sufficient reliability and validity to provide useful information about clinical competence. Furthermore, the quality and process of data collection used for the ratings is critically important. We will examine some of the psychometric challenges in using evaluation forms. An excellent review of the psychometric issues was performed by Gray.[5] A brief review of the key issues follows.

Reliability

High inter-rater agreement is a desirable property for rating scales, especially if the forms are completed during a similar time period by more than one evaluator. The results from various studies, however, are conflicting. Haber and Avins[29] reported a mean inter-rater agreement of 0.87, and Thompson reported an average reliability score of 0.64 among attendings in separate internal medicine training programs.[30] Among pediatric residents, Davis found substantially lower inter-rater agreement.[31] Rating of general medical knowledge had the highest agreement at a disappointing 0.36, and the ratings for a category concerning relationship with senior medical staff produced a paltry inter-rater agreement of just 0.06. Maxim and Dielman,[32] in a rating study of third- and fourth-year medical students, found the inter-rater reliability coefficients ranged from 0.14 to 0.31 among 13 items on their 7-point rating scales. However, faculty members were not trained in effective evaluation strategies or use of the forms in any of the above-mentioned studies. The most straightforward solution to improve reliability is simply to increase the number of evaluations. Reliability is a measure of reproducibility, and the more one does anything, the more "stable" the measurement becomes (e.g., the "error" around the mean narrows).

Validity

As we learned earlier in the chapter, a gold standard is required to adequately assess validity. Unfortunately, no definitive standard exists for important areas of interest, such as professionalism, attitudes, and clinical judgment, to name just a few. Therefore, we need to assess different types of validity. Haber and Avins[29] in a

1994 study found construct validity across several internal medicine programs. Residents in more competitive training programs received higher performance ratings from their attendings and program directors than residents from a less competitive program. They also found the ABIM rating form possessed reasonable inter-rater reliability to detect global differences. Ramsey and associates[33] found that ratings from professional peers regarding clinical skills among practicing physicians also correlated highly with ABIM certification status. Thus there is some evidence for construct validity of evaluation forms used in the medical setting.

Studies have also investigated the use of a concurrent (criterion) validity of rating scales. Knowledge as determined by examination has also been frequently used to assess concurrent validity. In a recent review faculty rating of knowledge among pediatric residents correlated with resident scores on their In-Training Examination (ITE). A similar study with family practice residents found that the ability to correctly predict scores on the In-Training Examination was dependent on the faculty's years of teaching experience. Conversely, a study of surgery residents found no correlation between the American Board of Surgery In-Training Examination and a 12-item, 7-point ward evaluation rating form.[34] Finally, a study at a military internal medicine residency found that faculty members were unable to predict which tertile of performance residents scored on their ITE despite having worked closely with the residents.[35] Thus, use of knowledge-based examinations may serve as a reasonable reference standard for knowledge ratings, but little has been done to validate other important domains on the rating scales such as professionalism, humanism, and physical examination skills. Interestingly, a more recent study found modest correlations between a 25-item rating scale for interns completed by residency program directors and their interns' performance in medical school. These authors identified five factors from the rating scale that accounted for the majority of the variance: interpersonal communication, clinical skills, population-based health, record-keeping skills, and critical appraisal skills.[36] Thus, ratings from medical school appear to have some predictive validity when compared to program director ratings.

Rating Errors

One goal of rating scales is to produce an evaluation of specific areas of clinical competence independently of each other. For example, one resident may possess substandard knowledge as evidenced by other measures (e.g., the in-training examination), but display extraordinary humanistic skill. Such a resident should receive high marks under humanistic qualities, but should receive a lower rating for medical knowledge if the attending has effectively evaluated the resident. Unfortunately, most raters have difficulty discriminating between dimensions of competence and tend to use a limited range on the rating scale.[37] The majority of problems with rating scales are mostly due to how faculty members use them, not due to major defects in the scales themselves.

Medical educators commit the same types of *rating errors* noted in all types of performance appraisal. There are two main categories of rater errors: distributional errors and correlational errors.[25] Two common distributional errors are due to range restriction and leniency/severity issues:

1. *Range restriction* is the failure to utilize the entire range of the scale. "Central tendency" error is a subtype of range restriction error in which the rater uses just the midportion of the scale. However, in medicine, attendings usually restrict the marks to the upper ends of the scale (see later in the chapter). An exception to this was seen by Battistone, who reported a shift of the grading curve to the left (away from the inflation) when the behavioral terms based on the RIME scheme (observer-reporter, interpreter, manager, educator) were substituted for numerical ratings.

2. *Leniency/severity error* is a type of distributional error in which the faculty is being either too kind (a "dove") or too harsh (a "hawk"), respectively. Most would argue there are few "hawks" in medicine.

Correlational error occurs when faculty members give similar ratings to each aspect of a trainee's performance regardless of what dimension of competence is being assessed, even when the dimensions are clearly separate. As Cleveland notes, "the result is an inflation of the inter-correlations among the dimensions."[25] When rating inflation occurs, this result is commonly known as *halo error*. This is a common problem in medical education, a field in which everyone is always above average or better. Having the entire list of desirable attributes of the candidate present, at one time, is intended to minimize the chance that teachers will confuse the different domains of evaluation, but caution is needed. The increasing length and complexity of forms may in themselves make the teachers less able, or willing, to use it as intended by the form's author(s). Therefore, increasing the number of domains, rating criteria, or items on a form may aggravate the halo effect. Despite our hopes in differentiating many different aspects of competence, factor analysis has shown that forms often reduce to two basic items: cognitive and noncognitive.

Thompson and colleagues noted in an internal medicine program that 96% of 1039 ratings for 85 residents were between 6 and 9 on a 9-point scale.[30] Both Haber and Avins[28] and Thompson[30] concluded from factor analysis that the rating form cannot reliably discriminate among the 9 listed dimensions of clinical competence used on their evaluation forms. Two other studies, one with first-year residents and another with medical students, found similar results through factor analysis.[32,33] In both studies, two factors accounted for the majority of the variance: the first factor was associated with procedural and cognitive skills and the second with interpersonal skills. The same was true for the two studies with internal medicine residents; cognitive skill and personality attributes accounted for the majority of the variance in resident evaluations.[29,30]

A more recent study that used a rating form incorporating the new ACGME general competencies found again that the form could not "discriminate" between the six general competencies.[38] In all these studies halo error was felt to be highly prevalent. What are the reasons for halo error? For one, raters may rely more on their global impressions when rating trainees on specific dimensions of competence. A second reason, one we all recognize, is the unwillingness of so many faculty members to give lower ratings on any dimension of competence. This has been called the "there goes my teaching award syndrome." Other possible causes of halo error include confirmation bias ("That's how I would do it, so it must be right"), ignoring discordant or inconsistent information or observations about the trainee, and the simple lack of enough observation or information about performance.[25,39] Box 3-3 provides a list of possible reasons for halo error.

One important caveat should be noted about all of the previous studies. The analytical strategy used was factor analysis, a statistical technique purposefully designed to *maximize* correlation and therefore "reduce" the data as much as possible. Using factor analysis to determine whether faculty can discriminate between categories of competence may fail to uncover modest differences between ratings.[40]

Rater Accuracy

Another issue is *rater accuracy*. How well does the rating match the actual performance? There are two distinct types of accuracy measures. The first are behavior-based measures. These types of measures allow the rater to specifically focus on whether the behavior did or did not occur. Checklists are the most common type of "rating scale" used on evaluation forms for behaviorally based measures. They are particularly useful for

structured, controlled assessments such as standardized patients. By definition, they tend to be less "global" because they target more specific behaviors. Second, behaviorally based rating scales are limited in their use for longitudinal assessment, mainly because only so many behaviors or incidents can be specified on the form. However, when used to assess specific trainee-patient encounters, the RIME framework can classify and document behaviors observed in an individual trainee's care of each in a series of patients as consistent with reporting, interpreting, managing, and educating.

The other type of accuracy involves judgmental measures. As the name implies, the rater must apply judgment when providing a rating. Accuracy in judgment is particularly important for rating scales and evaluation forms used in longitudinal educational experiences. There are several types of judgmental accuracy measures: accuracy in whether a trainee has attained a level of performance (criterion accuracy); accuracy in distinguishing among trainees (differential or normative accuracy); and accuracy in discriminating between specific performance or competence dimensions (stereotype accuracy). For evaluation in medical education, accuracy measures are important because defining key behaviors at various levels of competence facilitates better judgment.

Unfortunately, little work has been done with rating scales in medical education to address these issues. In industry, companies have adopted a number of approaches to improve the quality of evaluations.

Faculty Development and Evaluation Forms

The quality of the information on evaluation forms depends mostly on the individual completing the form, not the form itself. For too long medical educators have been looking for the holy grail of evaluation forms. Landry and Farr called for a moratorium on this "quest" over 25 years ago, arguing instead for an increased emphasis on training the evaluators.[24] As noted in the section Written Assessment, even simple approaches to faculty development such as observation cards can modestly improve the quality of information on evaluation forms. However, to realize the full potential of evaluation forms, more structured faculty training is needed.

Throughout this chapter we have highlighted the importance of an evaluation framework to guide the evaluation process. This is a critical first step to getting all faculty members "on the same page." Studies have shown specific types of training can improve inter-rater agreement using a simple three-step process:

1. Standardize the observation of the behavior of interest.
2. Reach agreement on common nomenclature for the desired expectations of interest.

BOX 3-3	**Possible Reasons for Halo Error**

1. Global impression drives the rating for all dimensions of competence
2. Unwillingness or inability to discriminate among different dimensions
3. Reluctant to give negative evaluations
4. Insufficient observation or information about a trainee's performance
5. Confirmation bias
6. Discounting conflicting or discordant information, observations
7. Level of familiarity with trainee
8. Level of familiarity with medical knowledge, skills, and attitudes
9. Dimensions of competence are in fact not completely independent

3. Agree on the relative importance of the different components of behavior being assessed.

Steps 1 and 2 in this process are called performance dimension training (PDT). PDT provides raters with the expected performance standards for each level of performance. Many have argued that such agreement about performance dimension standards is lacking in graduate medical education. Step 3 is known as frame of reference (FOR) training. These techniques have been applied in training faculty to use the RIME framework.

Performance Dimension Training and RIME

The Uniformed Services University of the Health Sciences (USUHS) has incorporated PDT and FOR training as part of the evaluation for medical students rotating on an internal medicine clerkship. Raters participate in evaluation sessions with clerkship directors and descriptive evaluations are collected. Clerkship directors use these evaluation sessions to train preceptors about expected levels of performance for each category of rating and how the student's performance should be documented on the rating scale form. The evaluation system goes one step further by incorporating the student's performance in multiple domains of competence into an overall performance level. Goals for each level of performance are divided into performance categories with defined expectations. Because reporter skills are introduced in first year (see Appendix 3-1), it is felt that that making proficiency in them is a reasonable, non-negotiable level for advancing to the next level of responsibility, yielding this conversion of observations into grades:

Reporter (Pass)
Interpreter (High Pass)
Manager/Educator (Honors)

Appendix 3-2 provides a more comprehensive description of the model and a copy of the performance matrix used at USUHS. The descriptions and criteria are more applicable for residents than for students, because no accommodation distinguishing "reasonable" (student level) from "accurate" (resident level) needs to be made.

Murphy and Cleveland[1] also make several important points about performance appraisal training pertinent to the use of rating scales:

1. Define performance dimensions in behavioral terms and be sure to communicate these terms to the resident and the faculty. It may even be helpful to use a blank evaluation form at the beginning of a rotation as a template to discuss goals and expectations before the evaluation process actually starts.

2. Ratings will more likely correspond with actual rater judgment if training programs support distinctions between house staff on the basis of *performance*, the raters perceive a strong link between the rating they give and specific outcomes, and the raters believe that outcomes should be based on *present* performance.

3. What the rater chooses to communicate through the form depends heavily on the rater's goals and contextual factors. Therefore, raters need to communicate goals directly to the residents and raters must be cognizant of both internal and external environmental factors affecting the context of the evaluation.

Conclusion

Evaluation forms should possess several desirable properties, being "user-friendly," unobtrusive, flexible, and "quantifiable." Correlation has been noted consistently with knowledge-based assessment instruments. The teacher's acceptance of the scale and its framework are prerequisites of consistent use. To some extent, there is an emotional barrier for teachers that has to be bridged: they often see themselves (and certainly describe themselves) as "giving" the student a grade, rather than making a diagnosis, reflecting their observations (something they would never do with a serious medical condition). The teacher may have emotional difficulty in "giving" a grade if contaminated by their acceptance of "subjective-objective" distinctions and by an intuitive, clinical fear of inadequate sampling of the student's abilities. Therefore, they see each observation as not just evaluation but as grading with premature or incomplete data.

Many questions remain regarding reliability, validity, and the ability to discriminate among different aspects of clinical competence, most notably "soft areas" such as humanism, attitudes, professionalism, and judgment. Research has also clearly demonstrated that rater training is crucial to the effective use of rating scales. The optimal approach to rater training in graduate medical education remains to be defined, but the general principles discussed throughout this chapter are an excellent place to begin.

ANNOTATED BIBLIOGRAPHY

1. Gray JD: Global rating scales in residency education. Acad Med 1996;71:S55.
   This excellent review provides a comprehensive overview of the major research work and educational issues about the use of global rating scales and includes an extensive reference list. Dr. Gray also outlines the major research questions for global rating scales, still pertinent today.

2. Hauenstein NMA: Training raters to increase the accuracy of appraisals and the usefulness of feedback. In Smither JW (ed): Performance Appraisal. San Francisco, Jossey Bass, 1998.
   This chapter provides valuable detail on the rater training techniques of performance dimension training and frame of reference training. The context is industry and business, but the general principles apply equally well to evaluation training in medical education. We recommend this chapter for educators responsible for training faculty in evaluation.

3. Pangaro LN: Evaluating professional growth: A new vocabulary and other innovations for improving the descriptive evaluation of students. Acad Med 1999;74:1203–1207.
   This article provides additional background and detail about the RIME framework. This paper would be useful for all faculty members involved in evaluating trainees in any setting.

4. Holmboe ES, Fiebach NF, Galaty L, Huot S: The effectiveness of a focused educational intervention on resident evaluations from faculty: A randomized controlled trial. J Gen Intern Med 2001;16(7):427–434.

This study describes a simple, straightforward approach to enhance, modestly, the quality of the written comments on evaluation forms. The brief faculty intervention described in the article also led to modest benefits in perceived feedback by the trainees in two residency programs. A copy of the simple pocket card is provided with the article.

5. Battistone MJ, Milne C, Sande MA, et al: The feasibility and acceptability of implementing formal evaluation sessions and using descriptive vocabulary to assess student performance on a clinical clerkship. Teach Learn Med 2002;14(1):5–10.
6. Hemmer P, Hawkins R, Jackson J, Pangaro L: Assessing how well three evaluation methods detect deficiencies in medical students' professionalism in two settings of an internal medicine clerkship. Acad Med 2000;75:167–173.
7. Hemmer PA, Pangaro L: Using formal evaluation sessions for case-based faculty development during clinical clerkships. Acad Med 2000;75:1216–1221.

These three articles provide valuable data and insight into the value of using formal evaluation sessions to enhance the evaluation process and improve the consistency of the evaluation process by providing ongoing, longitudinal faculty development. The third article provides specific guidance of how to use evaluation sessions for ongoing faculty development. This is a very important concept: the need to embed faculty development into ongoing educational activities and to move away from using only the workshop approach to faculty development.

REFERENCES

1. Turnbull J, van Barnveld C: Assessment of clinical performance: In-training evaluation. In Norman GR, van der Vleuten CPM, Newble DI (eds): International Handbook of Research in Medical Education. Dordrecht, Netherlands, Kluwer Academic, 2002.
2. Lockyer J: Multi source feedback in the assessment of physician competencies. J Cont Educ Health Prof 2003;23(1):4–12.
3. Streiner DL: Global rating scales. In Neufeld VR, Norman GR (eds): Assessing Clinical Competence. New York, Springer, 1985.
4. Devellis RF: Scale Development: Theory and Applications. Newbury Park, CA, Sage Publications, 1991.
5. Gray JD: Global rating scales in residency education. Acad Med 1996;71:S55.
6. Pangaro L: A new vocabulary and other innovations for improving the descriptive evaluation of students. Acad Med 1999;74:1203–1207.
7. Jamieson T, Hemmer P, Pangaro L: Legal aspects of failing grades. In Fincher R-M (ed): Guidebook for Clerkship Directors, 3rd ed. Washington, DC, Alliance for Clinical Education, 2005.
8. Bloom BS: Taxonomy of Educational Objectives, Handbook I, Cognitive Domain. New York, Longman, 1956.
9. Dreyfus SE, Dreyfus HL: Mind Over Machine. New York, Free Press, Macmillan, 1986, pp 16–51.
10. Pangaro L: Definitions and important distinctions in evaluation. In Fincher R-M (ed): Guidebook for Clerkship Directors, 2nd ed. Washington, DC, Association of American Medical Colleges, 2000, pp 81–84.
11. Pangaro L: Investing in descriptive evaluation: A vision for the future of assessment. Med Teacher 2000;22(5):478–481.
12. Epstein RM, Hundert EM: Defining and assessing professional competence. JAMA 2002;287(2):226–235.
13. Pohl CA, Robeson MR, Veloski J: USMLE Step 2 performance and test administration date in the fourth year of medical school. Acad Med 2004;79(10 Suppl):S49–S51.
14. Roop S, Pangaro L: Measuring the impact of clinical teaching on student performance during a third year medicine clerkship. Am J Med 2001;110(3):205–209.
15. Lavin B, Pangaro L: Internship ratings as a validity outcome measure for an evaluation system to identify inadequate clerkship performance. Acad Med 1998;73:998–1002.
16. Durning S, Pangaro L, Denton GD, et al: Inter-site consistency as a standard of programmatic evaluation in a clerkship with multiple, geographically separated sites. Acad Med 2003;78:S36–S38.
17. Noel G: A system for evaluating and counseling marginal students during clinical clerkships. J Med Educ 1987;62:353–355.
18. Hemmer PA, Pangaro L: Using formal evaluation sessions for case-based faculty development during clinical clerkships. Acad Med 2000;75:1216–1221.
19. Hemmer P, Hawkins R, Jackson J, Pangaro L: Assessing how well three evaluation methods detect deficiencies in medical students' professionalism in two settings of an internal medicine clerkship. Acad Med 2000;75:167–173.
20. Battistone MJ, Milne C, Sande MA, et al: The feasibility and acceptability of implementing formal evaluation sessions and using descriptive vocabulary to assess student performance on a clinical clerkship. Teaching Learning Med 2002;14(1):5–10.
21. Battistone MJ, Pendleton B, Milne C, et al: Global descriptive evaluations are more responsive than global numeric ratings in detecting students' progress during the inpatient portion of an internal medicine clerkship. Acad Med 2001;76(10 Suppl):S105–S107.
22. Ogburn T, Espey E: The R-I-M-E method for evaluation of medical students on an obstetrics and gynecology clerkship. Am J Obstet Gynecol 2003;189(3):666–669.
23. Hemmer P, Pangaro LN: The effectiveness of formal evaluation sessions during clinical clerkships in better identifying students with marginal funds of knowledge. Acad Med 1997;72:641–643.
24. Landy FJ, Farr JL: Performance rating. Psychol Bull 1980;87:72–107.
25. Murphy KR, Cleveland JN: Understanding Performance Appraisal. London, Sage Publications, 1995.
26. Hauenstein NMA: Training raters to increase the accuracy of appraisals and the usefulness of feedback. In Smither JW (ed): Performance Appraisal. San Francisco, Jossey Bass, 1998.
27. Holmboe ES, Fiebach NF, Galaty L, Huot S: The effectiveness of a focused educational intervention on resident evaluations from faculty: A randomized controlled trial. J Gen Intern Med 2001;16(7):427–434.
28. Norman GR, Van der Vleuten CP, De Graaff E: Pitfalls in the pursuit of objectivity: Issues of validity, efficiency and acceptability. Med Educ 1991;25(2):119–126.
29. Haber RJ, Avins AL: Do ratings on the American Board of Internal Medicine Resident Evaluation Form detect differences in clinical competence? J Gen Intern Med 1994;9:140.
30. Thompson WG, Lipkin MJ, Gilbert DA, et al: Evaluation: Assessment of the American Board of Internal Medicine Resident Evaluation Form. J Gen Intern Med 1990;5:214–217.
31. Davis JK, Inamdar S, Stone RK: Interrater agreement and predictive validity of faculty ratings of pediatric residents. J Med Educ 1986;61:901–905.
32. Maxim BR, Dielman TE: Dimensionality, internal consistency, and interrater reliability of clinical performance ratings. Med Educ 1996;21:130–137.
33. Ramsey PG, Carline JD, Inui TS, et al: Predictive validity of certification by the American Board of Internal Medicine. Ann Intern Med 1989;110:719–726.
34. Schwartz RW, Donnelly MB, Sloan DA: The relationship between faculty ward evaluations, OSCE and ABSITE as measures of surgical intern performance. Am J Surg 1995;169:414–417.
35. Hawkins RE, Sumption KF, Gaglione M, Holmboe ES: The In-Training Examination (ITE) in Internal Medicine: Resident perceptions and correlation between resident ITE scores and faculty predictions of resident performance. Am J Med 1999;106:206–210.
36. Paolo AM, Bonaminio GA: Measuring outcomes of undergraduate medical education: Residency directors' ratings of first year residents. Acad Med 2003;78:90–95.
37. Verhulst SJ, Colliver JA, Paiva REA, Williams RG: A factor analysis study of performance of first-year residents. J Med Educ 1986;61:132–143.
38. Silber CG, Nasca TJ, Paskin DL: Do global rating forms enable program directors to assess the ACGME competencies? Acad Med 2004;79(6):549–556.
39. Holmboe ES: The importance of faculty observation of trainees' clinical skills. Acad Med 2004;79:16–22.
40. Feinstein A: Principles of Medical Statistics. Boca Raton, Chapman and Hall/CRC, 2002.

APPENDIX 3-1
The RIME Evaluation Framework: A Vocabulary of Professional Progress

We describe performance goals for trainees using the following progression: reporter, interpreter, manager/educator (RIME). The framework emphasizes a developmental approach and distinguishes between basic and advanced expectations. Each step represents a synthesis of skills, knowledge, and attitude, forming a final, "common pathway" of professional competencies, and is useful for setting *minimal* expectations for a learner. A learner's progress toward higher steps is usually apparent in the basic stages. Trainees might function at a "reporter" level for a complex problem, and at a higher level for problems that are simpler or more familiar. RIME can be applied to single patient encounters or to overall level of consistency.

Reporter

The learner can accurately gather and clearly communicate the clinical facts on his/her own patients, and can answer the questions asking "what?" Proficiency in this step requires the basic skill to do a history and physical examination and the basic knowledge of what to look for. The step emphasizes day-to-day reliability, for instance, being on time, or follow-up of a patient's test results. Implicit in the step is the ability to recognize normal from abnormal and the confidence to identify and label a new problem. This step requires a sense of responsibility and achieving consistency in "bedside" skills in dealing directly with patients. These skills are often introduced to students in their preclinical years, but by the third year they must be mastered as a "passing" criterion. This level is a non-negotiable expectation for all interns.

Interpreter

Transition from "reporter" to "interpreter" is an essential step in the growth of a third-year student, and often it is the most difficult. At a basic level, students must prioritize among problems they have identified. The signs of diagnostic reasoning, such as active use of pertinent positives and negatives, and key findings that imply differential diagnosis, become apparent, and penetrate the process of reporting. Problem lists give syndromes and not merely repetition of findings. The next step is to offer an explicit differential diagnosis and supportive reasoning. Because a public forum can be intimidating to beginners, and third-year students cannot be expected to have the right answer all the time, we define student success as offering at least three reasonable diagnostic possibilities for new

problems, but they must take public ownership of the process of clinical reasoning. Follow-up of tests provides another opportunity to "interpret" the data (especially in the clinic setting). This step requires a higher level of knowledge and more skill in stating the clinical findings that support possible diagnoses and in applying test results to specific patients. A learner has to make the transition, emotionally, from "bystander" to an active participant in patient care, and can answer the questions asking "why?" Interns should be able to interpret, though for unusual problems, their knowledge may limit them.

Manager

Managing patient care takes even more knowledge, more confidence, and more judgment in deciding when action needs to be taken, and to propose and select among options; to answer the "how?" questions for getting things done. We can't require novices to be correct with each suggestion, so we ask students to include at least three *reasonable* options in their diagnostic and therapeutic plan, but they must take ownership of the process of clinical decision making. Finishing interns should be able to manage common problems they will see; advanced residents should be proficient at managing atypical and complex cases and using the full resources of the specific practice setting. An essential element is work with each particular patient's circumstances and preferences, that is, to be patient-centered, which depends upon interpersonal skills and the ability to educate patients.

Educator

This is part of being a manager, and the action is focused on a learning plan for the physician and the patient. Success in each prior step depends on self-directed learning, and on a mastery of basics; but to be an educator in the RIME scheme means to go beyond the required basics, to read deeply, and to share new learning with others, in other words, to take ownership of the process of self-evaluation and improvement. Having the drive and time-management skills to look for hard evidence on which clinical practice can be based and knowing whether current evidence will stand up to scrutiny are qualities of an advanced trainee; to share leadership in educating the team (and even the faculty) takes maturity and confidence. Systematically learning from one's own practice experience and being an educator are abilities generally expected of residents.

Adapted from Pangaro, LN: Evaluating professional growth: A new vocabulary and other innovations for improving the descriptive evaluation of students. Acad Med 1999;74:1203–1207.

APPENDIX 3-2

USUHS Medicine Curriculum Matrix for the Development of Clinical Skills—A Synthetic System (Reporter-Interpreter-Manager-Educator) for Setting Goals and Evaluation Criteria

Aspect of Professional Growth	Year in Training						
	I	II	III	IV	Intern	Residency	Fellowship
Reporter	I	R	P				
Interviewing	I	R	P				
Physical examination	I	R	P			P*	
Written H&Ps		I	R	P			
Oral case presentations		I	R	P			
Reliability, responsibility	I	R	P				
Respect for patient's values	I	R	P				
Interpreter		I	R	P			
Problem lists		I	P				
Differential diagnosis		I	R	R	P		
Interpreting basic ECG, lab tests		I	R	R	P		
Interpreting advanced studies			I	R	R	P	P*
Manager			I	R		P	
Diagnostic plans		I	I	R	P		
Therapeutic plans			I	R	R	P	
Benefit/risk decision making			I	R	R	P	
Basic procedures (IVs, etc.)			I	R	P		
Advanced procedures				I	R	P	
Incorporates patient values in plan			I	R	P		
System-based practice			I	R	R	P	P*
Educator	I		R			P	
Reflective, self-directed learning	I	R	P				
Critical reading skills			I	R	R	P	
Practice-based learning & improvement			I	R	R	P	

I, introduced in the curriculum; R, repetition, practice; P, proficiency sufficient for the next level of independence; P*, sophisticated, complex situations or procedures.

Typically, by a skill's third year in the curriculum, it becomes a passing criterion, or prerequisite for advancement. For each level of performance, examples are given to illustrate the framework, but they do not exhaust the category. The matrix illustrates how the RIME terminology can be used to frame progressively higher expectations across the training continuum.

Using Written Examinations to Assess Medical Knowledge and Its Application

Richard E. Hawkins, MD, and David B. Swanson, PhD

The acquisition and measurement of medical knowledge have received relatively little attention in recent years. Much interest on the part of medical educators and assessment experts has been focused on patient safety and medical errors, the teaching and assessment of clinical skills, teamwork and professionalism, and emerging simulation technologies. Nonetheless, a sound fund of medical knowledge, as well as the ability to apply it in a wide range of clinical contexts, remains the foundation upon which clinical competence is built.[1] Indeed, the breadth and organization of an individual's knowledge form the most important component of the clinical reasoning process and are essential to the development of sound critical thinking skills and expertise.[2,3]

The AAMC Medical School Objectives Project (MSOP) and the Accreditation Council for Graduate Medical Education (ACGME) Outcomes Project define medical knowledge as a core objective/competency in undergraduate and graduate medical education, respectively.[4,5] The MSOP states "physicians must be knowledgeable" as one of its four fundamental attributes, and it delineates a set of related learning objectives for graduating medical students. Knowledge-based learning objectives are also defined within the context of the other fundamental attributes. For example, knowledge and understanding of the economic, psychological, social, and cultural factors that relate to health and illness are essential to being "dutiful"; knowing about the clinical, laboratory, roentgenologic, and pathologic findings associated with common diseases allows the student to be "skillful."[4] Similarly, the ACGME General Competencies include medical knowledge as a specific competence; in addition, specific knowledge objectives are included within the other competencies. For example, knowledge of study design and statistical methods facilitates practice-based learning and improvement, and understanding the differences among various medical practice and delivery systems is critical to competent systems-based practice.[5]

The purpose of this chapter is to present an overview of the written assessment methods used to test medical knowledge and its application; other methods for assessing medical knowledge (computer- and patient-based clinical simulations, real-work observation) are discussed elsewhere in this volume. The authors prefer to consider the term "application" in a broad sense that encompasses a range of cognitive processes implicitly related to the retrieval and use of medical knowledge in problem solving and clinical reasoning. These cognitive processes include interpretation, analysis, synthesis, and inference; typically, an examinee varies in his/her ability to apply knowledge as a function of familiarity and experience with the specific clinical content and problem to be solved.[1,6] Here, the term "application" refers to the use of one or more of these processes in solving a clinical problem or test question (item), and it is distinguished from simple recall of isolated factual information.

Roles for Testing Before, During, and After Clinical Instruction

Clerkship and resident instruction has long been very diverse, occurring in a widely distributed, heterogeneous network of hospital and ambulatory settings. Most instruction is provided in a master-apprentice format, with both faculty and residents serving as masters. Instructional objectives, content, and quality vary extensively from training site to training site and from preceptor to preceptor. The patient mix at individual sites does not necessarily include the broad cross-section of clinical problems that educational common sense suggests is desirable and years of research on medical problem solving[7,8] and clinical competence assessment[9,10] have indicated is necessary. In a very real sense, each medical student and resident experiences a different curriculum.

Even if the overall patient mix at a training site fits well with the goals of instruction, it is difficult to plan and coordinate instructional activities in complex clinical environments that are primarily devoted to patient care. More than 40 years ago, Kerr White raised serious questions about the suitability of the limited and biased educational experience that the hospital setting provides for medical students.[11] More recently, changes in the hospital environment—diagnostic workup prior to hospitalization, early discharge, and the reduced lengths of stay and sicker patient population that have resulted—have made the hospital environment even less suitable educationally. This, among other factors, has increased recognition of the need for training in the ambulatory environment and has hastened development of ambulatory experiences to supplement hospital-based instruction. However, further decentralization of clerkship and resident education into ambulatory settings has increased the need for coordination of educational experiences. Thus, faculty and trainees participating in clinical clerkships and residency rotations face a difficult educational problem. There is typically a huge amount of material to be learned,

the learning environment is complex and unstructured, and, in addition to responsibility for their own learning, trainees often are expected to support the learning activities of peers and more junior trainees, concurrently playing a service role in provision of patient care.

Within the complex environment in which clinical instruction takes place, assessment has many potential roles to play in relation to individual trainees, including motivating them to learn, monitoring achievement of learning outcomes, aiding in plans for individualized remediation, assigning grades, and determining readiness for the next level of training and patient care responsibility. Similarly, assessment has multiple potential roles to play in relation to groups of trainees and the program as a whole, including determining the pace of group instruction, informing selection of instructional methods and topics, and providing evaluative feedback on the quality of individual instructional units and the overall program. Following Cronbach,[12] Table 4-1 provides a summary of the various roles that evaluation can play in relation to individual trainees and groups of trainees before, during, and after instruction.

Because instructional experiences can vary extensively from one trainee to the next, ongoing formative assessment to monitor learning outcomes is particularly important. It is in this area that high-quality written examinations can be most useful; because these examinations can cover a broad range of content efficiently, they can be used to identify areas of strength and weakness so that trainees and programs can capitalize on the former and remediate the latter, providing a basis for trainees and programs to monitor achievement of key learning outcomes. In particular, as discussed in a later section, well-written national standardized in-training examinations (ITEs) can be used to obtain and periodically update a portrait of trainees' clinical knowledge and their ability to apply that knowledge to simulated patient care situations, such as the last vignette illustrated in Box 4-1. The precision (reliability), accuracy (validity), and specificity of this portrait will vary as a function of the format, length, and quality of the assessment methods used, as discussed in the next two sections.

Methods for Assessment of Knowledge with Written Examinations

Over the years, literally dozens of different item formats have been developed for use in written examinations. For examples of multiple-choice formats in the medical field, see Case and Swanson,[13] particularly Appendix A, and Levine.[14] With the advent of computer-based testing, the number of item formats has continued to grow.[15] In general terms, though, most formats can be categorized along two dimensions based on the *response format* and the *stimulus format*.

Table 4-1 **Roles of Three Kinds of Evaluation in Improving Clinical Instruction**

Preparative Evaluation		Formative Evaluation		Summative Evaluation	
To determine the attribute possessed by trainees before instruction begins		To provide ongoing feedback to trainees and faculty on their effectiveness as they proceed through instruction		To assess the degree to which instructional objectives have been attained by the end of instruction	
Roles in Relation to Individual Trainees					
P1	Identifying and remediating deficiencies in a trainee's readiness for next units of instruction	F1	Diagnosing learning difficulties of individual trainees; planning remedial instruction	S1	Providing feedback on deficiencies in attainment; making grading and promotion decisions
P2	Planning individualized instruction	F2	Providing reinforcement for mastery	S2	Motivating and directing effort during instruction
P3	Shifting a trainee to an alternative unit of instruction	F3	Pacing the work of an individual trainee	S3	Providing reinforcement for attainment of objectives
Roles in Relation to Groups of Trainees and Programs as a Whole					
P4	Locating an appropriate starting point for group instruction	F4	Identifying areas in which group attainment of objectives is less than desired; planning remedial instruction	S4	Evaluating the effectiveness of a unit of instruction
P5	Planning remedial instruction	F5	Planning subsequent instruction for the current group of trainees	S5	Comparing learning outcomes in different groups of trainees
P6	Selecting instructional methods	F6	Evaluating effectiveness of the unit of instruction	S6	Providing information for preparative evaluation in subsequent instruction for the same group of trainees
P7	Assigning trainees to instructional groups	F7	Providing quality control over the unit of instruction	S7	Certifying the knowledge and skills attained by the group of trainees
P8	Gathering information on the effectiveness of previous instruction	F8	Maintaining uniform grading of trainees each time a unit is presented	S8	Predicting success in subsequent training activities

Adapted from Cronbach LJ: Educational Psychology, 3rd ed. New York, Harcourt Brace Jovanovich, 1997, p 688.

Response Formats

Traditionally, response formats are divided into two categories: constructed response and selected response. In turn, the latter can be broken down into true/false and best-answer formats. Examples of both constructed and selected response formats are shown in Box 4-2. Constructed-response formats range from those requiring examinees to fill in only a word or phrase to those requiring examinees to write a multipage essay. They also vary in the amount of structure provided to guide examinee response, with some formats requiring specific components (e.g., following a description of a patient presentation, preparing a SOAP note, or detailing lists of the diagnostic studies to be done and medications to be given) and others very broad and unstructured (e.g., identifying considerations in the care of patients after a myocardial infarction).

Stimulus Formats

Stimulus formats are best viewed as varying along a continuum from low to high "authenticity" (similarity to real-world clinical tasks), with formats requiring only recall of isolated facts at one end of the continuum and various forms of written clinical simulations at the other end. The first entry in Box 4-1 provides an example of the kind of "factoid" item stem that has given examinations using multiple-choice questions (MCQs) a bad name because they only require examinees to recall a fact in isolation. In contrast, the second and third patient vignettes in Box 4-1 illustrate the kinds of MCQs that challenge examinees to apply their knowledge to make a clinical decision. These vary in the amount of patient information provided and the extent to which it is provided in more or less interpreted form ("ascites" versus "abdominal distention

BOX 4-1	Testing Recall of Isolated Facts versus Application of Knowledge

No Vignette
What is the most common renal abnormality in children with nephrotic syndrome and normal renal function?

Short Vignette
A 2-year-old boy has a 1-week history of edema. Blood pressure is 100/60 mm Hg, and there is generalized edema and ascites. Serum concentrations are creatinine 0.4 mg/dL, albumin 1.4 g/dL, and cholesterol 569 mg/dL. Urinalysis shows 4+ protein and no blood. What is the most likely diagnosis?

Long Vignette
A 2-year-old African-American child developed swelling of his eyes and ankles over the past week. Blood pressure is 100/60 mm Hg, pulse 110/min, and respirations 28/min. In addition to swelling of his eyes and 2+ pitting edema of his ankles, he has abdominal distention with a positive fluid wave. Serum concentrations are creatinine 0.4 mg/dL, albumin 1.4 g/dL, and cholesterol 569 mg/dL. Urinalysis shows 4+ protein and no blood. What is the most likely diagnosis?

Possible Option List for Multiple-Choice Question
1. Acute poststreptococcal glomerulonephritis
2. Hemolytic-uremic syndrome
3. Minimal change disease
4. Nephrotic syndrome due to focal and segmental glomerulosclerosis
5. Schönlein-Henoch purpura with nephritis

with a positive fluid wave''); depending upon the purpose of the test and background of trainees, both can be appropriate.

BOX 4-2	Examples of Constructed-Response and Selected-Response Item Formats

Constructed Response Formats
Completion/fill-ins
Short answer
Essays and other extended responses
Modified essay questions
"Show-your-work" word problems

Selected Response Formats
True/False Formats
Simple true/false
Multiple true/false
Written clinical simulations (e.g., patient management problems)

Best Answer Formats
Single best answer
Matching
Case clusters (series of multiple-choice questions following a paragraph-length clinical presentation)

Note that all of the stems in Box 4-1 could be presented in selected- or constructed-response format. An option list that might be appropriate for advanced students and graduate trainees is shown in the bottom panel of Box 4-1. Alternatively, the items could be administered in a short-answer format without providing an option list from which examinees would choose; a structured essay format could also be used for any of the stems by asking examinees to justify their responses.

Selection of Stimulus and Response Formats

Research within medical education[16] and in education more generally[17,18] has shown that choice of response format has little impact on the rank order of examinee scores: after controlling for score reliability, the same examinees do well and poorly. However, this does not mean that the choice of response format is arbitrary; as discussed in the next section, a response format can have a large impact on testing time requirements, as well as the logistics and cost of scoring. Unless valid measurement of a trait requires production of a writing sample (e.g., measuring proficiency in preparing SOAP notes), use of extended-response formats such as essays is generally not advisable because so much testing time is required to obtain a reproducible score.[19,20] Though the clinical reasoning process may be easier to judge in an essay, it is better to use formats that allow the outcomes of that reasoning process across a larger number of problems.

From a logistical perspective, scoring of other constructed-response formats typically requires substantial time from content experts, and the subjectivity involved in grading often reduces reproducibility of scores without increasing the validity of score interpretation.[16,17] Among the selected-response formats, the various one-best-answer formats generally yield more information per unit of testing time[21] and appear more suitable than true/false formats for assessment of clinical decision-making skills.[13] In addition, because the one-best-answer format requires only that examinees mentally rank-order the provided options from best to worst and select the best answer, it is possible to assess clinical judgment (e.g., selecting the most appropriate therapeutic choice from several drugs in the same class or subclass).

Regarding selection among stimulus formats, items should require examinees to use information to make clinical decisions, rather than recall isolated facts—there is little reason to assess knowledge of facts independent of their application in common and critical patient care situations. In general, test items should focus on the key features of the situations—the critical, essential elements that are most crucial to provision of effective patient care or most likely to lead to errors and poor patient outcomes.[22] As illustrated by the sample item in Box 4-3, item stems should generally be structured as patient vignettes that provide realistic, rich, fairly

---

BOX 4-3	Multiple-Choice Questions as Low-Fidelity Clinical Simulations

A 53-year-old man is brought to the emergency department by emergency medical services after he crashed his car into a tree. He was not wearing a seatbelt. Upon arrival in the emergency department the patient is clearly drunk but he is cooperative during the examination. Vital signs are temperature 37.0°C (98.6°F), pulse 110/min, respirations 18/min, and blood pressure 110/75 mm Hg. Physical examination shows generalized tenderness over the lower abdomen and pelvis. Neurologic examination is normal. X-rays of the cervical spine, chest, and pelvis are normal, as is CT scan of the head. On reexamination 3 hours later, no urinary output has been recorded. The patient is unable to produce a urine sample. He has received 1400 mL of lactated Ringer solution since the accident. Foley catheter is placed and yields 5 mL of bloody urine. X-ray obtained after placement of a Foley catheter is shown in the accompanying figure. Which of the following is the most appropriate next step in patient care?

1. Foley catheter drainage for 10 days
2. Observation only
3. Percutaneous nephrostomy
4. Suprapubic catheter drainage
5. Surgical repair

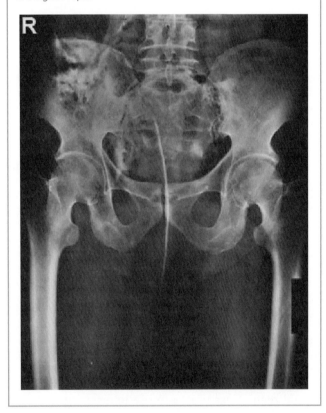

---

undigested descriptions of clinical situations.[23] This combination of stimulus and response formats provides, in effect, a low-fidelity patient simulation that can challenge examinees to apply their knowledge to make clinical decisions. This approach possesses so many advantages that use of other formats must be justified as measuring some attribute different from that measured by this one[14]—and many will not. Tests consisting of collections of such items can rapidly sample a broad range of important clinical decision-making situations within a reasonable amount of testing time. As discussed in the next section, posing sufficient numbers of clinical tasks in an assessment is a central issue if valid and reliable score interpretations are to result.

Reliability and Validity of Written Examinations

Reliability of Test Scores

The purpose of any assessment is to permit inferences to be drawn concerning the proficiency of examinees —inferences that extend beyond the particular questions included on the examination to the larger domain of questions from which the test includes but a sample. Performance on the sample provides a basis for estimating proficiency in the broader domain that is actually of interest. Depending upon the size and nature of the sample, those estimates can be more or less reproducible (reliable, precise, generalizable) and more or less accurate (valid). If the sample is too small, estimates of examinee proficiency will not be reproducible from one set of test questions to the next. If the sample is biased, performance may not be a good indicator of the proficiency of interest.

Several types of statistical indices have been devised to provide information about the reproducibility of test scores. One type of index is termed the test reliability. Indices of this type, which include Coefficient Alpha, two Kuder-Richardson formulas (KR-20 and KR-21), and other "internal consistency" indices, are all forms of intraclass correlations (generalizability coefficients) that indicate the strength of the relationship between the scores observed on the test and the score that would be observed on retesting with tests covering similar but not identical content. These are interpreted like other correlation coefficients: values near zero indicate retesting is likely to result in a score that is almost unrelated to the obtained score, and values near one indicate retesting is likely to yield a score that is strongly related. For tests on which high-stakes decisions (e.g., promotion, graduation, licensure, certification) are based, a test reliability greater than 0.8 (or, better yet, 0.9) is desirable: this value indicates that the score obtained on retesting should be correlated around 0.8 with the original test score. Well-written multiple-choice tests consisting of 100 to 200 one-best-answer items generally result in total scores with reliability coefficients in this range.

For most tests, regardless of assessment format, reliability indices increase as test length increases. The chart in Figure 4-1 illustrates the nature of the relationship for a hypothetical multiple-choice test that has a reliability of 0.8 at a test length of 100 items (a typical value for a well-designed end-of-clerkship examination) in a broad discipline such as internal medicine, surgery, pediatrics, or family medicine.

Another commonly used index of the reproducibility of test scores is the standard error of measurement (SEM).

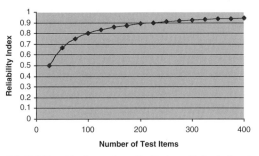

Figure 4-1 Relationship for a hypothetical multiple-choice test with reliability graph.

Unlike reliability indices that vary from zero to one regardless of the scale used for test scores, the SEM is expressed on the same scale as the scores, and it can be used to calculate confidence intervals around them. This makes interpretation of SEMs more straightforward. For example, suppose the mean and standard deviation (SD) for a 100-item final examination in a clerkship or residency rotation are 70% and 8% (on a percent-correct scale), the SEM is 3.5% (which corresponds to a reliability of roughly 0.8), and the pass/fail standard is 60% correct. If an examinee obtains a score of 58%, a 95% confidence interval around that score can be calculated by adding and subtracting twice the SEM from the obtained score. On retesting, one can expect that 95 times out of 100, the obtained score will fall between 51% (58% minus two times the SEM of 3.5%) and 65% (58% plus two times the SEM of 3.5%).

Because the SEM and confidence interval are expressed on the same scale as the score, it is easier to judge the adequacy of score precision in relation to the precision needed to make reproducible pass/fail decisions. In this instance, if a high-stakes decision (e.g., retention in the program) depends on the test score, it is clear that retesting might very well result in a score that is higher than the pass/fail standard of 60%, and use of a longer, more reliable test might be desirable. Continuing the example in Figure 4-1, the graph in Figure 4-2 depicts the relationship between the SEM expressed on a proportion correct scale and test length (number of items). For multiple-choice tests, the SEM generally varies

inversely with the square root of the test length: in order to halve the SEM, it is necessary to quadruple the number of items on a test.

Validity of Score Interpretations

A general discussion of validity and the validation process is beyond the scope of this chapter; see Clauser and associates (Chapter 2) in this volume for more information and Kane[24] for an extended discussion. But, in general terms, validity refers to the accuracy of inferences drawn from test performance—the extent to which the inferences from the scores on an assessment mean what they purport to mean. Assessment instruments themselves do not possess validity as an inherent quality, however; validity is a property of the inferences and decisions that are based on assessment results, and the same assessment instrument can be valid for one purpose and invalid for another. For example, a test of factual recall can be valid as a measure of whether or not a trainee has read and understood a chapter in a medical text, but completely invalid as a sole measure of whether or not a trainee can manage the care of a patient with the clinical problem discussed in that same chapter. Similarly, a well-designed measure of clinical skills administered at a U.S. medical school may provide a valid basis for inferring the quality of history-taking skills for trainees with English as a native language but not for students with English as a second language. Thus, the same instrument can have multiple validities, depending upon the inferences to be drawn and the groups to be assessed.

Evaluation of validity always involves judgment. As discussed in Clauser and associates, test validation can be viewed as the process of collecting evidence to support the intended interpretations of test scores. Generally, this will require development of an argument with several components. Kane[24,25] provides a structure for this validity argument that outlines four links in the inferential chain from the test administration to the final decision or interpretation. He labels these four components *scoring, generalization, extrapolation*, and *interpretation/decision*. Support for the *scoring* component of the overall argument includes evidence that the test was administered properly, examinee behavior was captured correctly, and scoring rules were appropriate and applied accurately. The *generalization* component requires evidence that the test items are appropriately sampled from the universe of test items that could have been used on the test and that the sample is large enough to produce scores with an acceptable level of precision. The *extrapolation* component of the argument requires evidence that the test score is relevant to the proficiency targeted by the test. This requires a demonstration that the observations are relevant to the interpretation and that scores are not unduly influenced by sources of variance irrelevant to the intended interpretation. The *decision/interpretation* component of the argument requires evidence in support of the pass/fail standard (cut-score) for

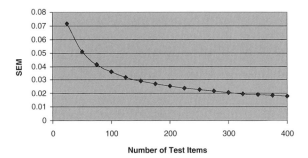

Figure 4-2 Standard error of measurement (SEM) relationship graph.

Table 4-2 **Questions Associated with Each of the Four Components of Kane's Argument-based Approach to Validity**

Component	Questions
Scoring	1. Were the observations made or stimulus materials administered under standardized conditions? 2. Were the scores recorded accurately? 3. Were the scoring algorithms applied correctly? 4. Were appropriate security procedures implemented?
Generalization	1. What are the sources of measurement error that contribute to the observed scores on the assessment? 2. How similar would scores be across replications of the measurement procedure? 3. How similar would classification decisions be across replications of the measurement procedure? 4. To what extent are test forms constructed using a systematic process?
Extrapolation	1. To what extent do the scores correspond to real-world proficiencies of interest? 2. Are there factors that interfere with assessment of the proficiencies of interest? 3. Do scores predict real-world outcomes of interest? 4. Are there artificial aspects of the testing conditions that impact the scores?
Decision	1. Was the standard established through implementation of a defensible and properly implemented procedure? 2. Do examinees identified for remediation improve to meet the standard or benefit more from a remediation program than would those who were not identified?

the test. The components are like links in a chain, and users of test scores can have confidence in a score interpretation only if evidence exists for each component of the argument—the chain is only as strong as its weakest link. The types of evidence required will vary with the purpose and characteristics of an assessment; Table 4-2, reproduced from Clauser and associates (Chapter 2), provides examples of some of the kinds of questions that arise at each stage of the argument.

For written examinations consisting of MCQs, the scoring and generalization links are typically both quite strong. Assuming the items have been carefully written and reviewed, the scoring link is very strong, though verifying the accuracy of the answer key by conducting a preliminary scoring of a test form is always desirable to identify items with aberrant statistical characteristics for review by content experts. Typically, tests of 100 or more items built to meet content specifications will provide reasonably reproducible scores (longer if high-stakes decisions such as promotion or graduation depend on the results), satisfying the generalization link. Good methods have been developed for standard setting, and the decision/interpretation link should be strong if one of those methods has been carefully used. The weakest link for MCQ-based tests is generally the extrapolation link: it clearly requires a leap of faith to infer that an examinee will perform well in real-world clinical tasks based on scores on a written test. However, it is more believable that an examinee who performs poorly on a well-constructed written examination will also perform poorly on real-world clinical tasks, particularly if the test comprises items written in the patient vignette format discussed in the previous section. If an examinee cannot apply his/her knowledge to clinical situations described on a written examination, performing well on similar tasks in the clinical environment seems

unlikely; good test performance can reasonably be viewed as a necessary but not sufficient condition for making real-world clinical decisions.

The validity of other written examination formats depends on the format and how well it is used. Tests consisting of "simple" MCQs of the nonvignette variety and true-false items will also tend to have strong scoring and generalization links, assuming the items have been carefully written and reviewed. However, because such items do not directly pose clinical tasks, the extrapolation link is apt to be weaker than that for MCQs framed as patient vignettes.[23] Unless care is used in writing items and developing and applying the scoring keys, scoring and generalization links can be weaker for tests consisting of short-answer and short-essay questions. Intuitively, it seems like the extrapolation link may be stronger for these formats because responses are not "cued" by option lists, but most research comparing MCQ and short-answer formats has indicated that correlations between scores on the two formats are very high.[16,23] The generalization link is typically very weak for tests consisting of long essays: they almost never include a sufficient number of essays to satisfy the generalization link,[19–20,23] and often the scoring and extrapolation links are weak as well.

Use of Written Examinations within Educational Programs

The majority of written examinations used in medical education can be viewed conceptually as achievement tests; they intend to measure at a certain point in time the knowledge acquisition of trainees within a specific or general content area. They are commonly used to inform students, residents, and their teachers about progress made toward defined educational objectives. Depending upon the intended purpose and length of the examination, more specific diagnostic information can be provided regarding particular topical areas within the broader content coverage. Additionally, aggregate data from individual performances on written examinations are often useful for providing feedback to educators about the success of a given educational program and may inform curriculum planning or modification.

Written examinations used in undergraduate and graduate medical education may be developed locally by course or program directors and faculty, with or without the assistance of individuals trained in education or assessment. Alternatively, educators may avail themselves of national standardized tests for use in their academic programs. National standardized tests are often developed by organizations with expertise in test development and administration (such as the NBME, ABMS boards, or medical societies). These organizations work with subject matter experts in a range of content areas to ensure that test items are clinically accurate and relevant, and the test as a whole is appropriately representative of the knowledge domain being examined. National standardized examinations are generally well constructed and provide educators with reliable information for comparing the performance of their programs and trainees with that of a national cohort of similar trainees and programs.[26–28] Educators should understand the differences between locally developed and national standardized tests and when to use each in their programs.

Locally Developed Examinations

Locally developed examinations are generally tailored more specifically to the educational objectives and curricula of the local program. National standardized examinations are generally more reflective of core knowledge objectives shared across settings and institutions; often, these objectives are explicitly developed by national clerkship or residency training organizations. In a sense, locally developed examinations and standardized tests may be viewed as complementary in that educational leaders need to assure that trainees meet institutional goals, as well as national standards for licensure and certification. Given potential limitations in resource support for educational programs, educators should be clear on the intended purpose of testing when deciding whether to develop their own examinations or use standardized examinations. Locally developed tests may include a variety of item formats, including multiple-choice items, true/false items, matching items, short-answer questions, and essay questions.

Although locally developed examinations may serve a useful purpose in determining trainee progress in achieving learning objectives and in serving as a basis for the provision of feedback to learners to aid in prioritizing learning efforts, inconsistency in test quality may detract from their ability to adequately serve such purposes. Educators should be aware of the time commitment involved in writing good test items, as well as the challenges involved in selecting appropriate content for testing (developing an examination blueprint) and in administering and scoring examinations (and setting a standard if pass/fail decisions are to be made based upon test results). A recent analysis of multiple-choice question examinations at three U.S. medical schools demonstrated that items developed by local faculty were inferior to items written by faculty members who had formal training in writing items for the licensure examination.[29] Items written by faculty specifically trained in item-writing were more likely to contain vignettes and less likely to contain flaws that compromised the ability of the test material to differentiate learners of varying proficiency.

Although the above study did not show that the locally developed examinations were unable to distinguish more capable from less capable trainees per se, there is reason to suspect that some local examinations may suffer from important validity flaws. One study, reviewing four examinations from first- and second-year medical school courses, found that 36% to 65% of the items were flawed, resulting in a significant impact on percent-correct scores and pass-fail results. Certain item flaws, such as use of multiple true/false (K-type) items, unfocused and negatively worded stems, and "all/none of the above" as options, were common and generally increased examination difficulty, resulting in incorrect pass/fail classifications for as many as 10% to 15% of the students.[30]

The threats to validity that arise in such examinations may include construct-irrelevant variance (CIV) and construct under-representation (CUR).[31] CIV describes the influence of factors unrelated to an examinee's knowledge base on test scores. Sources of CIV include poorly written test items that favor "test-wise" examinees or confuse well-informed ones. Examinations that are given each year, course, or rotation without alteration in test content may allow trainees with access to information about prior tests to perform better than expected based upon their actual fund of knowledge. Tests that have a limited number of items or a large number of flawed items may have low reliability, undermining the defensibility of pass/fail decisions or other important consequences based upon test results.[31]

Construct under-representation may result when tests do not provide for an adequate sample of the content and skills in a domain to allow for meaningful interpretations of test scores. The inclusion of trivial questions or questions reflecting instructors' "pet topics" may result in scores that do not reflect a trainee's actual mastery of the relevant knowledge domain. Finally, faculty who "teach to the test" by focusing their instruction on material contained in the examination can create a situation in which performance on the sample of items is not reflective of examinees' actual knowledge or skills in a given content area, thus inhibiting valid interpretation of test scores.[31]

It is often argued that tests used to determine whether examinees have passed a course or rotation need not be subject to the same psychometric standards as licensure or certification examinations. However, it is difficult to defend the opinion that tests used primarily to provide feedback to learners to inform educational interventions or influence patient care practices do not need to meet reasonable reliability and validity standards. It is possible to prevent most sources of irrelevant variance and inadequate or uneven content coverage through attention to sound item and test development practices (Box 4-4).

Materials are available to guide faculty and other item writers in improving the quality of their items.[13,32] Depending upon educational and assessment priorities, clerkship and program directors and other educational leaders should consider the implementation of faculty development and peer review activities to improve the quality of local examinations. Item-writing workshops provided for core faculty can provide a cadre of individuals who are able to write high-quality items and serve as a peer review committee to appraise and enhance the quality of items prepared by other faculty members.[13] The peer review committee can also review test content to ensure that items follow a consistent format and that content coverage is adequate relative to curricular objectives.[29,31] Faculty development and peer review activities require time and effort, but can be well worth the investment if decisions based on locally developed examinations have significant impact on trainee progress or clinical performance.

National Standardized Examinations

USMLE and NBME Subject Examinations

The most commonly used national standardized examinations in U.S. undergraduate medical education (UME) are the United States Medical Licensing Examination (USMLE) and the subject examinations developed by the National Board of Medical Examiners (NBME). In educational settings, these examinations are used for three primary purposes: assessment of individual students, evaluation of educational programs, and selection of residents for graduate medical education (GME) programs. In each of these areas examination results can contribute valuable information; however, if incorrectly applied, confusing or potentially harmful interpretations may result.[33-37]

Opinions vary regarding the use of the preceding examinations in educational programs. Some think that a separate examination for licensure assures the public that physicians have attained at least a minimal standard for knowledge and skills important for safe and effective patient care, allowing individual medical schools latitude in developing educational programs, including use of novel and innovative assessment methods to meet unique mission requirements. Others, in consideration of the important external audit role

---

BOX 4-4	Summary Guidelines for Developing and Using Multiple-Choice Question Examinations in Educational Programs

Developing Local Examinations

Ensure that test content is consistent with educational objectives and congruent with curriculum

Provide test development and item writing instructions/ workshops to core faculty

Provide item writing guidelines to all faculty writing test items

Appoint committee to review test content and refine items submitted by faculty

Encourage faculty to
  Write items in clinical vignette form, whenever possible
  Write items using a common format; avoid common item writing flaws
  Allow time to write items when preparing instructional content and materials
  Avoid teaching solely or preferentially on material on the examination

Using National Examinations

Consider the following in interpreting and acting on the performance of local examinees on external examinations
  Similarity in content of external test to local educational objectives and curriculum
  Item formats and level of difficulty
  Comparison group of test takers in relation to local examinee characteristics
  Information about course/rotation timing and duration on examination scores
  Reliability of the external examination
For program assessment
  Avoid complicated or expensive changes in curriculum based on small fluctuations in mean scores
  Consider structural factors on test scores (e.g., faculty ratio, course length, clinical workload), as well as curriculum content, when designing educational interventions
For individual assessment
  Remediation plan should be based on diagnostic information regarding explanation for low or decreased score

---

played by these examinations and their use as criteria in the accreditation process, feel pressured to thoroughly cover licensure examination content in their educational programs and to incorporate similar measures into internal assessment programs. The purpose of the following discussion is not to weigh the philosophical pros and cons for incorporating USMLE and NBME subject examination results into educational programs but to provide some guidance regarding their appropriate application for those who decide to use them.

A word of caution is appropriate here. Whenever any assessment method is used for something other than its intended purpose, it is essential that users be aware of the assessment's primary intended purpose and pertinent characteristics, as they may (or may not) relate specifically to anticipated alternate applications (see Box 4-4). The use of the NBME subject examinations or the licensing examination for assessment within educational programs is appropriate only to the extent that the examination content and format are reasonably congruent with the goals and objectives of the educational program and setting in which it is being used. The subject examinations are constructed according to content outlines that are discipline specific and designed for end-of-clerkship administration. The content of USMLE Step 2 is more interdisciplinary; it is designed to assess whether examinees have the requisite knowledge and understanding of clinical science considered to be important for the provision of safe and effective care under supervision (readiness for internship).[27]

Users of USMLE and NBME subject examination results should become familiar with the content of these examinations to ensure relevance to student and program assessment objectives and should fully understand any limitations or qualifications on interpretations of test scores. Content outlines provided in the USMLE Bulletin of Information or contained within NBME subject examination materials should be reviewed to gauge conformity with educational program objectives. As an example, a recent study found that the content coverage of the NBME obstetrics and gynecology subject examination was congruent with the Association of Professors of Gynecology and Obstetrics Medical Student Educational Objectives, with 99% of the items judged appropriate for medical students.[38]

Additionally, it would be useful for course or clerkship directors to review the items included in these examinations to ensure that they are congruent with instructional goals and objectives and are targeted at an appropriate level of difficulty. These examinations contain only single-best-answer multiple choice and extended matching items that are imbedded in clinical vignettes to measure application of knowledge beyond simple recall. They generally include more challenging items than those found in locally developed examinations, though whether or not this translates into lower pass rates will vary as a function of the standards set by clerkships, both for the subject examinations and locally developed tests.[33]

Perceived advantages of using USMLE or NBME subject examinations for assessing student performance include participation of national groups of content experts in development and review of test blueprints and items, the high level of quality control over test material and scoring, availability of multiple test forms, relatively high reliability, and provision of national norms and grading guidelines.[27,39,40]

Educators should be aware that students with equivalent abilities may perform differently on certain subject examinations depending upon when they take them and the duration of the relevant clerkship. Setting a passing standard based upon end-of-the-year performance criteria may not be fair to those taking the same examination several months earlier. Subject examination scores in broad-based disciplines such as internal medicine and surgery increase significantly over the course of the academic year.[39,41] This is not unexpected given the general nature of the knowledge base in these specialty areas and a reasonable

expectation that knowledge acquired in other clinical rotations may supplement or be reinforced by knowledge gained during these rotations. To a lesser extent, incremental improvements in scores on the obstetrics and gynecology subject examination have been reported.[40,42,43] Timing was not an independent factor in influencing psychiatry examination performance, but longer clerkships were associated with better performance. Students who had 8-week rotations in psychiatry scored better than those who had 6-week rotations, with the most pronounced differences in performance observed at the beginning of the academic year.[40] Similar complex relationships between clerkship timing and duration were described for the surgery and obstetrics and gynecology examinations.[39,43,44] The observed link between duration of training and knowledge acquisition should not be surprising. Performance on USMLE Step 2 and the Cardiology Board Certification Examination is directly associated with duration of the clinical clerkships in medical school and length of fellowship training programs.[45,46]

Faculty should be aware that students may perceive some degree of unfairness when there is a lack of congruence between what is tested by the external standardized examination and what is taught within the educational program. The use of national medical school faculty as subject matter experts in developing the NBME examinations provides some reassurance that examination content is relevant to educational programs, but there will always be instances in which course content or local educational objectives are not covered by the external test. For this reason, it is important *not* to use external examination scores as the sole measure of performance in a given educational program; they should be viewed as complementary to and supplements for faculty-developed assessments that include unique course or program objectives.[34] Additionally, most faculty members are becoming increasingly attentive to the adverse effects of using cognitive examinations as the sole measure of academic achievement, and global ratings of clinical performance, clinical skills examinations, portfolios, and other assessment approaches are increasingly being used to broaden coverage of other important skills and behaviors.

USMLE and NBME subject examination scores are also commonly used for evaluation of educational programs in medical schools.[35] Incorporating performance on these examinations into local program evaluation provides faculty with some assurance that they have been successful in achieving course objectives related to development of a broad knowledge base and mastery of the cognitive skills essential for provision of safe and effective patient care. The existence of an external monitor allows faculty to engage in curricular modification/reform and educational innovation while tracking potential positive or negative side effects. Recent studies described the use of NBME subject examinations in gauging the effectiveness of a range of curricular innovations and structural changes in clerkships. Pre- and post-intervention subject examination scores were used to monitor the impact of reducing clerkship duration, measure the result of introducing clinical correlation teaching and clinically relevant assessment into a basic science course, gauge the effect of introducing a multidisciplinary medicine-surgery clerkship, and assess the influence of a new problem-based learning approach on knowledge acquisition.[43,44,47–49] Subject examination scores were used to compare cohorts of students participating in ambulatory rotations at community practice sites or hospital-based clinics with those participating in a traditional in-patient experience.[50,51]

As in the use of external examinations for individual trainee assessment, incorporation into program evaluation systems should be based on a thorough understanding of the content and qualities of the external examination and congruence with the goals and objectives of the educational program. External assessments should not be applied in isolation but should be combined with aggregate data from other assessment methods, including other written examinations and clinical skills examinations. Course or clerkship directors should know the standard error of the mean for their school in order to fully understand the implications of year-to-year shifts in mean scores. Because student proficiency, as well as congruence between educational experiences and examination content, may fluctuate from year to year, it is generally not a good idea to implement or continue inconvenient and costly curricular modifications unless shifts in mean scores persist for more than one class (year). One sensible approach might require a change in examination mean scores to exceed 2 standard errors for 2 years in a row before permanent course adjustments are made or additional changes are introduced.[35]

Use of USMLE scores for selection of residents is both common and controversial. Given that performance on written standardized examinations often remains consistent over time, it is not unreasonable for residency program directors to be reluctant to accept candidates with low scores, because performance on board certifying examinations is an important outcome indicator for residency programs.[52] It seems appropriate for residency program directors to be concerned about allocating considerable resources and effort to educate a resident who may never be licensed. Also, there is a correlation between licensure and certification examination scores and various performance measures in residency and beyond.[36,53,54] So the use of licensure examination performance as one source of information in residency selection is justified. However, using such examinations as the sole criterion for residency selection and basing decisions on relatively small differences in test scores are not appropriate. Using a knowledge-based examination as the sole criterion for residency selection neglects the importance of other components of clinical competence such as communication and interpersonal skills and professional behaviors; indeed, in some studies measures of these attributes have predictive value for subsequent performance.[55,56] Establishing rank orders for residency selection based upon small differences in

scores is not sensible, as they may not relate specifically to differences in clinical performance.[57] As we move forward in this era of evidence-based and outcomes-focused education and assessment, it would be useful for program directors and institutional GME officials to systematically compile information about the relationship between selection criteria and resident performance at their institution in order to improve the process used locally for residency selection.[36]

In-Training Examinations

Resident in-training examinations (ITEs) are available in many specialties and subspecialties. Generally, they are designed to assess the knowledge and cognitive skills of residents for the purpose of monitoring and providing feedback on progress toward mastery of the knowledge base for the specialty. More specifically, they are intended to serve as a formative evaluation, providing feedback on a trainee's cognitive skills at particular points in training relative to national peer groups. ITEs also are intended to provide program directors with a measure of program effectiveness in promoting the attainment of knowledge objectives relative to other programs nationally. Most sponsors of ITEs discourage or prohibit the use of this examination, particularly in isolation, for making retention or promotion decisions.[28,58–62]

ITEs have two qualities that are important to program directors: high reliability and predictive validity for board certification examinations.[28,58–65] For example, reliability coefficients for the internal medicine ITE have been consistently greater than 0.90 for PGY-2 residents. Reliability coefficients for subscores in individual subspecialty areas are lower and more varied, ranging from 0.54 to 0.80 for the 1993 examination, reflecting the smaller number of and variation in the number of questions in each area.[28] Results from ITEs in other specialties are similar, generally providing highly reliable total scores and less reliable subscores for individual examinees.[58,62]

One of the intended, if not always expressed, uses of ITEs is the identification of trainees who may have difficulty passing the board certification examination. Ideally, in addition to early identification of such individuals, the profile of subscore performance would make it possible to determine specific areas of strength and weakness for targeted remediation (including adjustments to rotation schedules, assignments to sites and preceptors, supplemental reading, etc.). (See later discussion regarding the subscores.) Performance on the ITEs in the various specialties (family medicine, general surgery, internal medicine, radiology, orthopaedic surgery, psychiatry) has been shown to predict subsequent performance on the associated specialty board certifying examinations.[58,60,61,63,64,66–68]

The correlation between ITE and board certifying examination scores is consistent with prior studies evaluating performance on written examinations across the continuum of education and practice. For example, both Part I and Part II scores for the former NBME examination have been shown to correlate with American Board of Internal Medicine Certifying Examination (ABIMCE) performance. Sosenko found that NBME Part I scores were highly predictive of later performance on the ABIMCE.[69] Norcini demonstrated an even higher correlation between NBME Part II and ABIMCE performance.[70] More recent studies show similarly high correlations between USMLE Step scores and performance on ITEs in obstetrics and gynecology and orthopaedic surgery, as well as on the ABIMCE.[71–73] Similar results have been observed for the osteopathic licensing examination; strong correlations exist between performance on all three levels of the Comprehensive Osteopathic Medical Licensing Examination (COMLEX-USA), the three annual American College of Osteopathic Internists (ACOI) in-service examinations, and the American Osteopathic Board of Internal Medicine (AOBIM) certifying examination, with each one predicting over 60% of the variance of any other in the series.[74]

We do not think it is surprising, then, that future behavior on certifying examinations is predicted well by past behavior on the ITE. Both ITE and certifying examination performance depend upon detailed medical knowledge accrued over years of training. Success in a marathon is not primarily a matter of getting lucky on the day of the race: it also depends on training. Two important conclusions can be inferred from the pattern of results seen in the studies linking examination performance over time. First, performance is not explained simply by generic test-taking abilities, but is primarily determined by acquisition and retention of specific knowledge content. Although research has shown that examinees' scores on licensing and board certification examinations are significantly correlated, the relationship is substantially influenced by mastery of specific, related knowledge. For example, performance on the American Board of Orthopaedic Surgery Certification Examination is more strongly correlated with licensing examination subscores in anatomy and surgery than with scores in behavioral science and preventive medicine.[52] Similarly, performance on USMLE Step 2, intended to encompass broad and interdisciplinary content, is more closely associated with NBME subject examination scores in internal medicine than in psychiatry.[27]

Second, future examination performance is not explained solely by previous examination scores; program and individual examinee characteristics contribute an important fraction. Similar to the findings described earlier from comparing the osteopathic licensing and internal medicine examinations, Norcini found that prior licensing examination performance contributed importantly (40% of the explained variance) to subsequent ABIMCE performance. However, 60% of the explained variance was explained by characteristics of the particular residency program: 13% by program qualities alone and 47% by the interaction between the program and licensing examination performance.[70] Therefore, although the knowledge base

that the resident brings to the program is important in predicting his/her future performance, the quality of the educational program and the resident's engagement in the educational experience influence whether acquisition of knowledge continues in a consistent manner.

In deciding upon how to use ITEs in educational programs, including how frequently to administer them, information regarding the utility of other commonly used assessment methods for evaluating knowledge competence may be helpful. It is intuitive that resident performance as measured by standardized patients, medical record audit, direct observation of patient interactions, and patient satisfaction surveys will not provide as reliable and thorough an assessment of knowledge as ITEs. Numerous studies demonstrate highly variable correlations between knowledge-based and performance-based assessment methods (including faculty evaluations and standardized patient–based assessments).[65,75–80] For example, Dupras found that objective structured clinical examination (OSCE) performance by PGY-2 internal medicine residents correlated "moderately" with ITE scores, suggesting that different aspects of competence were being assessed.[80] Schwartz found that the ITE in general surgery and a residency OSCE were more likely to identify specific competence deficiencies than faculty evaluations.[75] The ITE measures primarily knowledge and cognitive skills, whereas other tools assess different aspects of clinical competence and performance. A low-to-moderate correlation with other measures of clinical competence, particularly performance-based assessment methods, would not exclude the ITE as a useful tool; different evaluation methods may simply assess distinct facets of clinical competence.

Despite evidence that faculty evaluations of cognitive skills do not correlate well with ITE scores, it is useful to know whether faculty members are able to specifically predict performance on such examinations. The potential added value and optimal frequency of use of an ITE will depend to some extent on faculty ability to identify residents who have deficient cognitive skills and are at risk for failing their board certification examination. Taylor found wide variability in family practice faculty members' accuracy in predicting residents' performance on the ITE.[81] Another study evaluated the accuracy of faculty predictions of internal medicine ITE performance and found that full-time, institutionally based faculty members were able to predict into which tertile residents would score only 50% of the time. Perhaps more important, faculty were able to identify residents who would score in the lower tertile at chance levels of accuracy.[82] Similar results were described for the radiology ITE. Faculty predictions of resident ITE performance were only modestly correlated ($r = 0.34$) with actual performance on this examination.[78] Unfortunately, residents are no more accurate in identifying their own knowledge deficits as measured by ITEs. Two studies from family medicine residency programs found that resident predictions for their own ITE performance varied considerably among residents, but were particularly poor in predicting poor performance.[83,84] These findings have obvious implications for our ability to identify residents with deficient knowledge competence, particularly those at risk for failing the board certification examination. They underscore the potential benefit of having an objective measure of knowledge with established validity for predicting success on specialty certification exams.

Although ITEs across specialties are reliable and support valid interpretations of knowledge competence, and the feedback regarding examination performance is generally considered to be of high quality relative to national norms, there remains considerable uncertainty, and even controversy, regarding appropriate use of ITE scores.

The use of external data for evaluating educational program effectiveness is essential and is required for accreditation by the ACGME.[85] Given the requirement that residency training programs meet common educational objectives, feedback regarding program performance may be useful in identifying patterns of curricular or assessment weaknesses in attaining shared objectives.[86] In fact, program directors do use ITE performance to evaluate their programs, focus teaching exercises, modify lectures, change curriculum content, and provide structured review for residents.[28,87,88] A variety of interventions has been tried in order to increase ITE scores. The efficacy of such interventions has been inconsistent between, and within, studies. However, several themes emerge from review of these studies: (1) efforts that engage the resident in active learning are more likely to be successful than simply adding or increasing didactic presentations; (2) multipronged interventions, employing a combination of approaches, are more likely to be successful in improving program performance; and (3) tactics that are successful at the program level may not necessarily prove effective for selected individual residents.[89–99]

Using feedback on ITE performance to increase or adjust conference schedules alone is not particularly effective in improving ITE performance.[89–93] This is consistent with other studies that found low correlation between conference attendance and performance on locally developed tests and certification examinations.[71,100] Systematic or structured reading programs, including those developed by the residents themselves, based on ITE feedback, combined with periodic written examinations, resident presentations or problem-based discussions, or using commercial self-assessment programs, have been associated with improved ITE scores.[93–98] Multipronged interventions may influence residents' motivation and study habits by communicating the importance of ITE performance to program faculty.[101,102]

Interventions successful at the programmatic level may not necessarily improve the ITE performance of all residents in that program, particularly low scorers. Although self-directed learning efforts led to increasing mean scores on the American Board of Surgery ITE, based upon experience with several specific remediation methods (repeated multiple-choice examinations,

monitored reading assignments, preceptor guidance, and formal review courses), Wade was unable to recommend a standard, effective format for improving low ITE scores.[90] An intensive 4-week intervention that included resident reading and presentation assignments, and answering questions based upon prior ITE content topics, did not improve ITE scores for family medicine residents with low ITE scores compared with peers with higher scores. In fact, improvement in ITE performance for the small number of intervention residents was similar to the previous annual incremental score increase for that PGY group.[103] It is unlikely that brief interventions, regardless of intensity, will be as effective as sustained activities in improving acquisition and retention of knowledge.

The inconsistency of study results regarding interventions to improve ITE performance is not surprising. It seems unlikely that a single remediation method can be successfully applied to all trainees with low ITE scores to increase the probability of successfully passing a certification examination. Successful remediation of any competence deficiency depends to a large extent on identifying the primary underlying problem. For residents who perform poorly on the ITE, potential contributing factors include inconsistent educational experiences, poorly developed study habits, limited intellectual capacity, accumulated knowledge deficiencies, inability to apply knowledge in clinical situations, and a wide variety of personal factors.

One potentially useful approach to initial diagnostic evaluation of a low ITE score would begin by comparing current with previous test performance. If the current ITE score is significantly different from prior standardized examination scores, one should certainly review the adequacy of recent educational experiences. However, if there is no indication of deficient educational opportunities, then it may be reasonable to consider whether secondary personal or professional factors are affecting performance(see Chapter 13). If examination scores were low or marginal in the past, review of study habits and learning style and preferences may be beneficial in designing an individualized remedial program.[104–105]

Whether to initiate specific administrative action (such as probation, delayed promotion, or dismissal) based on ITE results is an even more perplexing issue, especially since ITE sponsors generally prohibit its use for such purposes. Although there are studies linking ITE scores to certifying examination performance, in general there is uncertainty regarding what constitutes a meaningful knowledge deficiency as measured by these examinations. In an attempt to define a national ''remediation indicator'' for the obstetrics and gynecology ITE, the Committee on In-Training Examination for Residents in Obstetrics and Gynecology Task Force on Standard-based Scoring polled OB-GYN faculty members. The mean standard (percent correct) for PGY-3 residents recommended by university faculty (59%) was similar to that recommended by community faculty (57%) and both were close to a score (59%) that was two standard deviations below the mean score for that resident year group. The task force authors urged caution regarding action based solely upon ITE scores and suggested that these results be considered in the context of the remainder of a trainee's performance in deciding upon the need for remediation.[106] Program directors in general surgery varied widely in how they use ITE scores for evaluating individual residents and in the basis for taking administrative or academic actions based on results. Almost half (45%) of 197 surgery program directors surveyed would initiate counseling, ongoing evaluation, or referral to a review committee if a resident failed to meet the required ABSITE score. In addition, 28% of program directors indicated that they would place a resident on probation, 13% would have the resident repeat the year or consider dismissal, and 10% would initiate some other adverse action if the expected ITE score is not achieved.[87] In one surgery training program, setting a passing standard at the 35th percentile led to a significant decrease in the number of residents falling below that standard.[107] However, success does not necessarily justify such action, and the authors of this study suggest policy decisions to set a criterion standard should be individualized and should involve clear communication to residents regarding the rationale for such action and plans to support their learning needs. One should be aware that the use of a tool designed to support formative assessment as a summative tool may have deleterious effects, including induction of cheating and tension between program directors and residents.[108,109]

Much of the work intended to identify means to improve residents' knowledge and cognitive skills has concentrated primarily on the content aspects of curriculum as identified in ITE performance feedback. However, there are program structure and process factors that may influence the acquisition of knowledge. Norcini found that resident workload impacted performance on the ABIM certifying examination.[70] Certifying examination scores decreased as the number of "beds" that the resident was responsible for increased and daily patient volume exceeded 25 per day (or fell below 10 per day). Examination performance improved as a function of the ratio of U.S. to international medical graduate residents and faculty to residents, and also increased in relation to time spent with medical students or on ambulatory or consultative rotations. In addition to focusing program educational efforts on specific content areas, it is certainly reasonable to consider the adequacy of residents' clinical experiences (including volume) and faculty supervision, at least in areas where examination scores are lower. The effect of decreasing work hours is, at present, unclear; a reduction in the time spent in patient care activity may increase time for study and reflection. Although the level of difficulty of rotation schedule in the short term and perceived availability of study time do not appear to have a significant impact on performance, preliminary evidence suggests a consistent decrement in work hours might have a salutary effect.[105,110,111] Findings are inconsistent regarding the impact of being on call the

night before an ITE administration. However, it seems likely that scores are impacted, and sufficient justification exists to avoid such practice.[102,113,114]

Regardless of program director and faculty efforts to improve ITE performance, residents' perceptions regarding ITE credibility may serve as a motivator for self-directed learning. In one study 35/36 (97%) residents surveyed before the 1995 and 1996 examinations responded that they thought the ITE was useful. Most residents (32/35, 91%) initiated some form of educational intervention based upon ITE results. The majority (28/35, 80%) targeted their reading in a specific area; 15/35 (43%) scheduled a specific elective rotation.[82] These results are similar to those from a nationwide survey of obstetrics and gynecology residents.[112] Cox reported that 58% of residents found the obstetrics and gynecology ITE to be an accurate measure of their cognitive skills and 59% of residents modified their study habits based upon the previous year's scores. It is unclear whether such self-directed activities are beneficial in the long run.

Advantages of Written Examinations as Assessment Tools

Written examinations can be applied to a wide variety of assessment objectives for the purpose of measuring knowledge and application of knowledge. Written examinations can assess broad areas of knowledge in an efficient and highly reproducible manner. They can be used for multiple purposes, including to assist in making decisions regarding an individual's success in attaining curricular objectives, and to provide feedback to an examinee regarding their knowledge relative to a defined standard or in comparison to a variety of peer groups. Aggregate results can be used formatively by individual programs to evaluate the quality of instruction and determine success in meeting programmatic objectives, facilitating program improvement. Aggregate results can also be used for summative evaluation by accrediting bodies to make decisions about the quality of specific programs. It is also possible to use results selectively from educational research and evaluation perspectives to gauge the impact of educational interventions or curricular modifications.

Administration of such assessments makes few demands on faculty time in comparison with other tools that must be applied in a more continuous manner; written examinations can be one of the most cost-efficient measures used in medical education. Although faculty members need not proctor test administration, selected faculty do need to become involved in conveying and interpreting results to their students and residents, including recommending and monitoring educational or remedial interventions.

The predictive value of ITEs for success on board certification examinations is an important strength as board certification has become increasingly relevant to employment and granting of privileges. Because of variability in resident experiences at the time of ITE administration, coupled with the lower reliability of

ITE subscores in subspecialty area, ITEs are generally less valuable in identifying specific knowledge deficits to be remediated prior to sitting for certification examinations.[64,67]

From an outcomes perspective, aggregate feedback from resident performance on ITEs can serve as a "barometer" for a program relative to a national standard. Because internal consistency and reliability for each examination are high, feedback on program or curriculum content may be considered of good quality.[28] The same information is obviously provided by board certification examination scores, though "after the fact" information is less useful for a given group of trainees.

Acquisition of a broad knowledge base and proficiency in applying it are of fundamental importance to the development of overall clinical competence. The ITE is felt by some authorities to represent an accurate assessment of "working" knowledge (rather than "learned" knowledge), because few residents actually prepare for the examination as they do for the NBME, USMLE, and specialty board certifying examinations. For this reason it may be a more accurate estimate of a trainee's fund of knowledge.[28] A study involving military family medicine residents suggests that interruption in training (for nonacademic reasons) does not significantly affect ITE scores, although residents had continued clinical activity in a primary care environment during their absence from training.[115]

Disadvantages of Written Examinations as Assessment Tools

Written examinations can measure only knowledge and related cognitive skills. Performance on written examinations does not always predict success in the application of knowledge in real clinical settings. In this respect, they may be viewed as necessary but insufficient for ensuring the appropriate exercise of cognitive skills, including problem solving and clinical reasoning in the care of actual patients. Written examinations should be supplemented with other measures of knowledge application within the context of patient encounters, such as chart-stimulated recall or structured observation tools.

Written examinations do not assess important clinical skills such as the technical and performance aspects of physical diagnosis, communication, humanism, and professionalism. Dependence on a standardized written examination score in isolation as the only measure of clinical competence can shift the focus of medical education away from patients. Inappropriate emphasis on written examinations as an assessment tool may have a negative influence on student or resident attention to other aspects of clinical competence such as communication skills, teamwork, and practice-based learning and improvement.

Written examinations, particularly ITEs, are not inexpensive for larger programs. Is the "value-added" worth the cost? Is administration of the ITE, particularly every academic year, *cost-effective*? Studies described here suggest that reliable and valid assessment of knowledge competence is not provided by other measurement tools commonly used in our training programs—suggesting that annual administration may be desirable. Certainly, programmatic data may be sought more frequently to gauge the impact of curricular modifications or interventions.

Conclusion

A well-developed knowledge base provides an important foundation upon which clinical competence and medical expertise are built. Written examinations assess medical knowledge and its application in a reliable and efficient manner. They are appropriately applied to assessing the proficiency of individual trainees and the overall success of educational programs in attaining important knowledge objectives. Thus, they remain an important tool for educators to use within the context of a multimodal approach to the assessment of clinical competence.

ANNOTATED BIBLIOGRAPHY

1. Case SM, Swanson DB: Constructing Written Test Questions for the Basic and Clinical Sciences, 3rd ed. (revised) Philadelphia, National Board of Medical Examiners, 2003.
   This item-writing guide focuses primarily on development of MCQs for basic and clinical science examinations in undergraduate medical education, but the item-writing principles generalize well to graduate medical education and health professions education more generally. The guide may be downloaded free of charge from www.nbme.org/.
2. O'Donnell MJ, Obenshain SS, Erdmann JB: Background essential to the proper use of results of Step 1 and Step 2 of the USMLE. Acad Med 1993;68:734–739.
3. Hoffman KI: The USMLE, the NBME subject examinations, and assessment of individual academic achievement. Acad Med 1993;68:740–747.
4. Williams RG: Use of NBME and USMLE examinations to evaluate medical education programs. Acad Med 1993;68:748–752.
5. Berner ES, Brooks CM, Erdmann JB: Use of the USMLE to select residents. Acad Med 1993;68:753–759.
6. Bowles LT: Use of NBME and USMLE scores. Acad Med 1993;68:778.
   Although somewhat dated, these papers provide an excellent overview regarding the use of the NBME subject examinations and the licensing examination in assessing individual academic achievement, evaluation of medical education programs, and selection of residents. Recommendations for the selection and application of these examinations and the appropriate interpretation and use of scores are provided.
7. Downing SM: Threats to the validity of locally developed multiple-choice tests in medical education: Construct-irrelevant variance and construct underrepresentation. Adv Health Sci Educ Theory Pract 2002;7:235–241.
   This article describes how construct-irrelevant variance and construct under-representation present threats to the valid interpretation of test scores on locally developed MCQ examinations. It also provides practical advice in how to avoid or control their impact.
8. Downing SM, Haladyna TM (eds): Handbook of Test Development. Mahwah, NJ, Lawrence Erlbaum Assoc., 2006.
   This book of readings provides a broad and deep introduction to test development, including chapters on designing a testing program, developing test specifications, writing and revising test items, building and publishing test forms, administering the test, and scoring and reporting scores. It also includes chapters on test security, standard setting, item banking, computer-based testing, and other important topics in educational testing.
9. Clauser BE, Margolis ME, Swanson DB: Issues of validity and reliability for assessments in medical education. In Holmboe ES,

Hawkins RE (eds): Practical Guide to the Evaluation of Clinical Competence. St. Louis, Elsevier, 2008.

This chapter provides more in-depth coverage of the reliability and validity issues that commonly arise in assessment in the health professions, along with considerations in conducting validation studies.

10. Garibaldi RA, Trontell MC, Waxman H, et al: The in-training examination in internal medicine. Ann Intern Med 1994;121: 117–123.

This article provides a comprehensive report on the development, administration, and psychometric properties of the in-training examination in internal medicine.

11. Levine HG: Selecting evaluation instruments. In Morgan and Irby (eds): Evaluating Clinical Competence in the Health Professions. St. Louis, CV Mosby, 1978.

Though published 30 years ago, this "oldie-but-goodie" remains up to date in its discussion of the strengths and weaknesses of a broad range of assessment methods that are commonly used in the health professions.

12. Millman J, Greene J: The specification and development of tests of achievement and ability. In Linn R(ed): Educational Measurement London, Longman, 1989, pp 335-366.

This chapter provides an excellent overview of the purposes that examinations serve and how the test specifications and item formats used on a test relate to those purposes and to the kind of score inferences to be drawn from test performance. It also provides an introduction to statistical indices commonly used to assess item quality and make decisions about item use and reuse.

13. National Council on Measurement in Education, Instructional Topics in Educational Measurement Series

This series of high-quality instructional modules provide a wealth of information and guidance about educational testing, including standard setting, item response theory, combining scores on tests, performance assessment, generalizability theory, and other topics. They can be downloaded free from http://www.ncme.org/pubs/.

14. Nitko A: Designing tests that are integrated with instruction. In Linn R (ed): Educational Measurement, Longman, London, 1989.

This chapter, in one of the classic references on educational testing, provides valuable background on a broad range of topics for those interested in designing an effective system for assessing trainees during their educational experience.

15. American Educational Research Association, American Psychological Association, National Council on Measurement in Education: The Standards for Educational and Psychological Testing. Washington, DC, AERA, APA & NCME, 1999.

This is viewed as the "bible" by educational testing organizations, addressing professional and technical issues in test development and use, and providing guidelines to promote the sound and ethical use of tests.

REFERENCES

1. Miller GE: The assessment of clinical skills/competence/performance. Acad Med 1990;65:S63–S67.
2. Gruppen LD, Frohna AZ: Clinical reasoning. In Norman GR, van der Vleuten CPM, Newbel DI (eds): International Handbook on Research in Medical Education. Dordrecht, Kluwer Academic Publishers, 2002, pp 205–230.
3. Norman GR: Critical Thinking and Critical Appraisal. In Norman GR, van der Vleuten CPM, Newbel DI (eds): International Handbook of Research in Medical Education. Dordrecht, Kluwer Academic, 2002, pp 277–298.
4. Association of American Medical Colleges (AAMC): Learning Objectives for Medical Student Education: Guidelines for Medical Schools. Medical School Objectives Project. Washington, DC, AMC, 1998. Accessed at http:\\www.aamc.org/meded/msop/msop1/pdf, Jan. 10, 2006.
5. Accreditation Council for Graduate Medical Education (ACGME): General Competencies. Chicago, ACGME, 2003. Accessed at http:\\www.acgme.org/outcome/comp/compFull.asp, Jan. 10, 2006.
6. Elstein AS: Beyond multiple-choice questions and essays: The need for a new way to assess clinical competence. Acad Med 1993;68:244–249.
7. Elstein AS, Shulman L, Sprafka S: Medical Problem Solving. Cambridge, Harvard University Press, 1978.
8. Swanson DB, Stillman PL: Use of standardized patients for teaching and assessing clinical skills. Eval Health Prof 1990;13:79–103.
9. Swanson DB, Norcini JJ, Grosso L: Assessment of clinical competence: Written and computer-based simulations. Assess Eval Higher Educ 1987;12:220–246.
10. Swanson DB: A measurement framework for performance-based tests. In Hart I, Harden R (eds): Further Developments in Assessing Clinical Competence. Montreal, Can-Heal Publications, 1987, pp 13–45.
11. White KL, Williams TF, Greenberg BG: The ecology of medical care. N Engl J Med 1961;265:885–892.
12. Cronbach LJ: Educational Psychology, 3rd ed. New York, Harcourt Brace Jovanovich, 1977.
13. Case SM, Swanson DB: Constructing Written Test Questions for the Basic and Clinical Sciences, 3rd ed. London: National Board of Medical Examiners, 2001. Accessed at http://www.nbme.org/publications/item-writing-manual/html, Jan. 11, 2007.
14. Levine HG: Selecting Evaluation Instruments. In Morgan I (ed): Evaluating Clinical Competence in the Health Professions. St. Louis, CV Mosby, 1978.
15. Sireci SG, Zeniski AL: Innovative item types in computer-based testing: In pursuit of improved content representation. In Dowing SM, Haladyna TM (eds): Handbook of Test Development. Mahwah, NJ, Lawrence Erlbaum Assoc., 2006.
16. Norman G, Swanson DB, Case SM: Conceptual and methodological issues in studies comparing assessment formats. Teaching Learning Med 1996;8:208–216.
17. Wainer H, Thissen D: Combining multiple choice and constructed response test scores: Toward a Marxist theory of test construction. Applied Meas Educ 1993;6:103–118.
18. Lukhele R, Thissen D, Wainer H: On the relative value of multiple-choice, constructed response, and examinee-selected items on two achievement tests. J Educ Meas 1994;31:234–250.
19. Norcini JJ, Diserens D, Day SC, et al: The scoring and reproducibility of an essay test of clinical judgment. Acad Med 1990;65:S41–S42.
20. Day SC, Norcini JJ, Diserens D, et al: The validity of an essay test of clinical judgment. Acad 1990;65:S39–S40.
21. Swanson DB, Case SM: Variation in item difficulty and discrimination by item format on Part I (basic sciences) and Part II (clinical sciences) of U.S. licensing examinations. In Rothman A, Cohen R: Proceedings of the Sixth Ottawa Conference on Medical Education. Toronto, University of Toronto Bookstore Custom Publishing, 1995, pp 285–287.
22. Bordage G, Brailovsky C, Carretier H, Page G: Content validation of key features on a national examination of clinical decision-making skills. Acad Med 1995;70:276–281.
23. Swanson DB, Case SM: Trends in written assessment: A strangely biased perspective. In Harden R, Hart I, Mulholland H (eds): Approaches to the Assessment of Clinical Competence: Part 1. Norwich, England, Page Brothers, 1992, pp 38–53.
24. Kane M: Validation. In Bernnan RL(ed): Educational Measurement, 4th ed. Westport, CT, American Council on Education/Praeger, 2006
25. Kane M: An argument-based approach to validation. Psych Bull 1992;112:527–535.
26. Strauss GD, Yager J, Liston EH: A comparison of national and in-house examinations of psychiatric knowledge. Am J Psychiatry 1984;141:882–884.
27. Ripkey DR, Case SM, Swanson DB: Identifying students at risk for poor performance on the USMLE Step 2. Acad Med 1999;74:S45–S48.
28. Garibaldi RA, Trontell MC, Waxman H, et al: The in-training examination in internal medicine. Ann Intern Med 1994;121:117–123.
29. Jozefowicz RF, Koeppen BM, Case S, et al: The quality of in-house medical school examinations. Acad Med 2002;77:156–161.
30. Downing SM: The effects of violating standard item writing principles on tests and students: The consequences of using flawed

test items on achievement examinations in medical education. Adv Health Sci Educ Theory Pract 2005;10:133–143.

31. Downing SM: Threats to the validity of locally developed multiple-choice tests in medical education: Construct-irrelevant variance and construct underrepresentation. Adv Health Sci Educ Theory Pract 2002;7:235–241.

32. Haladyna TM: Developing and Validating Multiple-Choice Items, 3rd ed. Mahwah, NJ, Lawrence Erlbaum Assoc., 2004.

33. O'Donnell MJ, Obenshain SS, Erdmann JB: Background essential to the proper use of results of step 1 and step 2 of the USMLE. Acad Med 1993;68:734–739.

34. Hoffman KI: The USMLE, the NBME subject examinations, and assessment of individual academic achievement. Acad Med 1993;68:740–747.

35. Williams RG: Use of NBME and USMLE examinations to evaluate medical education programs. Acad Med 1993;68:748–752.

36. Berner ES, Brooks CM, Erdmann JB: Use of the USMLE to select residents. Acad Med 1993;68:753–759.

37. Bowles LT: Use of NBME and USMLE scores. Acad Med 1993;68:778.

38. Hammoud MM, Cox SM, Goff B, et al: The essential elements of undergraduate medical education in obstetrics and gynecology: A comparison of the Association of Professors of Gynecology and Obstetrics Medical Student Educational Objectives and the National Board of Medical Examiners Subject Examination. Am J Obstet Gynecol 2005;193:1773–1779.

39. Ripkey DR, Case SM, Swanson DB: Predicting performances on the NBME Surgery Subject Test and USMLE Step 2: The effects of surgery clerkship timing and length. Acad Med 1997;72:S31–S33.

40. Case SM, Ripkey DR, Swanson DB: The effects of psychiatry clerkship timing and length on measures of performance. Acad Med 1997;72:S34–S36.

41. Widmann WD, Aranoff T, Fleischer BR, et al: Why should the first be last? "Seasonal" variations in the National Board of Medical Examiners (NBME) Subject Examination Program for medical students in surgery. Curr Surg 2003;60:69–72.

42. Manetta A, Manetta E, Emma D, et al: Effects of rotation discipline on medical student grades in obstetrics and gynecology throughout the academic year. Am J Obstet Gynecol 1993;169:1215–1217.

43. Smith ER, Dinh TV, Anderson G: A decrease from 8 to 6 weeks in obstetrics and gynecology clerkship: Effect on medical students' cognitive knowledge. Obstet Gynecol 1995;86:458–460.

44. Edwards RK, Davis JD, Kellner KR: Effect of obstetrics-gynecology clerkship duration on medical student examination performance. Obstet Gynecol 2000;95:160–162.

45. Norcini JJ Jr, Downing SM: The relationship between training program characteristics and scores on the cardiovascular disease certification examination. Acad Med 1996;71:S46–S48.

46. Vosti KL, Bloch DA, Jacobs CD: The relationship of clinical knowledge to months of clinical training among medical students. Acad Med 1997;72:305–307.

47. Vasan NS, Holland BK: Increased clinical correlation in anatomy teaching enhances students' performance in the course and National Board subject examination. Med Sci Monit, 2003;9:SR23–SR28.

48. Blue AV, Griffith CH III, Stratton TD, et al: Evaluation of students' learning in an interdisciplinary medicine-surgery clerkship. Acad Med 1998;73:806–808.

49. Curtis JA, Indyk D, Taylor B: Successful use of problem-based learning in a third-year pediatric clerkship. Ambul Pediatr 2001;1:132–135.

50. Pangaro L, Gibson K, Russell W, et al: A prospective, randomized trial of a six-week ambulatory medicine rotation. Acad Med 1995;70:537–541.

51. White CB, Thomas AM: Students assigned to community practices for their pediatric clerkship perform as well or better on written examinations as students assigned to academic medical centers. Teach Learn Med 2004;16:250–254.

52. Case SM, Swanson DB: Validity of NBME Part I and Part II scores for selection of residents in orthopaedic surgery, dermatology, and preventive medicine. In Gonnella JS, Hojat M, Erdmann JB, Veloski JJ (eds): Assessment Measures in Medical School, Residency, and Practice: The Connections. New York, Springer, 1993, pp 101–114.

53. Tamblyn R, Abrahamowicz M, Dauphinee WD, et al: Association between licensure examination scores and practice in primary care. JAMA 2002;288:3019–3026.

54. Ramsey PG, Carline JD, Inui TS, et al: Predictive validity of certification by the American Board of Internal Medicine. Ann Intern Med 1989;110:719–726.

55. Papadakis MA, Teherani A, Banach MA, et al: Disciplinary action by medical boards and prior behavior in medical school. N Engl J Med 2005;353:2673–2682.

56. Boulet JR, McKinley DW, Whelan GP, et al: Clinical skills deficiencies among first-year residents: Utility of the ECFMG clinical skills assessment. Acad Med 2002;77:S33–S35.

57. Rifkin WD, Rifkin A: Correlation between housestaff performance on the United States Medical Licensing Examination and standardized patient encounters. Mt Sinai J Med 2005;72:47–49.

58. Webb LC, Juul D, Reynolds CF III, et al: How well does the psychiatry residency in-training examination predict performance on the American Board of Psychiatry and Neurology? Part I. Examination. Am J Psychiatry 1996;153:831–832.

59. Holzman GB, Downing SM, Power ML, et al: Resident performance on the Council on Resident Education in Obstetrics and Gynecology (CREOG) In-Training Examination: Years 1996 through 2002. Am J Obstet Gynecol 2004;191:359–363.

60. Baumgartner BR, Peterman SB: 1998 Joseph E. Whitley, MD, Award. Relationship between American College of Radiology in-training examination scores and American Board of Radiology written examination scores. Part 2. Multi-institutional study. Acad Radiol 1998;5:374–379.

61. Biester TW: The American Board of Surgery In-Training Examination as a predictor of success on the qualifying examination. Curr Surg 1987;44:194–198.

62. Replogle WH: Interpretation of the American Board of Family Practice In-Training Examination. Fam Med 2001;33:98–103.

63. Waxman H, Braunstein G, Dantzker D, et al: Performance on the internal medicine second-year residency in-training examination predicts the outcome of the ABIM certifying examination. J Gen Intern Med 1994;9:692–694.

64. Replogle WH, Johnson WD: Assessing the predictive value of the American Board of Family Practice In-Training Examination. Fam Med 2004;36:185–188.

65. Leigh TM, Johnson TP, Pisacano NJ: Predictive validity of the American Board of Family Practice In-Training Examination. Acad Med 1990;65:454–457.

66. Garvin PJ, Kaminski DL: Significance of the in-training examination in a surgical residency program. Surgery 1984;96:109–113.

67. Grossman RS, Fincher RM, Layne RD, et al: Validity of the in-training examination for predicting American Board of Internal Medicine certifying examination scores. J Gen Intern Med 1992;7:63–67.

68. Klein GR, Austin MS, Randolph S, et al: Passing the boards: Can USMLE and Orthopaedic In-Training Examination scores predict passage of the ABOS Part I examination? J Bone Joint Surg Am 2004;86-A:1092–1095.

69. Sosenko J, Stekel KW, Soto R, Gelbard M: NBME Examination Part I as a predictor of clinical and ABIM certifying examination performances. J Gen Intern Med 1993;8:86–88.

70. Norcini JJ, Grosso LJ, Shea JA, Webster GD: The relationship between features of residency training and ABIM certifying examination performance. J Gen Intern Med 1987;2:330–336.

71. FitzGerald JD, Wenger NS: Didactic teaching conferences for IM residents: Who attends, and is attendance related to medical certifying examination scores? Acad Med 2003;78:84–89.

72. Bell JG, Kanellitsas I, Shaffer L: Selection of obstetrics and gynecology residents on the basis of medical school performance. Am J Obstet Gynecol 2002;186:1091–1094.

73. Carmichael KD, Westmoreland JB, Thomas JA, Patterson RM: Relation of residency selection factors to subsequent orthopaedic in-training examination performance. South Med J 2005;98:528–532.

74. Cavalieri TA, Shen L, Slick GL: Predictive validity of osteopathic medical licensing examinations for osteopathic medical

knowledge measured by graduate written examinations. J Am Osteopath Assoc 2003;103:337–342.

75. Schwartz RW, Donnelly MB, Sloan DA, et al: The relationship between faculty ward evaluations, OSCE, and ABSITE as measures of surgical intern performance. Am J Surg 1995;169:414–417.

76. Joorabchi B, Devries JM: Evaluation of clinical competence: The gap between expectation and performance. Pediatrics 1996;97: 179–184.

77. Adusumilli S, Cohan RH, Korobkin M, et al: Correlation between radiology resident rotation performance and examination scores. Acad Radiol 2000;7:920–926.

78. Wise S, Stagg PL, Szucs R, et al: Assessment of resident knowledge: Subjective assessment versus performance on the ACR in-training examination. Acad Radiol 1999;6:66–71.

79. Quattlebaum TG, Darden PM, Sperry JB: In-training examinations as predictors of resident clinical performance. Pediatrics 1989;84:165–172.

80. Dupras DM, Li JT: Use of an objective structured clinical examination to determine clinical competence. Acad Med 1995; 70:1029–1034.

81. Taylor C, Lipsky MS: A study of the ability of physician faculty members to predict resident performance. Fam Med 1990; 22:296–298.

82. Hawkins RE, Sumption KF, Gaglione MM, Holmboe ES: The in-training examination in internal medicine: Resident perceptions and lack of correlation between resident scores and faculty predictions of resident performance. Am J Med 1999;106:206–210.

83. Parker RW, Alford C, Passmore C: Can family medicine residents predict their performance on the in-training examination? Fam Med 2004;36:705–709.

84. Nathan RG, Mitnick NC: Using an in-training examination to assess and promote the self-evaluation skills of residents. Acad Med 1992;67:613.

85. ACGME Timeline, 2006. ACGME Web site, accessed on 3-31-2006. Electronic citation.

86. Mahour GH, Hoffman KI: The development and validation of a standardized in-training examination for pediatric surgery. J Pediatr Surg 1986;21:154–157.

87. Abdu RA: Survey analysis of the American Board of Surgery In-Training Examination. Arch Surg 1996;131:412–416.

88. Hall JR, Cotsonis GA: Analysis of residents' performances on the In-Training Examination of the American Board of Anesthesiology–American Society of Anesthesiologists. Acad Med 1990;65:475–477.

89. Moon MR, Damiano RJ Jr, Patterson GA, et al: Effect of a cardiac-specific didactic course on thoracic surgery in-training examination performance. Ann Thorac Surg 2003;75:1128–1131.

90. Wade TP, Kaminski DL: Comparative evaluation of educational methods in surgical resident education. Arch Surg 1995; 130:83–87.

91. Shetler PL: Observations on the American Board of Surgery In-Training examination, board results, and conference attendance. Am J Surg 1982;144:292–294.

92. Cacamese SM, Eubank KJ, Hebert RS, Wright SM: Conference attendance and performance on the in-training examination in internal medicine. Med Teach 2004;26:640–644.

93. Bull DA, Stringham JC, Karwande SV, Neumayer LA: Effect of a resident self-study and presentation program on performance on the thoracic surgery in-training examination. Am J Surg 2001;181:142–144.

94. de Virgilio C, Stabile BE, Lewis RJ, Brayack C: Significantly improved American Board of Surgery In-Training Examination scores associated with weekly assigned reading and preparatory examinations. Arch Surg 2003;138:1195–1197.

95. Dean RE, Hanni CL, Pyle MJ, Nicholas WR: Influence of programmed textbook review on American Board of Surgery In-Service Examination scores. Am Surg 1984;50:345–349.

96. Hirvela ER, Becker DR: Impact of programmed reading on ABSITE performance. American Board of Surgery In-Training Examination. Am J Surg 1991;162:487–490.

97. Itani KM, Miller CC, Church HM, McCollum CH: Impact of a problem-based learning conference on surgery residents' in training exam (ABSITE) scores. American Board of Surgery in Training Exam. J Surg Res 1997;70:66–68.

98. Hollier LM, Cox SM, McIntire DD, et al: Effect of a resident-created study guide on examination scores. Obstet Gynecol 2002;99:95–100.

99. Shokar GS, Burdine RL, Callaway M, Bulik RJ: Relating student performance on a family medicine clerkship with completion of Web cases. Fam Med 2005;37:620–622.

100. Picciano A, Winter R, Ballan D, et al: Resident acquisition of knowledge during a noontime conference series. Fam Med 2003;35:418–422.

101. Godellas CV, Hauge LS, Huang R: Factors affecting improvement on the American Board of Surgery In-Training Exam (ABSITE). J Surg Res 2000;91:1–4.

102. Godellas CV, Huang R: Factors affecting performance on the American Board of Surgery in-training examination. Am J Surg 2001;181:294–296.

103. Shokar GS: The effects of an educational intervention for "at-risk" residents to improve their scores on the in-training exam. Fam Med 2003;35:414–417.

104. Derossis AM, Da RD, Schwartz A, et al: Study habits of surgery residents and performance on American Board of Surgery In-Training examinations. Am J Surg 2004;188:230–236.

105. Riggs JW, Johnson C, O'Neill P, Berens P: Are residents' work schedules related to their in-training examination scores? Obstet Gynecol 1996;88:891–894.

106. Ling FW, Grosswald SJ, Laube DW, et al: The in-training examination in obstetrics and gynecology: An attempt to establish a remediation indicator. Am J Obstet Gynecol 1995;173:946–950.

107. Pofahl WE, Swanson MS, Cox SS, et al: Performance standards improve American Board of Surgery In-Training Examination scores. Curr Surg 2002;59:220–222.

108. Friedmann P: A program director's view of the In-Training Examination. Bull Am Coll Surg 1985;70:7–11.

109. Ballinger WF: The validity and uses of the In-Training Examination. Bull Am Coll Surg 1985;70:12–16.

110. Barden CB, Specht MC, McCarter MD, et al: Effects of limited work hours on surgical training. J Am Coll Surg 2002;195:531–538.

111. Vetto JT, Robbins D: Impact of the recent reduction in working hours (the 80 hour work week) on surgical resident cancer education. J Cancer Educ 2005;20:23–27.

112. Cox SM, Herbert WN, Grosswald SJ, et al: Assessment of the resident in-training examination in obstetrics and gynecology. Obstet Gynecol 1994;84:1051–1054.

113. Stone MD, Doyle J, Bosch RJ, et al: Effect of resident call status on ABSITE performance. American Board of Surgery In-Training Examination. Surgery 2000;128:465–471.

114. Jacques CH, Lynch JC, Samkoff JS: The effects of sleep loss on cognitive performance of resident physicians. J Fam Pract 1990;30:223–229.

115. Ellis DD, Kiser WR, Blount W: Is interruption in residency training associated with a change in in-training examination scores? Fam Med 1997;29:184–186.

Practice Audit, Medical Record Review, and Chart-Stimulated Recall

Eric S. Holmboe, MD

Critique of the medical record is a time-honored approach in the evaluation of trainees. Most faculty members have some experience evaluating student write-ups as part of their clinical clerkships. However, systematic review of the medical record is done much less frequently in residency and fellowship education. Medical records serve a number of important functions: (1) an archive of important patient medical information for use by other health care providers *and* patients; (2) a source of data to assess performance in practice such as treatment of specific chronic medical conditions (e.g., diabetes), postoperative care, or preventive services; and (3) the documentation of clinical decisions. One can readily see how these patient care functions of the medical record can be used for educational and evaluative purposes.[1]

In the United States, the Residency Review Committee (RRC) of the Accreditation Council for Graduate Medical Education (ACGME), the organization responsible for the accreditation of training programs, requires medical record audits as part of the training program's evaluation.[2] The accreditation requirements specifically state that the program director should ensure that a representative sample of trainees' medical records are audited for quality of documentation and information during resident inpatient and outpatient clinical rotations, with feedback given to residents. Medical record audits are an essential element in the evaluation of the new competency of *practice-based learning and improvement* (PBLI). PBLI requires that residents be actively involved in monitoring their own clinical practice and improving the quality of care based on a systematic review of the care they provide. The American Association of Medical Colleges also endorses the importance of skills in medical records for medical students.[3] Chapter 11 covers how and why the data from medical record audits are essential to evaluate a trainee's competence and performance in quality improvement. Medical records can also be used to assess clinical reasoning through a technique known as chart-stimulated recall, described in the section Chart-Stimulated Recall. Both activities promote self-reflection, an important skill needed for lifelong learning.

Sources of Data for Practice Audits

In this new era of information technology (IT), data are often available from other sources besides the "paper-based" medical record. Many hospitals, and to a much lesser extent outpatient clinics, are moving to electronic medical records to document visit encounters. However, the "written" medical record remains a vital component of the educational experience, whether in paper or electronic form. Other potential data sources for audit include computerized laboratory data and radiographic records, claims and pharmacy data, and other administrative databases. For example, quality improvement organizations (QIOs) use Medicare claims data to track the quality of care for Medicare beneficiaries who receive outpatient care for chronic conditions such as diabetes (eye examination rates, hemoglobin A_{1c} testing), prevention screening tests (mammography, colonoscopy), and immunizations.[4] Programs can work with their state QIO or health plans to obtain aggregate data on outpatient performance. Each particular type of data system has its own set of limitations, so it is important to ask your local QIO and IT department what types of data are available at your institution in your specific specialty.

Paper-Based Medical Records

The paper-based written medical record is still the most common format used to document clinical care activities and can provide valuable data to evaluate and provide feedback about the "quality" of care. However, most experts believe that there should be more rapid uptake of electronic medical records (EMRs); current data suggest only 10% to 15% of outpatient practices in the United States have fully operational EMRs.[5] Until EMRs are more widely adopted, medical educators will need to understand how to use and extract important information from paper-based medical records for education and evaluation. Audet showed that less than 30% of U.S. physicians are using any performance data to improve their care practices; our trainees must be better prepared.[5]

The major limitation of the paper-based, and even electronic, record is that the record is only as good as the information contained in it. First, research has shown that important aspects of the clinical encounter are often not documented (see Potential Disadvantages of Medical Record Audits),[6] and the quality of the written information is highly variable from trainee to trainee (assuming, of course, you can read it!). Second, paper sheets are like socks in a dryer; they tend to get lost all too easily. Third, paper records require an inordinate amount of personnel time to maintain. These aspects should be considered when deciding how to use paper-based records in your evaluation system.

The Electronic Medical Record

For years the term "medical record" referred to the collection of written information, including history and physical examinations, laboratory and radiology results, problem lists, and so on, contained in the patient's paper chart or file.

The introduction of EMRs is beginning to substantially alter the way patient clinical information is organized and used for the delivery of medical care.[7] As a result, the EMR can be expected to also alter the way in which we use the medical record for evaluation. The effect of computer-based record systems on documentation in training programs is not well known, but deserves further study as many institutions move to electronic records. To date, the main effect of EMRs has occurred in the inpatient setting, with many, but not all, studies showing improvement in patient safety and a reduction in medical errors.[8–10] A number of these EMRs provide the mechanism to enter the medical history and physical examination. Little is known on how EMRs affect the quality and nature of the medical trainee's documentation practices.[11,12] However, electronic records may be highly valuable in helping to determine the actual clinical experiences of trainees.[13,14] One study at a single hospital in Boston with a computer-based records system found that more information per each patient's problem was being entered into the computer record, as opposed to a paper record.[15] Although this study did not address the direct impact on assessment of competence through electronic record review, the study does suggest that computer records may provide a greater quantity of information about a patient encounter over the written medical record.

However, we have noted one serious documentation problem we call the "cut and paste" syndrome, in which trainees cut and paste previous notes for use in admission and daily progress notes, with or without adequate editing. In one of my previous hospital's internal quality improvement activities, we noted this was a common activity for "efficiently" completing daily progress notes. However, unless we've moved into a new time dimension, I found it hard to believe a patient was "postoperation day 1" for 7 consecutive days. In another review of inpatient electronic charts for a quality of care project on pneumonia, we uncovered a number of instances in which the "cut and pasted" information by trainees was both erroneous and failed to account for changes in a patient's clinical status. Educators should be particularly sensitive to this practice.

EMRs can potentially make the retrieval of specific types of clinical data for review much easier. Unfortunately, pulling data at the individual practitioner level for specific categories of patients is very difficult at this time for most inpatient and outpatient EMR products.[7] This "registry" function is important for several reasons. First, clinical data are necessary for performance assessments and quality improvement projects. Without robust clinical data targeted for specific populations of patients (e.g., those needing preventive services, patients with chronic disease such as diabetes), it is almost impossible to implement quality improvement. Second, trainees need to know what types of patients and conditions they are seeing in clinical practice. At the current time few programs have the capacity to track the clinical experiences of trainees. For educators who have EMRs as part of the clinical environment, we recommend approaching the information technology or quality improvement departments of your organizations to see what types of information can be retrieved from the EMR system for trainees.

Claims Data

At the residency and fellowship levels, trainees and office staff routinely use ICD and CPT codes for patient visits, especially in the outpatient setting.[13,14] This information can be a valuable source of information about the clinical practice of trainees. For example, claims data can be very helpful in identifying a cohort of patients. We used the claims database at National Naval Medical Center to identify the population of all diabetic patients seen in an internal medicine residency clinic. Using this data, we were able to then access the laboratory database to assess processes of care (measurement of hemoglobin A_{1c}, lipids, microalbumin) and the degree of glycemic control (hemoglobin A_{1c} level) and hyperlipidemia for each trainee's panel of diabetic patients. We also used this claims database to "track" the make-up of each resident's patient panel. Likewise, the claims database can be used to identify a group of patients admitted with conditions such as acute myocardial infarction (AMI) and pneumonia. This can then facilitate the pulling of charts for review. Because AMI and pneumonia are target conditions for Medicare, your quality improvement department may already be reviewing the quality of care for these groups of patients.

Several caveats should be noted about using claims data for evaluation. First, the use of claims data to measure "quality" is highly dependent on the quality of the coding. Poor coding practices can limit the value of the claims data. Second, claims data are essentially limited to the process of care and usually cannot provide specific detail about the care received.

Laboratory and Other Clinical Databases

For most hospitals, but to a much lesser extent for outpatient settings, the laboratory, pharmacy, and radiology data for groups of patients are available electronically.

Access to this type of electronic data greatly facilitates the systematic review of chronic illness care, cancer screening, etc. Unfortunately, for many training programs, patients often receive services from multiple locations, making it more difficult to track these services. Mammography is one example of a test for which the patient may have several options concerning where it is performed (offsite office, mobile van, hospital, etc.). In this situation, those using only the local hospital database are likely to significantly underestimate the use and receipt of certain services.

The Audit Process

Understanding the basics of the audit process is crucial to maximizing the utility of medical records as a tool for both formative and summative assessment. Because medical record audits can be time-consuming, you should not perform an audit until you are clear about the educational and evaluation purpose of the audit. The audit cycle is closely related to the PDSA (plan-do-study-act) quality improvement cycle developed by Shewart over 60 years ago.[16] The audit cycle (Fig. 5-1) highlights how information from a medical record audit can help trainees to improve and progress professionally.

The simple diagram in Figure 5-1 highlights the importance of clinical practice data as a catalyst for individual change. Without such data, it is nearly impossible to determine "quality" of performance and to measure progress. As we will see in Chapter 11 on practice-based learning and improvement and systems-based practice, data from medical record audits form an essential component. Trainees must not only understand this simple audit cycle, they must have the opportunity during training to perform all of its steps.

The value of the audit process is only as good as the information abstracted from the medical record. There are two main approaches to the conduct of an audit: "explicit" and "implicit" review. For years, the most common approach was implicit review. Implicit means the auditor does not have strictly defined criteria when reviewing a medical record. Instead, the reviewer relies on general guidelines to determine if care delivered, based on the medical record, was "good" or "bad." Implicit review was commonly used in the

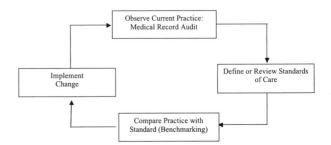

Figure 5-1 The audit cycle. (Adapted from Crombie IK, Davies HTO, Abraham SCS, Florey C du V: The Audit Handbook: Improving Health Care Through Clinical Audit. Chichester, UK: Johan Wiley & Sons, 1993.)

1980s for patients experiencing critical incidents or adverse events, to review complaints, or for routine peer review activities. In medical education, implicit review is a common technique for judging trainees' patient "write-ups" on clerkships or other clinical experiences. There are several important limitations to implicit review. First, there tends to be unacceptable inter-rater variation, resulting in low levels of reliability. Second, in the absence of reasonable and consistently applied criteria and standards, it is difficult for a reviewer to determine what constitutes good and bad care, especially for complex cases. Attempts to train reviewers to improve the quality of the implicit review approach have been mostly unsuccessful.[17,18]

Therefore, to determine what constitutes a high-quality trainee write-up; some basic structure with a minimal set of predetermined criteria is essential. In contrast, an explicit review approach uses detailed criteria to perform a medical record audit. Explicit review is now the preferred approach among most quality organizations. In explicit reviews, the quality measures are carefully chosen and defined to be sure they (1) can be measured with reliability and accuracy; (2) are generalized across clinical sites; and (3) can be aggregated for populations of patients. Likewise, the audit process is also carefully described with well-defined inclusion and exclusion criteria. Box 5-1 provides an example of a quality measure from the U.S. National Quality Forum (NQF), an organization working to standardize a set of quality measures for use by all interested organizations.[19]

For high-stakes decisions about quality of care delivered to groups of patients, the explicit review process is the current "gold standard."

Advantages of the Medical Record Audit

As an evaluation tool, audit of the medical record has a number of important strengths. Some form of medical record audit should be part of every training program's evaluation system. The specific advantages of medical record audit are described here.

Availability

Medical records or other clinical data are usually available and accessible. Getting to the record is usually not a major problem, but depending on the type of record (paper, electronic), pulling out specific aspects of care can be a challenge. Electronic patient registries are best for creating population-based reports for specific quality process measures, but even the use of flowsheets and problem lists can greatly facilitate the collection and analysis of the quality of chronic care, acute care, and preventive services.

Feedback

Medical records allow for corrective feedback centered on actual clinical care in a timely manner. Most faculty are required to review, and often co-sign, trainee notes on clinical rotations. Too often, faculty fail to take advantage of information obtained from the medical record for use in their evaluation of and feedback to the trainee. In fact, the written medical record can be used as a "guide" to query the resident about the choices of specific diagnostic or therapeutic approaches for the patient. This approach is known as chart-stimulated recall (CSR) and is discussed in greater detail later in the chapter.[20–23]

Changing Clinical Behavior

The majority of studies have shown that chart review can change trainee behavior through direct feedback such as that provided by "report cards" on performance of targeted clinical interventions (e.g., prevention measures).

Early studies demonstrated audits could be very effective when explicit criteria were used for data abstraction. Martin and associates[24] reported in 1980 that a group of residents subjected to continuous chart review demonstrated a 47% reduction in laboratory usage in comparison to a control group of residents receiving no review. In fact, chart review with feedback was more effective than a "financial incentive" (a textbook). Kern and associates[25] found that a chart review combined with feedback improved performance in record documentation and compliance with preventive care measures. Several other studies found that a structured chart review using explicit criteria coupled with written and verbal feedback led to substantial improvement in the delivery of three preventive health measures.[26,27] One study found that the audit of just three preventive care interventions was associated with substantial improvement in

---

BOX 5-1   Diabetes Process of Care Quality Measure*
Measure
Percentage of patients with one or more hemoglobin A$_{1c}$ tests
Numerator
One or more hemoglobin A$_{1c}$ tests conducted during the measurement year identified either by the appropriate CPT code, or at a minimum, documentation in the medical record must include a note indicating the date on which the Hgb A$_{1c}$ was performed and the result
Denominator
A systematic sample of patients age 18–75 years who had a diagnosis of either type 1 or 2 diabetes
Exclusions
Exclude patients with a history of polycystic ovaries, gestational diabetes, or steroid-induced diabetes during the measurement year
Data Source
Visit, laboratory, or pharmacy encounter data or claims; electronic data may be supplemented by medical record data

*From the U.S. National Quality Forum.

the delivery of six other nonaudited preventive care interventions ("spill-over" effect).[26]

A recent systematic review by Veloski and colleagues investigating the effects of audit and feedback found positive results in the training setting. Specifically, Veloski reviewed 29 studies that involved residents or a mixture of faculty and residents. Of the 29 studies, 18 (62%) reported positive effects of feedback on clinical care. However, the majority of the studies involved residents at multiple levels, making it impossible for them to comment about the effects of supervision.[28]

Several other systematic reviews have also found modest positive effects of audit and feedback on clinical care for all developmental stages of physicians.[29] Medical record audits appear to be most effective when the data feedback is *resident* (or physician) specific and the data are provided back to the individual resident for review. Data provided at the group level appear less effective; individuals looking at group data often remark, "I wish my colleagues would do a better job because I know I'm doing better than this!"[27]

Practicality

Medical record audits allow for a random or targeted selection of patients to be surveyed, and record reviews can be done without the patient physically being present. Furthermore, audits can be scheduled into clinical activities convenient for the training program and resident. We created a half-day rotation in quality improvement for our residents and used a portion of this time for residents to audit their medical records in diabetes and preventive care. Medical record audits are also unobtrusive as an evaluation tool and in this way may help to minimize the "Hawthorne effect."

Evaluation of Clinical Reasoning

Depending on the quality of the documentation, evaluation of skills in analysis, interpretation, and management is possible. In addition, evaluations of particular patients or conditions can be performed over time, and for many chronic conditions good evidence is available to develop key outcome and process metrics. We'll come back to this when we discuss chart-stimulated recall.

Reliability and Validity

When *explicit* criteria are used, a high degree of reliability is possible. This approach applies to such areas as appropriate use of the laboratory, preventive health measures, cost effectiveness, care of chronic illnesses such as diabetes, and the quantity of documentation. Explicit criteria are best suited for process of care measures (such as ordering a hemoglobin A_{1c} on a diabetic patient within a certain time frame) and some outcomes that are easily measured and do not require substantial time (e.g., measuring the level of hemoglobin A_{1c} as a surrogate outcome). Because the information contained in the record relates directly to actual patients, the results of medical record audits have excellent face validity and authenticity. Medical records provide documentation of performance, meaning what a trainee actually does.[30] Some studies have also found evidence of construct validity in that results of quality of care audits modestly correlate with cognitive expertise as measured by a secure examination or certification status.[31–33]

Learning and Evaluating by Doing

Medical record audits allow residents to directly participate in the process of peer review. Engerbretsen commented in 1977[34] on the positive impact of a peer review system at his family practice residency. Ashton[35] made the case for involving residents in hospital quality improvement programs over 10 years ago. Having the residents perform their own audit may be even more powerful; one study involving resident self-audit found the majority of trainees were surprised by results demonstrating they often failed to perform key quality indicators.[27] We call this the chagrin, or "a-ha," factor. A study of practicing physicians participating in a study examining a Web-based self-audit tool found identical reactions from the physicians.[36] The main power of self-audit is that the trainee cannot "hide" from the results, and cannot complain about the quality of the data or blame an abstractor for errors because they are the ones who entered most of the data and performed the audit. PGY-2 residents in the Yale Primary Care Internal Medicine Residency Program participated in self-audit as part of a quality improvement experience during their ambulatory block rotations. Residents used part of the time to review their own charts for quality of care in immunizations, cancer screening, and diabetic care. This relatively simple intervention led to meaningful changes in resident behavior and modest improvements in patient care.[27] Finally, benchmarking the resident's performance against some standard, whether internal or external, can also be helpful.[26,28,29]

Teaching effective medical record audit techniques is becoming increasingly important. Most health insurance companies routinely ask for copies of records to perform reviews of certain practice habits. The Center for Medicare and Medicaid Services (CMS) is also beginning to review the care of Medicare patients in both inpatient and outpatient settings with a goal of public reporting in the near future.[37] Accurate and reliable medical record audits are an essential component of many pay-for-performance programs. Thus, involving trainees in the medical record audit process is important for their future success as practicing physicians.

Self-Assessment and Reflection

When the trainee is incorporated into the audit process, the result can be a powerful tool to promote self-assessment and reflection. Given what was just stated about a likely future of public reporting and continual assessment, physicians-in-training must be prepared to effectively self-assess their own performance, reflect accurately on the results, and then use the results for continuous professional development.[38,39]

Medical record review can be a very useful educational tool, can potentially change behavior, and can provide useful information when explicit criteria for review are utilized. Such audits can be tracked and included as part of a comprehensive clinical competency record and can be easily incorporated into an evaluation portfolio. Finally, the result of a medical record audit across multiple trainees provides valuable information for program assessment. Audits can identify strengths and weaknesses in the actual care delivered to patients that should play a major role in program assessment and curriculum design. Some would argue that clinical training is only as good as the quality of the care given to the patients. Audits can also be used to assess the effectiveness of educational interventions in the clinical training setting.

Potential Disadvantages of Medical Record Audits

Despite the tradition of using the medical record as a tool for evaluation of competence, Tugwell and Dok lamented more than 20 years ago over the lack of good research using trainees' medical records for education and assessment. While the situation is modestly better today, much work remains to be done.[6] The challenges of the ever-changing and evolving organizational format used for medical records were highlighted in the section Sources of Data for Practice Audits. A few other issues should be highlighted. First, whereas the organizational format used for creating a medical admission or progress note receives a lot of attention in medical school, the same scrutiny seems to evaporate at the residency and fellowship levels. I often felt like I was trying to decipher the DaVinci code when reviewing the progress notes of too many trainees. I've seen more modifications of problem-oriented or SOAP (subjective-objective-assessment-plan) notes than I care to remember. Add to this situation the many different EMR vendors all using different organizational formats involving various combinations of templates, checklists, and free text. This new world has created a host of new problems for medical educators. As noted earlier, many educators have discovered trainees often use the "cut and paste" function to simply update progress notes or take information from other notes to complete admission workups. Poorly edited notes electronically copied worsen documentation accuracy and quality, may put patients at risk, and even more disturbing, may represent blatant plagiarism. Despite the obvious efficiencies, I believe the "cut and paste" function should be used sparingly and very carefully.

However, given the clear importance of EMRs for more effective, efficient, and safe health care delivery,[7] educators must prepare trainees to use EMRs more effectively in the future. This should include what functionality a trainee should look for when implementing an EMR system.[7] The other challenge is using the medical record as a "measure" of clinical competence. The most important question is, "What are we really measuring about competence in a medical record review?"

Quality of the Documentation

The quality of a medical record audit can only be as good as the quality of the documentation. Tugwell and Dok[6] noted, "the fact that records are used more as an aide-de-memoir rather than a documentation of the justification for management decisions, which continues to compromise the validity of the medical record." This situation may actually be worse today. When trying to assess more than whether certain processes of care were or were not delivered, important questions to ask are as follows:

- Does the record accurately reflect what occurred during the visit?
- Was all pertinent information that was collected during the patient encounter recorded?
- Are impressions and plans justified in the record?
- What facilitating tools (e.g., templates, problem lists, flowcharts) are provided with the medical record?

Do physicians record with completeness what they actually did during the encounter? Norman and associates[40] in 1985 found, using unannounced standardized patients, that physicians often failed to completely record information obtained and procedures performed. Certain areas, such as physical examination and clinical investigations, were recorded appropriately over 70% of the time. However, items such as diagnosis, patient education, and procedures were *undocumented up to 50% of the time*. A study that compared the written record with a videotape recording of patient encounters found that only 56% of medical history items were recorded in the chart. Psychosocial issues were even less likely to be recorded.[41] Leaf and colleagues found that chart audit correlated poorly with physician self-report in a study of cardiac risk assessment in an outpatient clinic.[42]

Two more recent studies have highlighted the potential problems using medical record audits to measure specific aspects of quality of care and performance. One study compared medical record audit with a standardized patient's (SP) completion of a checklist for quality-of-care items. Luck and associates found that the overall quality score from an SP was significantly higher than the chart audit. In this study, the medical record audit was only 70% specific when compared with the SP as the gold standard.[43] The same authors then compared clinical vignettes, SPs' scores, and medical record audits and again found that medical record audits detected the lowest number of quality criteria among a group of faculty and residents.[44] A study by Ognibene and colleagues[45] is one of the few to find a high rate of documentation: 81% of residents successfully documented 10 components of the physical examination in the medical record. At the present, the majority of studies using written records demonstrate that many important aspects of the medical encounter are not recorded in the medical record. Electronic medical records may improve documentation of items such as physical examination but this has yet to be proved, and nontechnical aspects of care, such as counseling, may still suffer from poor documentation.

A "good chart" does not necessarily equal "good care." For example, the chart may have a check box for smoking cessation counseling, but such a "check" does not provide much information about what was covered in the counseling session. More work is needed on examining the impact of quality charting with patient outcome. This may be especially important in an era when patient care is often fragmented among a number of doctors who "communicate" diagnostic and therapeutic choices through written records that include letters and e-mail. Lack of continuity is an especially pressing problem for residency training programs. These studies raise questions as to the best combination of methods to measure both trainees and program performance regarding quality of care.

Process versus Outcomes

Medical record audits are a reasonably good method to determine if specific processes of care have been performed, especially when explicit criteria are defined. However, the utility of using the medical record audit to determine causation for patient outcomes is very limited. Most often a surrogate outcome is used such as blood pressure, hemoglobin A_{1c} level, absence of a postsurgical complication, etc. Systematic approaches to reviewing critical incidents, such as root cause analysis,[46] will use information from the medical record.

Implicit Review

Reviewing a medical record without a minimal framework, structure, or especially well defined criteria results in low reliability and reduced validity. Much of chart review in quality improvement programs previously utilized implicit review by "experts." The reliability of implicit review, also known as peer review, came under attack because of low reliability and the resulting negative perceptions of these reviews by physicians. Goldman[47] reviewed 12 studies investigating quality of care and found agreement among reviewers was poor, and often only marginally better than chance. Hayward and associates[17] examined the quality of structured implicit review in evaluating the care of inpatients on a general medicine service. Reasonable agreement (kappa = 0.5) was seen only with overall assessment of care and prevention of death. They also noted that at least five reviewers per patient were necessary to achieve an accuracy of 90%. This poor interrater agreement was noted despite 15 hours of training for the select group of physician reviewers! They concluded implicit review, even with structured criteria linked to a rating scale, was "expensive, burdensome,

and untenable for many specific quality-of-care judgments." Because of these observations and others, the CMS abandoned the peer review approach to measuring quality of care.[48]

Although many faculty members probably do recognize a "poor chart" when they see one (the gestalt factor), the lack of defined criteria as to why the chart is poor is a disservice to the trainee, who needs specific feedback in order to improve. Furthermore, numerous studies in other settings have found that implicit reviews (e.g., those without predefined, explicit criteria for abstraction) contain too many errors. Thus, simply reviewing a chart for "quality" without predefined criteria and objectives will have low reliability and is much less likely to provide useful information about performance or for feedback to the trainee.

Assessment of Clinical Judgment

Resident analytic and integrative skills can be assessed only partially through record review, especially when one considers the problems in the quality of documentation. Furthermore, is the physician's judgment adequately recorded on the record? Did that judgment translate into an appropriate management plan? Gennis and Gennis[49] found that when a separate attending physician evaluated a patient independently from the resident, the faculty attending's recommendations for care management was different in nearly 33% of the resident's patients. A similar study in a military outpatient training clinic found a similar frequency of differences between attending and resident management decisions but the differences were less dramatic and the majority of the recommended changes from faculty were minor.[50] These two studies raise significant questions about the ability to accurately assess the appropriateness of management plans from medical record review. Chart-stimulated recall, discussed later, is a method to more effectively use the medical record to assess clinical judgment.

Time

Medical record review can be very time-consuming, especially if it is used for high-stakes decisions. Norman[40] and Ognibene[45] both found that audit of a large number of charts is needed to ensure reasonable reliability in the training setting. Researchers working with practicing physicians have found that at least 25 to 35 patient medical records are required for pass-fail decisions for a single condition (e.g., diabetes) in provider recognition programs.[51]

Audits require the development and testing of abstraction instruments, data collection and entry, data analysis, and then dissemination of the results to individual residents. However, several factors can help to minimize these limitations. First, I strongly recommend using standardized abstraction tools and quality measures already developed and field-tested whenever possible. In the United States, there is actually a Web-based clearinghouse for quality measures supported by the Agency for Healthcare Research and Quality (AHRQ).[52] The National Quality Forum systematically endorses quality measures; approved measures can be downloaded from their website.[19] An example of an abstraction form for preventive services and diabetes care developed and field tested by Qualidigm, a QIO in the United States, is provided in Appendix 5-1. Using existing well-defined measures and abstraction tools can save training programs substantial time. Second, consider having the trainees perform the actual audit. Not only does this save time for faculty and programs, but as previously discussed, the self-audit experience is valuable for the trainee.

Cost

Cost may be a factor in your program if the medical record audit is performed on archived records and the institution charges a fee for pulling the charts. Cost will also be a factor if you use faculty or other administrative personnel to perform the abstraction. For faculty, the usual cost is their time. If you use abstractors, they may charge a monetary fee for their services.

Faculty Development

We have found few current faculty members who have extensive experience with medical record audits. There are several key issues around faculty development: personal skill documentation, abstraction skills, and interpretation. Many faculty members exhibit the same behaviors as trainees when documenting the results of their own medical encounters. Furthermore, some faculty members are learning to use electronic medical records at the same time as the trainees. When faculty skills in using medical records are suspected to be problematic your first priority should be to train your faculty in the optimal use of the medical record at your institution. Second, reliable and accurate abstraction is a skill in itself, and most faculty members have little experience. While I do not advocate that faculty be the primary source for abstraction services, faculty members do need to understand how to conduct a proper audit, including how to use an abstraction manual and how to properly interpret the specifications of quality measures. Finally, the faculty needs to know how to interpret the results of an audit to help trainees improve. For example, what should a faculty member tell a trainee whose "quality report" shows poor compliance with several quality measures? Chapter 11 on practice-based learning and improvement provides guidance and suggestions. Brook and Lohr[18] make several critical points:

1. Explicit review will only be as good as the criteria developed for the review.
2. Physicians performing the review must be carefully selected and properly trained. This is particularly critical when utilizing implicit review. Tugwell and Dok[6] appropriately pointed out that when using chart review as an educational tool you must have committed faculty and the specific goals with explicit criteria. This is essential in any review process.
3. Ultimately, collection of data directly from the patient is important, especially when considering "quality of care."

This last point reinforces the need for a multifaceted approach to evaluation, highlighting how combining direct observation and patient surveys with medical record audit can be a potentially powerful combination for assessment.

Summary of Limitations of Medical Record Audits

1. Medical record review can be time-consuming, and to be reliable for "high-stakes" decisions, review of a substantial number of records (usually more than 25 medical records) per trainee is needed. A substantial commitment from faculty may be needed depending on local information systems and resources. As electronic medical records evolve with better search capabilities and registry functions, real-time audits may be able to provide continuous quality feedback.
2. The quality and completeness of documentation hamper validity of medical record review. The written record rarely records the physician-patient interaction comprehensively.
3. Medical record audits cannot assess the quality of important aspects of the encounter. For example, documentation of the cardiac examination says nothing about the skill of the examiner. Quality of patient instruction by the physician cannot be assessed.
4. It is difficult to adequately assess physician interpretive abilities and judgment without corroboration.
5. The current lack of consistency in medical record organizational format will continue to hamper the standardization of medical record audits.
6. Medical record review can be potentially costly if the audit is performed by trained individuals outside the training program.
7. Medical records may be better for assessing the process of care and be less useful when looking at patient outcomes. Specific measures (e.g., compliance with preventive health measures such as immunization) can help enhance the utility of chart review.
8. Implicit review, even if "structured," suffers from significant reliability problems. Furthermore, the investment required for training is significant.

Table 5-1 summarizes some of the key limitations of medical record audits with possible solutions.

Chart-Stimulated Recall

How can medical records be used to more effectively assess clinical judgment? Chart-stimulated recall (CSR)

Table 5-1 **Summary of Medical Record Audit (MRA) Limitations**

Limitation	Possible Solutions
Quality of documentation	Use problem lists and flowcharts for chronic conditions and preventive care Provide templates for medical history and physical examination Use electronic medical record (may or may not improve documentation; training required in effective use of EMRs) Combine MRA with direct observation
Time	Have trainees perform audit of their own charts or their peers' Seek assistance from hospital or clinic quality improvement department to generate performance reports, especially if have EMR Use other health care personnel (if available)
Implicit review	Provide minimal framework for medical record review and do not rely solely on the judgment of the reviewer Encourage explicit criteria whenever possible Provide auditor training
Cost	Have trainees perform audit of their own charts or their peers' Use existing reports, when available, from quality improvement departments
Assessing clinical judgment	Combine MRA with chart-stimulated recall

uses either a single medical note or multiple components of the medical record to assess a trainee's analytic, integrative, and clinical judgment skills. CSR enables a faculty rater to assess a trainee's rationale for diagnostic and treatment decisions, the other options that were considered but ultimately discarded, and the reasons these other options were ruled out. CSR also allows the rater to investigate any other factors that influenced the trainee's clinical decision making, such as patient, environmental, and microsystem factors (see Chapter 11). The medical note, including admission, acute encounter, daily progress, and routine outpatient follow-up notes, serves as a template for the examiner (e.g., faculty) to develop specific interview questions that probe a trainee's clinical decision making and judgment skills.

The American Board of Emergency Medicine (ABEM) performed pioneering work with this technique in the 1980s. The ABEM used CSR as a way of constructing an oral examination using emergency department records from the examinee.[20] The ABEM examiners used the examinee's charts to assess knowledge, clinical problem solving, and a "general measure of clinical competence." The ABEM ultimately found that the CSR was reliable and valid.[21] In fact, the ABEM found that three to six charts could provide sufficient reliability for CSR interviews. However, from a certification, high-stakes testing standpoint the CSR was too expensive and time-consuming. Despite their satisfaction with the approach, the ABEM discontinued CSR as part of its certification process.[20,21]

Jennett and Affleck provided a number of important recommendations and guidelines for performing CSR. First, the CSR interviewer should ideally be a medical faculty member and be trained to perform CSR consistently and reliably.[22] We recommend using the techniques and principles of performance dimension and frame of reference training described in discussion of direct observation (Chapter 9). Second, the medical

record of interest should be reviewed beforehand to develop the specific questions for the CSR interview. Third, the interview should begin with open-ended questions to minimize rater bias and to provide the rater with insight into the trainee's thought processes. All questions should be asked in a nonjudgmental, nonbiased approach. Depending on the intended use of the CSR, the session can be audiotaped for future analysis. Audiotaping also allows the rater to focus more on the interview and questions instead of taking the time to document the discussion and decisions. CSR can be performed in person or by telephone, if necessary.

At Yale University, we used CSR for formative assessment and as part of our diagnostic approach for residents in difficulty (see Chapter 13). In our CSR approach, we used single encounter notes (admissions, daily progress notes, outpatient notes, etc.) for two main purposes. First, we look at the basic "quality" of the notes with a simple framework. Questions for the reviewer were: Is the note legible? Does it follow a standard format (SOAP or problem-based)? Second, as part of the "quality" review, we examine notes for two specific deficiencies: lack of internal consistency and discordances. Internal consistency refers to whether an issue or problem noted in the history or physical examination section of the note is logically "carried through" the remainder of the note (see Appendix 5-2). For example, if the trainee lists and describes in the subjective or history section of the note chest pain as a symptom, then the physical examination, assessment, and plan sections should all contain pertinent information about that symptom. The physical examination should contain the appropriate components relevant to this symptom (e.g., cardiac examination) and the assessment and plan should provide a differential diagnosis and plan of action for the chest pain, respectively.

Discordance refers to a phenomenon that occurs when information in one section of the medical note is discordant with information or decisions documented in other sections of the note. Returning to our chest pain example, if a trainee lists chest pain with accompanying signs and symptoms that suggest evidence of ischemic disease but lists heartburn as the likely diagnosis without mention of coronary artery disease, the assessment is "discordant" with the history information provided.

Although problems with internal consistency and discordance may simply be related to documentation errors, deficits in knowledge and clinical decision making are more likely. The faculty member performing CSR can use these observations to probe a trainee's medical knowledge and clinical decision-making skills. The roster of questions developed for the Canadian physician assessment review (PAR) CSR is an excellent template to help guide faculty.[53] CSR can still be a useful technique even if a chart doesn't contain problems with internal consistency or a discordance. For example, a trainee may have appropriately diagnosed hypertension and chosen a "diuretic" for treatment. Choice of a diuretic would certainly be an evidenced-based choice. However, was the decision to prescribe a diuretic simply a "rote" choice or was the trainee aware of the related guidelines? Was a diuretic the best choice for this patient? Is the trainee aware of the side effect profile of the medication and how it may relate to the specific patient's risk factors and other comorbidities?

CSR can be "combined" with other evaluation tools to measure competence. For example, faculty members can combine a direct observation exercise, such as the mini-clinical evaluation exercise, with a CSR exercise. Information obtained from direct observation can be combined with the medical record documentation to assess deeper aspects of clinical decision making. Combining CSR with medical record audit can provide a very robust assessment of the quality of care at the individual patient level. A study in Canada found that a combined medical record audit and CSR interview for a small group of practicing family practitioners was a valuable experience for assessing and improving quality of care.[54] Also, in a number of continuing education settings CSR has been found to be a useful tool for both assessing the impact of a continuing medical education course and determining learning needs for practitioners.[22]

Conclusion

Medical record audits and data feedback can be valuable tools to assess clinical competence. Given the critical importance of performance data for quality improvement and the competency of practice-based learning and improvement, all trainees should receive individual performance data at a minimum during training. Medical records are also readily accessible. They allow the examination of a potentially large number of clinical encounters, and their use in assessment may be relatively unobtrusive, thereby minimizing the Hawthorne effect. When explicit criteria and end points are used, such assessments may yield important information about practice habits in specific areas of care (e.g., preventive health). Databases and EMR may provide a wealth of accessible information in a timely and ongoing manner. Furthermore, the Residency Review Committee requires medical record reviews. Use of the chart-stimulated recall technique helps educators to evaluate more complex skills such as clinical judgment. Given the new structure of the ACGME general competencies, more effective use of the medical record, whether paper or electronic, will be needed for program directors.

Involving trainees in medical record audit activities is strongly recommended. As the level of scrutiny for physicians increases through health care insurance organizations, Center for Medicare and Medicaid Services (CMS), and peer review organizations, to name just a few, physicians will need a good understanding of audit methodology, and chart review remains a cornerstone of most audit programs. Therefore, this skill should be incorporated into residency training. The quality of care audit provides a simple example of a program that can be incorporated into a residency program. This is also an excellent method to satisfy the requirements of the new *practiced-based learning and improvement* competency while simultaneously working to improve outcomes among patients cared for by the house staff program.

ANNOTATED BIBLIOGRAPHY

1. Veloski J, Boex JR, Grasberger MJ, et al: Systematic review of the literature on assessment, feedback and physicians' clinical performance: BEME Guide No. 7. Med Teacher 2006;28(2):117–128.
   This comprehensive review of the effects of medical record and feedback on physician behavior includes a valuable summary of studies from training settings. The authors used the rigorous methodology from the Best Evidence Medicine Education (BEME) initiative (see http://www.bemecollabroation.org/).Consistent with previous studies, medical record audit and feedback can produce modest changes in quality.
2. Holmboe ES, Prince L, Green ML: Teaching and improving quality of care in a residency clinic. Acad Med 2005;80:571–577.
3. Holmboe ES, Meehan TP, Lynn L, et al: The ABIM diabetes practice improvement module: A new method for self assessment. J Cont Educ Health Prof 2006;26:109–119.
   Little is known about the impact and value of trainees performing their own audits instead of simply receiving data from an external source. Both preceding studies found the process of self-audit was a powerful experience for residents and practicing physicians. Both groups experienced a ''surprise'' at the gap between knowing what to do and their actual clinical performance. Both studies provide guidance on how to set up self-audit. The abstraction instrument used in the resident study (article 2) is provided in Appendix 5-1.
4. Jennett P, Affleck L: Chart audit and chart stimulated recall as methods of needs assessment in continuing professional health education. J Cont Educ Health Prof 1998;18:163–171.
   This remains one of the best reviews of all the work done on chart-stimulated recall. This is a valuable article for any educator planning to implement chart-stimulated recall in their program.
5. College of Physicians and Surgeons of Alberta: The Physician Achievement Review (PAR) program. Accessed at http://www.cpsa.ab.ca/collegeprograms/par_program.asp.
   The PAR program in Alberta has developed a useful, practical form for conducting chart-stimulated recall. The form comes with clear instructions and provides a series of possible questions the reviewer can ask in a chart-stimulated recall. This form has been field tested and studied by investigators working with the College of Physicians and Surgeons of Alberta. I'd recommend educators download the pdf CSR form if they are considering implementing CSR in their program.

REFERENCES

1. Arnold CWB, Bain J, Brown RA, et al: Moving to Audit. Dundee, Scotland, Centre for Medical Education, University of Dundee, 1992.
2. Accreditation Council for Graduate Medical Education: Program requirements. Accessed at http://www.acgme.org, Oct. 15, 2007.
3. American Association of Medical Colleges: Accessed at http://www.aamc.org, Oct. 15, 2007.
4. Quality Improvement Organizations: Accessed at http://www.cms.hhs.gov/QualityImprovementOrgs/, Oct. 15, 2007.
5. Audet AM, Doty MM, Shamasdin J, Schoenbaum SC: Measure, learn, and improve: Physicians' involvement in quality improvement. Health Affairs 2005;24(3):843–853.
6. Tugwell P, Dok C: Medical record review. In Nefueld VR, Norman GR (eds): Assessing Clinical Competence. New York, Springer, 1985.
7. Kilo CM, Leavitt M: Medical Practice Transformation with Information Technology. Chicago, Healthcare Information and Management Systems Society, 2005.
8. Kaushal R, Shojania KG, Bates DW: Effects of computerized physician order entry and clinical decision support systems on medication safety: A systematic review. Arch Intern Med 2003;163(12):1409–1416.
9. Bates DW, Gawande AA: Improving safety with information technology. N Engl J Med 2003;348(25):2526–2534.
10. Longo DR, Hewett JE, Ge B, Schubert S: The long road to patient safety: A status report on patient safety systems. JAMA 2005;294(22):2858–2865.
11. Hier DB, Rothschild A, LeMaistre A, Keeler J: Differing faculty and housestaff acceptance of an electronic health record. Int J Med Informatics 2005;74(7–8):657–662, 2005.
12. O'Connell RT, Cho C, Shah N, et al: Take note(s): Differential EHR satisfaction with two implementations under one roof. J Am Med Informatics Assoc 2004;11(1):43–49.
13. Sequist TD, Singh S, Pereira AG, et al: Use of an electronic medical record to profile the continuity clinic experiences of primary care residents. Acad Med 2005;80(4):390–394.
14. Hripcsak G, Stetson PD, Gordon PG: Using the Federated Council for Internal Medicine curricular guide and administrative codes to assess IM residents' breadth of experience. Acad Med 2004;79(6):557–563.
15. Safran C, Rury C, Rind DM, Taylor WC: A computer-based outpatient medical record for a teaching hospital. MD Comput 1991;8:291–299.
16. Langley GJ, Nolan KM, Nolan TW, et al: The Improvement Guide. A Practical Approach to Enhancing Organizational PerformanceThe Improvement Guide. San Francisco, Jossey-Bass, 1996.
17. Hayward RA, McMahon LF, Bernard AM: Evaluating the care of general medicine inpatients: How good is implicit review? Ann Intern Med 1993;118:550.
18. Brook RH, Lohr KN: Monitoring quality of care in the Medicare program. JAMA 1987;258(21):3138.
19. The National Quality Forum: Accessed at http://www.qualityforum.org/, Oct. 15, 2007.
20. Munger BS: Oral examinations. In Mancall EL. Bashook PG (eds): Recertification: New Evaluation Methods and Strategies. Evanston, IL, American Board of Medical Specialties, 1994.
21. Munger BS, Krome RL, Maatsch JC, Podgorny G: The certification examination in emergency medicine: An update. Ann Emerg Med 1982;11:91–96.
22. Jennett P, Affleck L: Chart audit and chart stimulated recall as methods of needs assessment in continuing professional health education. J Cont Educ Health Prof 1998;18:163–171.
23. Hall W, Violato C, Lewkonia R, et al: Assessment of physician performance in Alberta: The physician achievement review. CMAJ Can Med Assoc J 1999;161(1):52–57.
24. Martin AR, Wolf MA, Thibodeau LA, et al: A trial of two strategies to modify the test-ordering behavior of medical residents. N Engl J Med 1980;303:1330.
25. Kern DE, Harris WL, Boekeloo BO, et al: Use of an outpatient medical record audit to achieve educational objectives: Changes in residents' performances over six years. J Gen Intern Med 1990;5:218.
26. Holmboe ES, Scranton R, Sumption K, Hawkins R: Effect of medical record audit and feedback on residents' compliance with preventive health care guidelines. Acad Med 1998;73:65–67.
27. Holmboe ES, Prince L, Green ML: Teaching and improving quality of care in a residency clinic. Acad Med 2005;80:571–577.
28. Veloski J, Boex JR, Grasberger MJ, et al: Systematic review of the literature on assessment, feedback and physicians' clinical performance: BEME Guide No. 7. Med Teacher 2006;28(2):117–128.
29. Jamtvedt G, Young JM, Kristoffersen DT, et al: The Cochrane Library, Issue 3. Audit and feedback: Effects on professional practice and health care outcomes. Chichester, UK, Wiley and Sons, 2003.
30. Miller G: Invited reviews: The assessment of clinical skills/competence/performance. Acad Med 1990;65:S63–S67.
31. Tamblyn R, Abrahamowicz M, Dauphinee WD, et al: Association between licensure examination scores and practice in primary care. JAMA 2002;2888(23):3019–3026.
32. Tamblyn R, Abrahamowicz M, Brailovsky C, et al: Association between licensing examination scores and resources use and quality of care in primary care practice. JAMA 1998;280(11):989–996.
33. Norcini JJ, Lipner RS, Kimball HR: Certifying examination performance and patient outcomes following acute myocardial infarction. Med Educ 2002;36:853–859.
34. Engerbretsen B: Peer review in graduate education. N Engl J Med 1977;296:1230.
35. Ashton CM: Invisible doctors: Making a case for involving medical residents in hospital quality improvement programs. Acad Med 1993;68:823.
36. Holmboe ES, Meehan TP, Lynn L, et al: The ABIM Diabetes Practice Improvement Module: A new method for self assessment. J Cont Educ Health Prof 2006;26:109–119.
37. Center for Medicare and Medicaid Services: Accessed at http://www.cms.gov, Oct. 15, 2007.
38. Davis DA, Mazmanian PE, Fordis M, et al: Accuracy of physician self-assessment compared with observed measures of competence. JAMA 2006;296:1094–1102.
39. Duffy FD, Holmboe ES: Self-assessment in lifelong learning and improving performance in practice: Physician know thyself. JAMA 2006;296:1137–1138.
40. Norman GR, Neufeld VR, Walsh A, et al: Measuring physicians' performances by using simulated patients. J Med Educ 1985;60:925.
41. Moran MT, Wiser TH, Nanda J, Gross H: Measuring medical residents' chart documentation practices. J Med Educ 1988;63:859.
42. Leaf DA, Neighbor WE, Schaad D, Scott CS: A comparison of self-report and chart audit in studying resident physician assessment of cardiac risk factors. J Gen Intern Med 1995;10:194–198.
43. Luck J, Peabody JW, Dresselhaus TR, et al: How well does chart abstraction measure quality? A prospective comparison of standardized patients with the medical record. Am J Med 2000;108:642–649.
44. Peabody JW, Luck J, Glassman P, et al: Comparison of vignettes, standardized patients, and chart abstraction. JAMA 2000;283:1715–1722.
45. Ognibene AJ, Jarjoura DG, Illera VA, et al: Using chart reviews to assess residents' performances of components of physical examinations: A pilot study. Acad Med 1994;69(7):583.
46. Battles JB, Shea CE: A system of analyzing medical errors to improve GME curricula and programs. Acad Med 2001;76(2):125–133.
47. Goldman RL: The reliability of peer assessments of quality of care. JAMA 1992;267(7):958.
48. Jencks SF, Wilensky GR: The Health Care Quality Improvement Initiative: A new approach to quality assurance in Medicare. JAMA 1992;268:900–903.
49. Gennis VM, Gennis MA: Supervision in the outpatient clinic: Effects on teaching and patient care. J Gen Intern Med 1993;9:116.
50. Omori DM, O'Malley PG, Kroenke K, Landry F: The impact of the bedside visit in the ambulatory clinic. Does it make a difference? J Gen Intern Med 1997;12(S1):96A.

51. Landon BE, Normand ST, Blumenthal D, Daley J: Physician clinical performance assessment prospects and barriers. JAMA 2003;290(9):1183–1189.
52. Agency for Healthcare Quality and Research: Quality information and improvement. Accessed at http://www.ahrq.gov/qual/qualix.htm, Oct. 15, 2007.
53. College of Physicians and Surgeons of Alberta: The Physician Achievement Review (PAR) program. Accessed at http://www.cpsa.ab.ca/collegeprograms/par_program.asp, Oct. 15, 2007.
54. Jennett PA, Scott SM, Atkinson MA: Patient charts and office management decisions: Chart audit and chart stimulated recall. J Cont Educ Health Prof 1995;15:31–39.

APPENDIX 5-1

Sample Medical Record Abstraction Form for Diabetes

Date of abstraction _____

Abstractor initials _____

Abstraction time (min) _____

Physician name _____

First visit with this MD?   YES   NO

First visit to this clinic?   YES   NO

Demographics

1. Patient Name (First, MI, Last) _____

2. Patient Identification (MRN) # _____

3. Gender (circle)   a. Male   b. Female

4. Race/Ethnicity   a. White
    (circle all that apply)   b. Black
                         c. Hispanic
                         d. Asian
                         e. Other
                         f. Not documented

5. Date of birth _____
    (MM/DD/YYYY)

Chart Information

6. Does the chart contain a problem list?   Yes   No

7. Does the chart contain a preventive services checklist?   Yes   No

8. Does the preventive services checklist have **any** entries?   Yes   No

Conditions Present

9. Hypertension   Yes   Not documented

10. Coronary artery disease   Yes   Not documented

11. Heart failure   Yes   Not documented

12. Conduction disorder/bradyarrhythmia   Yes   Not documented

13. Aortic stenosis   Yes   Not documented

14. Chronic obstructive pulmonary disease/asthma   Yes   Not documented

15. Cerebrovascular disease   Yes   Not documented

16. Peripheral vascular disease   Yes   Not documented

17. Chronic renal disease   Yes   Not documented

18. Chronic liver disease   Yes   Not documented

19. Diabetes mellitus   Yes   Not documented

20.	Dyslipidemia	Yes	Not documented
21.	Breast cancer	Yes	Not documented
22.	Colon cancer	Yes	Not documented
23.	Dementia	Yes	Not documented
24.	Bleeding disorder/risk	Yes	Not documented
25.	Peptic ulcer disease	Yes	Not documented
26.	Anemia	Yes	Not documented

Physical Examination

27. Height   _____ Inches Not documented

28. Date of most recent height   _ _/_ _/_ _ _ _ N/A

29. Weight   _____lbs Not documented

30. Date of most recent weight   _ _/_ _/_ _ _ _ N/A

Physical Examination

31. Record all blood pressures from the last three visits during the observation period (*insert period*).

Date	Blood Pressure	Date	Blood Pressure
1. _ _/_ _/_ _ _ _	_____/_____	7. _ _/_ _/_ _ _ _	_____/_____
2. _ _/_ _/_ _ _ _	_____/_____	8. _ _/_ _/_ _ _ _	_____/_____
3. _ _/_ _/_ _ _ _	_____/_____	9. _ _/_ _/_ _ _ _	_____/_____
4. _ _/_ _/_ _ _ _	_____/_____	10. _ _/_ _/_ _ _ _	_____/_____
5. _ _/_ _/_ _ _ _	_____/_____	11. _ _/_ _/_ _ _ _	_____/_____
6. _ _/_ _/_ _ _ _	_____/_____	12. _ _/_ _/_ _ _ _	_____/_____

Counseling/Prevention

32. Was an assessment of tobacco use performed?   Yes Not documented

33. Is patient a current smoker?   Yes No Not documented

33a. Was smoking cessation counseling offered?   Yes Not documented N/A

Counseling/Prevention

34. Was a foot exam performed? (*insert observation period*)   Yes Not documented

34a. Was a monofilament test for neuropathy performed?   Yes Not documented

35. Has the patient ever received pneumovax?   Yes Not documented

Labs/Diagnostic Studies:

For all questions pertaining to labs/diagnostic studies, review the record from 6/30/2001 back to 7/1/1999 (if necessary). Record the most recent date that the test was performed prior to 6/30/2001 and the value.

Lab Study	Test/Diagnostic Study	Test Performed	a. Date Performed	b. Value
36.	Blood urea nitrogen	36. Yes Not documented *If yes, record the date and value.*	36a. _ _/_ _/_ _ _ _	36b. _____ (Normal range 6–19 mg/dL)
37.	Creatinine	37. Yes Not Documented *If yes, record the date and value.*	37a. _ _/_ _/_ _ _ _	37b._____ (Normal range 0.6–1.4 mg/dL)
38.	Blood sugar	38. Yes Not documented *If yes, record the date and value.*	38a. _ _/_ _/_ _ _ _	87b. _____ (Normal range 70–105 mg/dL)
39.	Was blood sugar recorded as fasting?	39. Yes Not documented		

Labs/Diagnostic Studies—cont'd

Lab Study	Test/Diagnostic Study	Test Performed	a. Date Performed	b. Value
40.	Albuminuria test	40. Yes Not documented	40a. _ _/_ _/_ _ _ _	40b. Albumin present? Yes Not documented
41.	Hemoglobin A_{1C}	41. Yes Not documented *If yes, record the date and value.*	41a. _ _/_ _/_ _ _ _	41b. _____ (Normal range 3.0–6.5%)
42.	Total cholesterol	42. Yes Not documented *If yes, record the date and value.*	42a. _ _/_ _/_ _ _ _	42b. _____ (Normal range 120–220 mg/dL)
43.	HDL cholesterol	43. Yes Not documented *If yes, record the date and value.*	43a. _ _/_ _/_ _ _ _	43b. _____ (Normal range 44–55 mg/dL)
44.	LDL cholesterol	44. Yes Not documented *If yes, record the date and value.*	44a. _ _/_ _/_ _ _ _	44b. _____ (Normal range 40–170 mg/dL)
45.	Triglycerides	45. Yes Not documented If yes, record the date and value.	45a. _ _/_ _/_ _ _ _	45b. _____ (Normal range 40–150 mg/dL)
46.	Potassium	46. Yes Not documented *If yes, record the date and value.*	46a. _ _/_ _/_ _ _ _	46b. _____ (Normal range 3.3–5.1 mEq/L)
47.	EKG performed	47. Yes Not documented *If yes, record the date and findings.*	47a. _ _/_ _/_ _ _ _	47b. EKG findings: *(Select all recorded findings)* a. Myocardial infarction (any age) b. Atrial fibrillation c. LVH d. LBBB e. None of the above f. No interpretation

Treatment

48.   Does the chart contain a current list of medications?   Yes   Not documented

48a. Are the patient's medications documented at the last visit to this physician?   Yes   Not documented

49.   Record all medications that the patient was taking or that were prescribed at the end of the observation period (*insert observation period*). Use hospital discharge summaries, consultation notes, phone conversations, etc., if necessary.

50.   Does the chart contain a medication allergy section?   Yes   Not documented

Medication	**Dosage**
1. _____	_____
2. _____	_____
3. _____	_____
4. _____	_____
5. _____	_____
6. _____	_____
7. _____	_____
8. _____	_____
9. _____	_____
10. _____	_____

Office Visits (Measurement Year):

51.   Record all dates on which the patient was seen at this office (Chase) during the observation period.

1. _/_ _/_ _ _ _   11. _/_ _/_ _ _ _   21. _/_ _/_ _ _ _
2. _/_ _/_ _ _ _   12. _/_ _/_ _ _ _   22. _/_ _/_ _ _ _
3. _/_ _/_ _ _ _   13. _/_ _/_ _ _ _   23. _/_ _/_ _ _ _
4. _/_ _/_ _ _ _   14. _/_ _/_ _ _ _   24. _/_ _/_ _ _ _
5. _/_ _/_ _ _ _   15. _/_ _/_ _ _ _   25. _/_ _/_ _ _ _
6. _/_ _/_ _ _ _   16. _/_ _/_ _ _ _   26. _/_ _/_ _ _ _
7. _/_ _/_ _ _ _   17. _/_ _/_ _ _ _   27. _/_ _/_ _ _ _
8. _/_ _/_ _ _ _   18. _/_ _/_ _ _ _   28. _/_ _/_ _ _ _
9. _/_ _/_ _ _ _   19. _/_ _/_ _ _ _   29. _/_ _/_ _ _ _
10. _/_ _/_ _ _ _   20. _/_ _/_ _ _ _   30. _/_ _/_ _ _ _

Created by Qualidigm and the Yale Primary Care Internal Medicine Residency Training Program.

APPENDIX 5-2

Basic CSR Documentation Template

Chart-Stimulated Recall Note

Trainee: **Date**:

Level:

1.   Organization and clarity of note

     (*Is the note organized? Is the format appropriate and consistent? Is it legible?*)

2.   Note content

     (*Are clinical issues explained in sufficient detail? Is any essential information missing?*)

3.   Internal consistency

     (*Do clinical issues follow a logical sequence throughout the note?*)

4.   Discordances

     (*Are there any maneuvers or decisions that are discordant with other information provided in the note?*)

5.   Questions for resident

     (*Write up to five questions you would want to ask this resident with a focus on clinical reasoning and judgment.*)
     A.

     B.

     C.

     D.

     E.

Multisource Feedback (360-Degree Evaluation)

Jocelyn M. Lockyer, MHA, PhD, and Stephen G. Clyman, MD

Multisource feedback (MSF), often termed 360-degree evaluation/assessment, describes specific processes and instruments for information gathering, appraisal, and feedback in the workplace. Questionnaires designed to gather data about specific behaviors or professional constructs (e.g., communication skills, professionalism, team work) are administered on behalf of the assessee (i.e., the person being assessed).

In medical settings, the observers (i.e., assessors or raters) may include medical colleagues (e.g., peers or referring physicians, trainees), nonmedical co-workers (e.g., nurses, pharmacists, and psychologists), patients and their family members, and self. These observers, from various groups, have different perspectives and observations regarding physician performance based upon the context in which they interact. MSF is used along the continuum of medical education, although most of the published literature focuses on practicing physicians and postgraduate trainees.

MSF originated in industrial settings in which employees were not being observed closely or frequently enough by the supervisor for the employee to receive meaningful feedback. Others in the work group, in fact, were in a better position to provide work-related information about the employee. By having people in the work group complete surveys, information from several co-workers could be aggregated and used to provide feedback. MSF has been accepted in the industrial world because it uses information from multiple individuals (observers) and multiple sources (groups of observers), thus reducing the bias inherent in "one person, one perspective" (i.e., the supervisor) assessment systems. Observers in these settings include peers, direct-reports, supervisors, and occasionally patients.

MSF instruments comprise sets of items that can be constructed in different ways. Typically, items are brief comments, interrogatives, or categories of constructs that are associated with a multipoint rating scale (e.g., 1 to 5, 1 to 9) or a behavioral anchor scale (e.g., "usually late" to "on-time"). This allows information to be obtained on specific behaviors or more global categories/constructs, or both. Different sources (e.g., peers vs. patients) can respond to different items or to the same items. For example, Table 6-1 provides a selection of constructs, items, and sources taken from the College of Physicians and Surgeons of Alberta (CPSA) Physician Achievement Review (PAR) Program instruments for episodic care practitioners (e.g., emergency medicine, locum physicians).[1] These questionnaires address issues of communication and professionalism with each of their sources but have different items for each.

In MSF, patient surveys may provide information about the patient experience with the physician, often focusing on aspects of communication, patient care, and professionalism. Patient assessments can also include

Table 6-1 **Examples of Constructs, Sources, and Items**

Construct	Source	Examples of Items
Communication	Patients	This doctor listened to me This doctor answered my questions
	Nonphysician co-workers (e.g., nurses, pharmacists)	Verbally communicates with other health care professionals effectively Is accessible for appropriate communication about patients
	Medical colleagues (peers, referring and referral physicians)	Medical records are legible Provides valuable clinical advice to colleagues when approached about difficult clinical decisions
Professionalism	Patients	Treated me with respect Respected my privacy
	Nonphysician co-workers	Respects the professional knowledge and skill of co-workers Accepts responsibility for patient care
	Medical colleagues	Accepts an appropriate share of work Accepts responsibility for own professional actions

Adapted from College of Physicians and Surgeons of Alberta Physician Achievement Review Program. Accessed at http://www.par-program.org, Oct. 15, 2007.

the patient's observations about interprofessional collaboration and collegiality and office systems (e.g., telephone response systems, office wait times). Nurses and other health care professionals can provide data about patient care, interprofessional collaboration, professionalism, and communication. Medical colleagues (including peers) are often asked about these areas but also have the ability to provide information about medical knowledge, technical skills, advocacy, and use of resources. Table 6-2 provides examples of scales that might be used in MSF. There is no "right" number or type of response options on a scale, but there is information on the factors that can influence scale selection.[2]

Feedback on performance can vary. However, most often the data are aggregated for each source (e.g., peer group), by construct and by item. Feedback usually includes comparative data with others who were assessed as well as with the person's self-assessment data. Feedback reports frequently include both graphical and numerical data (e.g., ranges, means, medians). This approach to feedback (often coupled with mentoring and assistance in developing an action plan for performance enhancement) enables the assessee to examine his or her personal data from a number of perspectives.

It is important to note that with more traditional observational assessments (e.g., objective structured

clinical examinations [OSCEs] and "end of rotation" assessments) data and feedback come from individuals who have the hierarchical or organizational authority to assess. With MSF, feedback comes from a much broader group of observers working closely with the medical student or physician. In contrast to multiple-choice questions (MCQs), MSF is based on variable real-life observations; different observers will see different events. This leads to measurement and validity challenges in ensuring that appropriate inferences are made based on data sampling. As illustrated in Table 6-3, it is essential to keep in mind many other differences. With MCQs, materials are typically kept secure prior to administration because publicizing their content may invalidate the measures; with MSF, salutary effects can be achieved simply by letting participants know expectations for performance (in large part defined by the items). Potential sources of bias are higher with MSF than with MCQs because human judgments are inherent; with MCQs, "judges" are highly trained and once their judgments are codified, they are applied consistently. Although observers are often not highly trained for MSF, in the ideal they should have extensive orientation, training, and feedback on their performance as raters. Metrics for converting MCQ responses to a single measure have the benefit of half a century of theoretical development, commonly available analytic tools, and industry

Table 6-2 **Examples of Scales Used in Multisource Feedback**

Type	Range					
Agreement	Strongly agree	Agree	Neutral	Disagree	Strongly disagree	Insufficient information
Frequency	Always	Usually	Sometimes	Never	Not applicable	
Expectations	Exceeds expectations		Meets expectations		Does not meet expectations	
Quality	Excellent	Good	Acceptable	Unacceptable		

Table 6-3 **Traditional Formats: Multiple-Choice Questions (MCQs) versus Multisource Feedback (MSF)**

Factor	MCQs	MSF
Response options	Kept secure	Publicized
Sources of bias	Low	High
Training/orientation/expertise	High	Low
Metrics	Well developed	In development
Risks in feedback	Low	High
Risks in process deviation	Low	High

standards. MSF by comparison is not as advanced. Because the feedback from MSF can be construed to be of such a highly personal nature, risks in delivery of this information are high. As such, it can also have deleterious or overtly destructive consequences if deployed improperly, particularly for those who are rated negatively or whose ability to self-assess is poor. Finally, MSF requires introduction of processes that are not typically standardized centrally and may be interpreted differently by the many participants. As such, risks are greater for deviation in recommended processes that may threaten program integrity.

MSF is a unique form of assessment offering more than the aggregation of single-source feedback (SSF). MSF is based on surveys of different groups (e.g., peers, patients); additive value is accrued from *comparison* of multiple sources. When implementing SSF based on evidence from MSF and vice versa, some "upstream" processes and findings may be interchangeable. For example, data gathering and item/survey response characteristics observed with SSF may generalize to MSF because observers may not know whether the program is SSF or MSF. However, because MSF is built upon the premise that insights are gained from comparisons among different sources, some "downstream" findings may not apply. Assessees may respond differently to multiple sources of data than to single sources, particularly if they can triangulate data and meaning across surveys. Findings based on feedback and resultant effects may not generalize from SSF to MSF.

Using the MSF Tool in Educational Programs

MSF can be quite variable in its intent. In some cases, the intent is clearly focused on formative feedback. In these cases, assessees are expected to be informed through orientation and feedback sessions by the items and the constructs of interest as well as their specific feedback in developing a plan for the future. The organization that has developed the items and produced their scores may have as goals both quality improvement of whole groups and the improvement of individuals. In Alberta, Canada, for example, the CPSA wanted a formative quality improvement

program that would serve as a first-level screen for all physicians.[1] Although the CPSA-PAR program can trigger other levels of assessment, it is intended to help physicians form a plan for improvement. In the United Kingdom, the General Medical Council wanted an assessment for its postgraduate trainees that was aligned with its Best Medical Practice initiative. Both the Sheffield Peer Review Assessment Tool (SPRAT)[3,4] and the Pre-registration House Officers Appraisal and Assessment System (PHAST)[5] are designed to identify physicians at risk who may need remediation. Mini-PAT (a shorter version of SPRAT) is used for foundation trainees in the United Kingdom who are in their first two postgraduate years. Although the tool is intended to identify physicians at risk, it is part of a larger portfolio designed to help trainees identify educational needs, set goals, and plan how to achieve them.[6]

MSF has been used along the continuum of medical education, but based on published literature it appears to be less commonly used for undergraduates. Although there is literature on peer and self-assessment,[7–9] other sources do not seem to be included in conjunction with these assessments. Conversely, there are many examples of its use for residents.[3–6,10] For physicians in practice, MSF is being used for quality improvement of individuals and groups,[11–15] as part of a maintenance of certification program,[16] and to provide feedback to physicians about selected competencies.[11–15] As Evans and associates observed, even when MSF is developed as a formative tool, it may also be being used to identify physicians in difficulty.[17] Even in formative assessment, there is an ethical obligation to protect patients.

The current interest in assessing broad competencies—such as those found in the Accreditation Council for Graduate Medical Education (ACGME),[18] Royal College of Physicians and Surgeons of Canada's Canadian Medical Education Directions for Specialists (CanMEDs) roles,[19] and the United Kingdom's Good Medical Practice framework[20]—almost naturally leads to assessment tools like MSF. This is particularly the case for postgraduate trainees but also for practicing physicians as regulatory authorities and professional bodies move into revalidation. It is difficult, otherwise, to establish evidence for collegiality, professionalism, and communication skills if one does not obtain these data from those able to observe them directly. By contrast, those competencies related to medical knowledge and skill can be assessed by more traditional methods such as MCQ examination and OSCEs.

Getting Started

Introducing MSF within an organization is a major undertaking. It requires the full support of administration and buy-in at all levels of the organization for sustainability. Box 6-1 outlines many of the steps needed, although reference to other information sources is also recommended.[21–23]

The first step in MSF is to assess the organization's readiness for MSF. In particular, consideration needs to be given to how this type of assessment will meet evaluation needs, and complement or replace existing tools, policies, and processes. MSF has to be seen as a value-added program which will provide data to guide the development of the individual and fit within the value system of the organization's culture, curricula, and assessment procedures. Support from the leadership will be needed for sustainability. Very early, a leadership team will need to be identified to guide and monitor the process and ensure communication with all stakeholders. Successful teams will include leaders as well as those who will be participants (assessees and observers) in the process.

The intended use of this assessment tool must be determined. Of particular importance are decisions related to the formative versus summative nature of the assessment. It is important to identify whether the stakes associated with its use are high or low. Some instruments are designed for self-guided reflection and improvement; others are intended to monitor progress and even make promotion decisions or salary adjustments. These decisions need to be made early and without ambiguity. Knowing that an instrument is for formative rather than summative assessment will likely cause observers to respond differently and assessees to select different observers. For example, some participants may be less stringent if the MSF is for summative purposes.

MSF instruments are composed of a series of items. As such, it is a very flexible tool and can be used to measure almost any behavior in the workplace. A key step in development is deciding the domain(s) or construct(s) that will be measured. Instruments can assess professionalism or team-based behaviors. They can assess communication skills, clinical judgment, or almost any facet of medical practice. If the decision is to create an instrument for professionalism, care must be taken to ensure that it captures that construct and not something else. Available resources within the organization will guide buy versus "build" decisions. These latter decisions will need to be made in conjunction with information about validity and reliability of existing tools, the congruence between an organization's needs and existing instruments, and the work that would be required to create instruments that are specific to the organization's needs.

The team will need to decide about the group(s) to be assessed and their observers. It is important to decide which sources will be included based on the behaviors these sources actually can observe as well as the feasibility and acceptability of asking people from diverse backgrounds to assess physicians. Data may be difficult to collect from patients with emergency, psychiatric, or terminal illnesses. Similarly, patients whose literacy and language skills are limited will be difficult to include. Decisions will need to be made about whether people will select their own observers or have them assigned (e.g., by program director, unit administrator). The number of observers will need to be determined based on feasibility, the purpose of the assessment (e.g., identify physicians in difficulty versus quality improvement), and the psychometric robustness needed. The frequency of administration will be governed by feasibility, survey burden, and the importance of providing enough time between administrations so that assessees can address problems.

The instruments can be administered through paper and pencil, online, by telephone, or through hybrid approaches. Each medium has its drawbacks and advantages. If computer access by all respondents is uncertain (e.g., areas with low-speed connection or few computers) low technology solutions may be appropriate. Short surveys can be handled by phone key pad entry. Computer surveys require special IT support, for example, for data capture, survey transmission, reminder systems, and feedback reports.

The method by which feedback is provided needs to be considered before instruments are given a trial. The contents of the report require special attention. Some reports provide the assessee's own data along with comparator data. If observer comments are provided to the assessee, it will be important to determine whether they get screened or not. If comments are not screened, anonymity and confidentiality issues will need to be considered. The physical means for delivery of data will be another consideration. Options here include mail and e-mail as well as in-person communication by a mentor. Certainly, early consideration of mentoring around the feedback will be essential. These data may come from peers with whom the assessee may work in the future. If the purpose of the instrument is

BOX 6-1	Critical Steps in Implementing a Multisource Feedback Program

Communicate
- Assess organizational readiness
- Identify leadership team
- Determine intended use (formative vs. summative)
- Establish the constructs/domains and content
- Create, adapt, or purchase instruments
- Identify assessees and observers
- Establish frequency of administration
- Determine instrument delivery methods
- Create protocol for feedback, goal setting, and mentoring
- Test instruments
- Implement program
- Evaluate and modify program

individual development, an essential piece of the feedback process is explicit goal setting.

Consideration of the consequences of data delivered, whether suboptimal, average, or excellent, needs to be taken into account early. For those whose data might be perceived as particularly negative, the consequences of hearing the feedback and need for remedial action should be considered before program implementation. In particular, it is critical that *a priori* determination of information that might trigger other institutional processes be considered, such as in the case of unprofessional behavior. Even programs that are formative in nature have an ethical responsibility to redirect data indicating possible risk to patients and the workplace.

Instruments should be tested before implementation. This may involve a small group who test the instruments before full implementation. This would allow an assessment of the delivery system as well as perceptions of all participants. These data could then inform full implementation. How the overall program will be evaluated is also important. There may need to be several aspects of the evaluation including how well the program works, perceptions of participants, and the psychometric quality of the data generated.

Communication is an absolutely critical component. It needs to be frequent and clear. It will be necessary throughout the entire process from initial stages which announce the program and its intent, through testing, implementation, and evaluation. Communication vehicles might include e-mail, newsletters, departmental meetings, rounds, and scholarly activities. Messages need to be consistent. Clarity about the formative and summative nature of the assessment is critical, particularly around any consequences for participants.

Reliability and Validity

MSF is a survey-based method. Accordingly, each instrument needs to be developed and assessed based on generally accepted standards for survey instruments[24] to ensure there is evidence for the validity and reliability of the inferences made. Analysis of the whole instrument and its factors or subscores is important. Additionally, though, each item on the surveys can be important in guiding the assessee's self-improvement plan; therefore, the validity argument must also extend to the item level.

In assessments using MSF instruments, the evidence for validity needs to be built up to establish the instrument's ability to measure what it is supposed to measure with inferences supported by evidence and reconsideral when new validity threats are raised over time. Therefore, the validity investigation becomes a continuous one rather than a single study. Generally, the higher the stakes for the assessment, the greater is the need to demonstrate sound argument and evidence for validity and reliability.

As shown in Box 6-2, in the initial stage, the argument for validity is built up from intended inferences or decisions. In this work, it is important to be clear about

BOX 6-2	Building the Argument for Validity: Initial Questions

- What inferences or decisions are intended based on the information obtained?
- How was the instrument created? Who created it?
- What domains or constructs are being assessed?
- What literature was referenced to support development?
- How did the developers assess the content and format of, and the proposed feedback provided by, the instrument? What group of experts or end-users was consulted and how was their feedback used?
- Is there a blueprint for content sampling or coverage?
- How are observers trained? Do they all understand the meaning of the items?
- What communication vehicles are used to disseminate the purpose and goals of this type of assessment?

the purpose of the instrument and the determination of constructs to be measured. The items themselves must align with the construct and preferably be based upon a theoretical underpinning. Because this is about people and their judgments about themselves and others, input from end-users through focus groups or questionnaires is important. These actions will help to ensure that there is coherence between the objectives of the assessment and the intended inferences about behavior and competence. Adjustments need to be made along the development path. Items may be changed as observers provide more in-depth feedback after working with the instrument for longer periods.

In published accounts of MSF work and technical reports, it is common to see the initial design group described or acknowledged, the use of focus groups or questionnaires to test the instruments with end-users (both assessees and observers), and reference to other instruments and literature. For example, in work to develop the PAR program in Alberta,[1] the published descriptions reveal how the attributes to be assessed and sources of data were determined as well as how each physician to be assessed was consulted about the questionnaires.[11-15] Similarly, in the United Kingdom, SPRAT and mini-PAT were based on components of practice determined by the General Medical Council and the Royal College of Paediatrics and Child Health and field tested.[3,4] Similar procedures were followed by the American Board of Internal Medicine.[16,25,26] It is less common in these publications and reports to determine the quality and quantity of information provided to the observers and assessees about the purpose and intent of the MSF program or the training provided to ensure people were interpreting items in a consistent manner.

When empirical data from testing or use of the instrument are available, the focus shifts to other aspects of instrument integrity and the effects of its use. Sample questions are provided in Box 6-3.

In published accounts, survey response rates are generally high. For residents and undergraduates, these data are required as part of the overall assessment. For practicing physicians, for programs such as

---

BOX 6-3   Continuing the Validity Investigation

- What was the response rate? Was it possible to recruit a sufficient number of observers to provide feedback that is acceptable to the assessee?
- What is the range of scores? Are they normally distributed or skewed?
- What is the correlation with measures from other instruments (e.g., another multisource feedback assessment of professionalism or communication skills or an objective structured clinical examination)?
- What affects the scores? Is the variance in scores affected by gender, years in training/practice, ethnicity, or familiarity between assessee and observer?
- If a factor analysis is done, did it identify intended factors?
- How are the data used by feedback recipients, the supervisor, or the organization? Do they believe the data are credible? Did behavior change based on the feedback? Did that behavioral change translate into improvement in patient care?
- Were there any unintended as well as intended consequences from the assessment or program?

---

the PAR program in Alberta, the program is run under the auspices of a regulatory authority and participation is mandatory, at least for the physicians. In the case of the American Board of Internal Medicine (ABIM) program, it is an elective part of the recertification program and those who elect it have a vested interest in the data. Typically the range of scores appears to be positively skewed for practicing physicians for both the PAR and ABIM programs.[11-16] It appears to be less skewed for residents when the goal of the program has been to identify those in difficulty such as provided by PHAST, SPRAT[3] and mini-PAT.[6]

Correlations between scores derived from the MSF instrument and those of other instruments can be calculated to establish whether the same construct is being assessed and provide evidence of criterion-related validity. For example, Johnson and Cujec[27] correlated cognitive knowledge tests with ratings by physicians and nurse observers. Lipner and associates[16] correlated their data with previous assessments by program directors of overall clinical competence. The intent with such analyses may be to eliminate an assessment or to confirm that this new assessment taps into areas that have previously not been measured. Additionally, correlations are often used to assess whether data from different observer groups provide identical or complementary information. Self and peer ratings are frequently compared as are ratings from peers and nurses. Correlation studies in medicine have shown that self-other MSF ratings have low or nonsignificant correlations (i.e., $r < 0.25$), but other-other group correlations are usually moderate ($r = 0.30$ to 0.50).[11,26,27] These data provide evidence for both convergent and divergent validity and confirm the importance of maintaining data from different groups (sources) separately.

In MSF work, linear regressions may be used to assess the importance of phenomena that may affect the variance in scores. One of the biggest concerns arises when assessees get to select their own observers. For practicing physicians, there is often no other practical solution to the identification of observers when physicians are spread throughout a large geographic region. Ramsey and associates' analysis demonstrated that observers chosen by people being assessed do not provide significantly different evaluations from those chosen by a third party.[26] Often familiarity between the observer and the assessee is examined. Some studies have shown that this accounts for less than 10% to 15% of the variance in ratings.[12,13,28] To ensure instrument robustness, it can be helpful to determine whether and how the variance in ratings is affected by phenomena such as full- or part-time status,[3] hospital type (e.g., teaching versus general),[3] patient health status,[16] patient gender or age,[16] physician gender,[16] or years of training.[3]

Factor analyses may be conducted to determine whether the individual items on the instruments align in the intended directions (i.e., to create a factor). When items are identified for a domain of interest or a factor (e.g., communication skills, professionalism), it is assumed they will correlate more with the items in that factor than with items in another factor. The factor analyses will show which items align and how much they account for the total variance. Generally an internal consistency reliability (Cronbach's Coefficient Alpha) will be calculated for each factor as well as the scores from the whole instrument.

In MSF work, an essential part of the validity chain has to do with perceptions of the end-users and those assessed, and the ultimate effects of use of MSF processes, instruments, and feedback. Studies show that most observers and assessees feel this is an important tool for assessment.[5,25] Further, most studies show that physicians are reasonably comfortable with the data provided, although it has been shown that the questions (survey items) had to be appropriate for that source.[25] Physicians may be more comfortable with nurse assessments of their communication skills but not their clinical skills.[25]

Studies show that many physicians will use the data that is provided to make changes,[11,16,29,30] although use of the data may be affected by internal and external factors. Internal factors include physician self-perception of performance, emotions, personal expectations and beliefs, and abilities to make the change. External influences that affect the physician include the nature of the feedback, the credibility of the feedback, the specificity of the feedback, the consistency of the feedback with other feedback, and barriers to change.[30] In this work, it is important to have realistic expectations about change as there is considerable variability in how informative the data will be to the person as well as the person's perceived need for change. No one has published longitudinal studies in medicine examining the impact on scores over two or more time periods. However, this work has been done in industrial settings and a meta-analysis of 24 longitudinal studies, in which people were measured on two or more occasions, showed that improvement was generally small but was more likely for some recipients than for others.[31] Improvement was more likely when the data suggested change was necessary, recipients had a positive feedback orientation, perceived a need to change their behavior, reacted positively to the feedback, believed change was feasible, set appropriate goals to regulate their behavior, and took actions to improve their skill and performance. These types of analyses of assessee use of data are important in further establishing evidence of instrument validity. If people disregard their feedback data, it is difficult to make an argument for validity.

Having established that the test measures what it is intended to measure, it is important to consider the instrument's reliability. Although approached in a variety of ways, it generally includes an assessment of the overall instrument's internal consistency reliability using Coefficient Alpha (Cronbach's Coefficient Alpha) initially. These reliability coefficients can be used to estimate a standard error of measurement (SEM) for a survey in total or for individual scores on items, factors, or subscores. As MSF studies may report on specific items or groups of items within a survey, item response theory (IRT) approaches to reliability may be appropriate as individual item characteristics, including individual item SEMs, are estimated. IRT also provides advantages when MSF is used to classify individuals into categories that represent dividing lines in a continuous measure as standard errors for each individual and classification of individuals measure can be estimated more readily than with classical test theory for different points on the ability continuum.

Generalizability theory is often applied as a second level of assessment employing the generalizability coefficient (Ep^2). This approach investigates the number of raters and the numbers of items that are sufficient to provide stable data to the individual being assessed.[11–16,26] Alternately, the calculation of a 95% confidence interval for mean ratings using generalized theory by varying numbers of raters is done to determine the number of raters needed to achieve a stable score if the intent is to determine whether the person is satisfactory.[3] The confidence interval method allows developers to measure the effect of increasing the size of observer groups. There are trade-offs between costs and administrative difficulties, on the one hand, and improving the precision at the decision point on the rating scale on the other.

Medical applications of MSF show that data derived from these instruments can achieve high levels of internal consistency reliability. For example, the instruments developed for the CPSA PAR Program have demonstrated high Cronbach Coefficient Alpha levels > 0.90.[11–15]

Generalized analyses have been undertaken in MSF work for two purposes. In the first set of studies, G studies were done to establish whether the combination of raters and items produces reliable data for the assessee. In this work, studies show that it is possible to achieve $Ep^2 \geq 0.70$ with reasonable numbers of observers.[10,11,13–16,26] For example, Ramsey and

colleagues achieved 0.70 with an 11-item global instrument and 10 to 11 peer physician raters.[26] When the same group of physicians was assessed by nurses, Wenrich and colleagues found 10 to 15 nurses were required to achieve 0.70 with their 13-item global instrument.[25] G studies have also been done to ensure whether the number of observers was adequate to be confident that physicians in difficulty were identified. For example, in the assessment of the SPRAT instrument for pediatricians in training, Archer and associates determined that four raters using a 24-item survey provided a 95% confidence interval for the rating to be within ±0.5 on a 6-point scale.[3]

Strengths and Weaknesses of MSF as a Tool for Assessment

Strengths

MSF was developed with the assumption that it could enhance the information available to the supervisor and individual, would yield unique information as compared with simulated testing, and could provide information more indicative of current and perhaps future job performance and success. But there are other strengths as well. MSF is based on the work the individual does rather than his or her potential to perform. It uses self-awareness to facilitate change. MSF makes the values and professional expectations explicit to the assessee and to observers. It allows multiple points of view, which are sometimes required to ensure that assessees receive the message(s). It can be used by the organization as a tool to assess its own intraorganizational cultures and expectations, particularly if comparisons across sites/programs are available. MSF is relatively inexpensive and flexible.

Much of MSF is rooted in an approach that develops competencies that support job success, identifies excellence, or predicts superior job performance. The items and constructs are typically assembled through group processes in which participants (organizational leaders, observers, and assessees) have an opportunity to participate in determining the foci and the questions to be addressed. Therefore, from a validity standpoint, MSF might be among the more transparent forms of assessment in linking items and job performance.

Another strength of MSF is that it capitalizes on and facilitates the development of awareness, reflection, and insight of the assessee. Typically, the assessee completes a self-assessment as part of an MSF process. By using the self-assessment data along with data from others, the assessee focuses on discrepancies and similarities. Preceptors or mentors who are working with the assessee can use these data to help the person. Studies from industrial settings suggest that the direction and the amount of discrepancy between self and others affect use of the data. For example, people who rate themselves significantly higher than others rate them can be de-motivated by the experience.[32–35] These studies have not been replicated in medical settings.

One of the distinct advantages of MSF is that the very process of building the instrument forces articulation not only of job-relevant criteria for performance but also of other aspects of the "rules" in the culture and environment that are often unspoken. In contrast to traditional standardized assessment wherein content and knowledge domains are well described, MSF often focuses on behaviors and values for which there are less well defined content outlines. As such, it requires that participants explicate and codify their values, policies, and curricula in this regard. Feedback is optimally provided when everyone agrees to clear definition of items and behaviors, and expectations for performance. The discussions that evolve from this process can be extremely productive and informative. An extension of this same point is manifested through MSF process planning and implementation, in that those participating as observers and assessees become aware of expectations. An additional side effect of MSF use is that it sends a message that everyone has, as part of their professional role, the responsibility of providing constructive, supportive, and professionally presented feedback to peers and others within the system.

By definition, MSF includes perspectives of others in addition to that of the assessee's direct supervisor. This diversity may include the full range of medical trainees and practitioners, other health care professionals, other staff working in the same setting, and patients and family members. A complaint with commonly used assessment relying on the supervisor alone is that it is subject to accusations of limited information at best and bias at worst when the recipient disagrees with unfavorable feedback. MSF can circumvent complaints that feedback is biased by a problematic relationship with a single individual. MSF expands necessarily and significantly the numbers of raters, the number of samples, and the occasions across which samples are taken. Additionally accusations of bias and other complaints based on "a bad day," a faulty administration, or a "misinterpretation" of a single event or performance might be averted.

As with any assessment of individual performance, MSF data can be aggregated across individuals to provide information about groups of people. Depending on the content of the MSF, this might provide useful information for policy or curricular revision that is different from that obtained by other formats. For example, individual surveys that focus on professionalism might in the aggregate highlight aspects of the culture with which groups were dissatisfied, or specific topics for which there is a range of opinion worthy of investigation. Much work has been done in the study of organizational culture; surveys of worker performance might in the aggregate provide information about unit performance, workplace satisfaction, or other indicators of how the local environment is doing as a whole. Even though supplemental surveys might get at this information more directly, the aggregated individual data might add quite a bit.

Survey instruments administered within MSF processes have advantages in that they might be modified easily, administered through multiple different media, and provide feedback relatively quickly as compared to other forms of assessment. Modification can occur relatively flexibly, particularly when MSF instruments are used for lower stakes applications. In those instances, items can be inserted or whole surveys can be modified quickly and easily. Surveys can be administered by paper, phone, fax, or computer—whatever is of greatest ease to the person completing it. Of course, use of different media will affect survey design and speed of data processing. But for patients, for example, the ability to respond by paper or phone may increase response rates and circumvent limitations of literacy, time pressure for response, or computer technology access. Finally, surveys lend themselves to rapid turn-around time from survey completion to delivery of feedback to the assessee. If feedback is strictly formative and the data does not need to be processed, then feedback can be instantaneous. If data analyses or other steps are needed for quality control, surveys may have the same turnaround time as other formats.

Weaknesses

MSF has inherent weaknesses. A number of features distinguish MSF from other forms of assessment. In contrast to typical standardized assessment, MSF stimuli are daily, real events during which observations take place. They are random and different for every observer. The lack of standardization can create challenges in data interpretation and reliability analyses. Also, in contrast to more standardized formats, MSF may be extremely sensitive in that slight variations in implementation can make big differences in the quality of the information collected. For example, lack of trust that the information will be used only for low-stakes formative feedback may lead to observer over-rating or under-commenting. In contrast to knowledge and skills assessments, feedback that focuses on behaviors and values can be extremely delicate, and miscommunicated feedback may have both immediate and long-term implications. Physicians typically work together for the years of their residency program and in practice. Learning that their medical colleagues or that nurses and pharmacists feel performance is suboptimal may come as a surprise and may cause unintended reactions for a considerable time after the feedback has been transmitted. Inattention to the setting, the respondents, and the manner in which feedback is delivered can seriously reduce the utility of MSF.

MSF may not work in some settings. First, it requires an organizational culture that is trusting and that views active participation in feedback as a professional expectation and not an unnecessary administrative burden. But legitimate concerns might impede widespread acceptance. Some of these concerns include the assurance of confidentiality of observers; legal implications for use of inaccurate, harmful or misused information;

and professional embarrassment.[36] Also, successful MSF implementation typically requires buy-in from key decision makers and leaders to ensure widespread acceptance and participation and to ensure that use of the information is consistent with organizational goals and related interventions.[37] Introduction of survey instruments alone in the absence of robust MSF processes or MSF processes without broader buy-in is extremely difficult.

There may be certain work settings, however, wherein even widespread buy-in and good intent are insufficient. For example, MSF relies on input from multiple observers. In small rural practices, or in settings where an individual works in isolation or with very few people, the number of observers may be too small to yield reliable data, or the risks to the social network may be too great if confidentiality of responses is breached. In small residency programs, implementation may be difficult if there is no mechanism to influence the participation of other observers (e.g., medical students, nurses).

Once agreement is reached about the individuals who will complete the instrument, there are still threats to the quality of data gathering. It seems intuitive that observer training for familiarity with the observational task, the instrument, and item meaning would be central to the success of an MSF approach. However, there are few studies within medical education on the effects of training physician raters,[38,39] although studies outside medicine point toward beneficial effects.[40] Obtaining large numbers of independent observations is one way to address the concern about reproducibility of responses. Those who can be trained about MSF, the items, and the rating scales should be. As Norcini[41] notes, for peers assessment criteria must be developed and communicated and participants should receive training.

Feedback should be distinguished from assessment, and thought should be paid to which is intended. Basic guidelines for providing feedback are available.[42,43] MSF can differ from other types of feedback in fundamental ways. When the feedback about knowledge is negative, there is an inherent belief that it is remediable through study, tutoring, or other means, and therefore only a temporary and fixable deficit. With MSF, behavioral or values feedback can be seen as reflecting flawed character traits both by the person communicating the information and by the person receiving it. As a result, lack of preparedness of the feedback provider or recipient can cause miscommunication or worse. As well, the information in MSF reports can in fact have messages that may be extremely difficult to hear (e.g., your peers have strongly disagreed that "this physician accepts an appropriate share of work"). If free text input (i.e., comments) is allowed by the instrument, thought should be given to how it is to be presented and the circumstances under which it might be edited.

Depending on the purpose of MSF, the appropriate person to provide the feedback may vary. For example, impartial counselors may be preferable to direct supervisors. Nonetheless, the person providing the feedback should be trained in this regard, including understanding the expectations of the recipient. Indeed, perceptions of the process and feedback can influence whether feedback is used at all for improvement.[30]

Conclusion

MSF provides a unique tool to examine aspects of physician competence. Bracken and associates caution, however, that MSF processes are challenging. MSF operates in uncontrolled environments with "a large number of feedback providers (of questionable skill and motivation) using instruments of marginal quality and spurious linkages to existing initiatives, under conditions of large-scale data collection that require 100 percent accuracy. MSF is a complex combination of all these elements operating in a real-time environment in uncontrolled settings"(p xxvi).[22]

Good MSF processes require the support and commitment of the organization's leaders; good communication plans to ensure that participants understand goals, purpose, and data use; and a steering group to lead and manage the program. These instruments can produce measures that are reliable, generalized, and valid.[11–16,25–28] Studies show that physicians will use the data to make changes but that there will be variability in how; they won't embrace it equally.[16,29–31]

In developing MSF systems, it is important to recognize that MSF is not a single tool but a set of processes; each questionnaire that is developed needs to be psychometrically assessed for robustness. Further, reliability and validity are influenced by many dynamic variables. As instruments are used over time, it is important to continue to monitor their utility, along with the reliability and validity of measures. There is certainly room for future work. Where data exist from other sources, it will be important to assess criterion validity. Evans[17] reminds us that insufficient construct validity work has been undertaken. There may be a stronger role for using MSF approaches to assess domains where observable behaviors are the most convenient and important primary manifestation (e.g., communication skills, professionalism, and collaboration). Aspects of clinical competence reflecting physician knowledge and skills may be more accurately obtained through other methods (e.g., performance databases, chart reviews, and traditional examinations).

ANNOTATED BIBLIOGRAPHY

1. Archer JC, Norcini J, Davies HA: Use of SPRAT for peer review of paediatricians in training. BMJ 2005;330:1251–1253.
   This study assessed the feasibility and reliability of a MSF instrument to inform the record of in-training assessment for pediatric senior house officers and specialist registrars.
2. Bracken DW, Timmreck CW, Church, AH (eds): The Handbook of Multisource Feedback: The Comprehensive Resource for

Designing and Implementing MSF Processes. San Francisco, Jossey-Bass, 2001.

This extensive textbook provides a broad base of information about MSF as adopted in industrial settings. North American authors provide information about the history and development of MSF, considerations for adoption of MSF (organizational readiness, instrument selection, organizational needs, and working with vendors), instrument design, rater selection, reliability and validity, reports, and measuring impact.

3. Evans R, Elwyn G, Edwards A: Review of instruments for peer assessment of physicians. BMJ 2004;328:1240–1245.

Evans and associates conducted a systematic review of the literature to identify existing instruments for rating peers (professional colleagues) in medical practice and to evaluate these instruments in terms of how they were developed, their validity and reliability, and their appropriateness for use in clinical settings.

4. Fidler H, Lockyer JM, Toews J, Violato C: Changing physicians' practices: The effect of individual feedback. Acad Med 1999;74:702–714.

This study assessed the responses of 255 physicians who received MSF data from peer physicians, referring/referral physicians, co-workers (e.g., nurses), and patients about 55 aspects of their medical practices.

5. Hesketh EA, Anderson F, Bagnall GM, et al: Using a 360° diagnostic screening tool to provide an evidence trail of junior doctor performance throughout their first postgraduate year. Med Teach 2005;27(3):219–233.

This study describes the development and assessment of an MSF tool based on four of the domains of the United Kingdom General Medical Council's Good Medical Practice for physicians in the first postgraduate year (i.e., pre-registration house officer).

6. Lipner RS, Blank LL, Leas BF, Fortna GS: The value of patient and peer ratings in recertification. Acad Med 2002;77(10 Suppl): S64–66.

This study describes an assessment of the American Board of Internal Medicine's patient and peer assessment module used by practicing physicians as part of its recertification program. The assessment focused on instrument reliability, the relationship of ratings to demographic and other variables, and the perceived value of the assessment by diplomats.

7. Ramsey PG, Wenrich MD, Carline JD, et al: Use of peer ratings to evaluate physician performance. JAMA 1993;269:1655–1660.

This study describes a seminal American Board of Internal Medicine study in which physicians and nurses assessed physicians using an 11-item questionnaire.

8. Sargeant J, Mann K, Ferrier S: Exploring family physicians' reactions to multisource feedback: Perceptions of credibility and usefulness. Med Educ 2005;39(5):497–504.

This qualitative study was undertaken to explore physicians' reactions to MSF, perceptions influencing these reactions, and the acceptance and use of feedback.

9. Smither JW, London M, Reilly RR: Does performance improve following multisource feedback? A theoretical model, meta-analysis and review of empirical findings. Personnel Psychol 2005;58:33–66.

This article provides a review of important industrial (organizational) literature related to MSF along with a meta-analysis of 24 longitudinal studies showing that improvement from direct report, peer, and supervisor ratings over time is small. Their theoretical model suggests that improvement is most likely to occur when feedback indicates change is necessary, recipients have a positive feedback orientation, perceive a need to change their behavior, react positively to the feedback, believe change is feasible, set appropriate goals, and take actions that lead to skill and performance improvement.

10. Violato C, Lockyer JM, Fidler H: Assessment of pediatricians by a regulatory authority. Pediatrics 2006;117(3):796–802.

This article describes the development and assessment of a set of MSF instruments developed for patients, medical colleagues, nonmedical co-workers (e.g., nurses, pharmacists), and self to assess pediatricians.

11. Woolliscroft JO, Howell JD, Patel BP, Swanson DB: Resident-patient interactions: The humanistic qualities of internal medicine residents assessed by patients, attending physicians, program supervisors and nurses. Acad Med 1994;69(3):216–224.

In this study, the humanistic qualities of 70 first-year internal medicine residents were assessed by patients, attending physicians, program supervisors, and nurses.

REFERENCES

1. College of Physicians and Surgeons of Alberta, Physician Achievement Review Program. Accessed at http://www.par-program. org, Oct. 15, 2007.
2. Cox EP: The optimal number of response alternatives on a scale. J Marketing Res 1980;17:407–422.
3. Archer J, Norcini J, Davies HA: Peer review of paediatricians in training using SPRAT. BMJ 2005;330:1251–1253.
4. Davies HA, Archer JC: Multisource feedback using Sheffield Peer Review Assessment Tool (SPRAT): Development and practical aspects. Clin Teach 2005;2(2):77–81.
5. Hesketh EA, Anderson F, Bagnall GM, et al: Using a 360 degree diagnostic screening tool to provide an evidence trail of junior doctor performance throughout their first postgraduate year. Med Teach 2005;27(3):219–233.
6. Archer J, Norcini J, Southgate L, et al: Mini-PAT (peer assessment tool): A valid component of a national assessment programme in the UK? Adv Health Sci Educ 2006. Accessed at http://www.springer-link.com/content/v8hth3h06507ph56/fulltext.pdf, Oct. 15, 2007 (subscription required).
7. Bryan RE, Krych AJ, Carmichael SW, et al: Assessing professionalism in early medical education: Experience with peer evaluation and self-evaluation in the gross anatomy course. Ann Acad Med Singapore 2005;4(8):486–491.
8. Shue CK, Arnold L, Stern DT: Maximizing participation in peer assessment of professionalism: The students speak. Acad Med 2005;80(10 Suppl):S1–S5.
9. Sullivan ME, Hitchcock MA, Dunnington GL: Peer and self assessment during problem-based tutorials. Am J Surg 1999;177(3):266–269.
10. Woolliscroft JO, Howell JD, Patel BP, Swanson DB: Resident-patient interactions: The humanistic qualities of internal medicine residents assessed by patients, attending physicians, program supervisors and nurses. Acad Med 1994;69(3):216–224.
11. Violato C, Marini A, Toews J, et al: Using peers, consulting physicians, patients, co-workers and self to assess physicians. Acad Med 1994;72(Suppl 10):57–63.
12. Hall W, Violato C, Lewkonia R, et al: Assessment of physician performance in Alberta: The Physician Achievement Review Project. CMAJ 1999;161(1):52–57.
13. Violato C, Lockyer JM, Fidler H: Multisource feedback: A method of assessing surgical practice. BMJ 2003;326:546–548.
14. Violato C, Lockyer J, Fidler H: The assessment of pediatricians by a regulatory authority. Pediatrics 2006;117:796–802.
15. Lockyer JM, Violato C, Fidler H: A multisource feedback program for anesthesiologists (Un programme de rétroaction multisources pour les anesthésiologists). Can J Anesth 2006;53:33–39.
16. Lipner RS, Blank LL, Leas BF, Fortna GS: The value of patient and peer ratings in recertification. Acad Med 2002;77(10 Suppl): 64–66.
17. Evans R, Elwyn G, Edwards A: Review of instruments for peer assessment of physicians. BMJ 2004;328:1240–1245.
18. Accreditation Council for Graduate Medical Education Competencies. Accessed at http://www.acgme.org/outcome/comp/compFull.asp, Oct. 15, 2007.
19. Royal College of Physicians and Surgeons of Canada CanMEDS Competencies. Accessed at http://rcpsc.medical.org/canmeds/index.php, Oct. 15, 2007.
20. General Medical Council (UK): Good Medical Practice. Accessed at http://www.gmc-uk.org/guidance/good_medical_practice/index.asp, Oct. 15, 2007.
21. British Psychological Society: Search: 360 degree feedback. Accessed at http://www.psychtesting.org.uk/, Oct. 15, 2007.
22. Bracken DW, Timmreck CW, Church AH (eds): The Handbook of Multisource Feedback: The Comprehensive Resource for Designing and Implementing MSF Processes. San Francisco, Jossey-Bass, 2001.
23. Tornow WW, London M: CCL Associates: Maximizing the Value of 360-Degree Feedback: A Process for Successful Individual and Organizational Development. San Francisco, Jossey-Bass, 1998.
24. Streiner DL, Norman GR: Health Measurement Scales: A Practical Guide to Their Development and Use. Oxford, Oxford University Press, 2000.

25. Wenrich MD, Carline ID, Giles LM, Ramsey PG: Ratings of the performances of practicing internists by hospital-based registered nurses. Acad Med 1993;68:680–687.
26. Ramsey PG, Carline JD, Inui TS, et al: Use of peer ratings to evaluate physician performance. JAMA 1993;269:1655–1660.
27. Johnson D, Cujec B: Comparison of self, nurse and physician assessment of residents rotating through an intensive care unit. Crit Care Med 1998;26:1811–1816.
28. Sargeant JM, Mann KV, Ferrier SN, et al: Responses of rural family physicians and their colleagues and coworker raters to a multi-source feedback process: A pilot study. Acad Med 2003; 78(Suppl 10):42–44.
29. Fidler H, Lockyer J, Toews J, Violato C: Changing physicians' practices: The effect of individual feedback. Acad Med 1999; 74:702–714.
30. Sargeant J: Multi-source feedback for physicians learning and change. Doctoral dissertation. The Netherlands, Maastricht University, 2006.
31. Smither JW, London M, Reilly RR: Does performance improve following multisource feedback? A theoretical model, meta-analysis and review of empirical findings. Personnel Psychol 2005;58:33–66.
32. Atwater LE, Roush P, Fischtal A: The influence of upward feedback on self and follower rating of leadership. Personnel Psychol 1995;48:35–59.
33. Atwater LE, Yammarino FJ: Does self-other agreement on leadership perceptions moderate the validity of leadership and performance predictions. Personnel Psychol 1995;45: 141–164.
34. Atwater LE, Ostroff C, Yammarino FJ, Fleenor JW: Self-other agreement: Does it really matter? Personnel Psychol 1998; 51:577–598.
35. Van Velsor E, Taylor S, Leslie J: An examination of the relationship among self-perception accuracy, self-awareness, gender, and leader effectiveness. Hum Res Manage 1993;32:249–264.
36. Bowie P, McKay J, Dalgetty E, Lough M: A qualitative study of why general practitioners may participate in significant event analysis and educational peer assessment. Qual Saf Health Care 2005;14:185–189.
37. Church AH: Do higher performing managers actually receive better ratings? A validation of multirater assessment methodology. Consulting Psych J Pract Res 2000;52(2):99–116.
38. Newble DI, Hoare J, Sheldrake PF: The selection and training of examiners for clinical examinations. Med Educ 1980;14: 345–349.
39. Noel GL, Herbers JE Jr, Caplow MP, et al: How well do internal medicine faculty members evaluate the clinical skills of residents? Ann Intern Med 1992;117:757–765.
40. Woehr DJ, Huffcutt AI: Rater training for performance-appraisal: a quantitative review. J Occup Organ Psychol 1994;67:189–205.
41. Norcini JJ: Peer assessment of competence: Med Educ 2003;37(6):539–543.
42. Ende J: Feedback in clinical medical education. JAMA 1983;250(6):777–781.
43. Katz PO: Providing feedback. Gastrointest Endosc Clin North Am 1995;5(2):347–355.

USEFUL WEB SITES

College of Physicians and Surgeons of Alberta
 http://www.par-program.org
 This website provides copies of the questionnaires being used in Alberta for family physicians, surgeons, anesthesiologists, medical/pediatric/psychiatry specialists, episodic caregivers (e.g., emergency room physicians, locum physicians, hospitalists), and radiologists along with background information about the program and the feedback report.

Foundations Program (United Kingdom)
 http://www.foundationprogramme.nhs.uk
 Copies of the questionnaires used are contained within the pdf for the Physician Learning Portfolio document.

British Psychological Society. Gray A, Lewis A, Fletcher C, et al: 360 degree feedback: Best practice guidelines, 6/6/2003.
 http://www.psychtesting.org.uk/.
 At this Web site, search for ''360 degree feedback'' to retrieve the pdf. This pdf provides an excellent overview to developing and understanding multisource feedback.

Portfolios

Eric S. Holmboe, MD, Margery H. Davis, MD,
and Carol Carraccio, MD

Portfolios are receiving increasing attention as a more robust method to assess performance and professional development in this era of increasing focus on clinical competence. A key reason for this alignment is that many of the principles underlying portfolio assessment also form the foundation of competency-based education (Fig. 7-1).

Portfolios have been used for many years at all stages of education.[1-6] Portfolio uses include a range of assessment activities, from a single student clerkship experience to encompassing the entire clinical years of training.[7-9] There are many definitions of portfolios ranging from a compilation of "best" work to a purposeful collection of materials to demonstrate competence. Box 7-1 provides four portfolio definitions used for medical education from the student to the practicing physician level.

A synthesis of the preceding definitions, along with others, suggests portfolios are typically collections of work, evaluations, products, and similar material of the learner collected over time that reflects professional development, annotated by the trainee's reflection on what has been learned in terms of learning outcomes.[1,2,9-12] Such reflection is the critical difference between a portfolio and a log book. The purpose of the assessment determines the content and creation of the portfolio, and how the "evidence" in the portfolio will be interpreted and judged.[1] Regardless of the ultimate purpose, the trainee must have

an active role and responsibility in creating and managing the portfolio. In some instances, the content of the portfolio may be mostly or wholly determined by the trainee. However, if one of the major goals of a portfolio assessment in medical training is reliable and valid determination of competence and performance, the portfolio in medical training will need to be a collaborative effort between the educators and the trainee. Before discussing important considerations in determining how to use a portfolio, let's first examine some of the important strengths of portfolio assessment.

Strengths of the Portfolio Process

Portfolios contain a number of potential advantages as part of a robust evaluation system. Many of these are nicely described in a systematic review by Friedman and colleagues[1]; they are displayed in Box 7-2. Several points should be highlighted. First, by definition portfolios require the active engagement of trainees in their own education through reflection. This is an essential lifelong learning skill. It is important to remember that the majority of a physician's career will be spent in "independent" practice and not a structured educational environment. Given the evidence that a physician's performance may decline over time, the

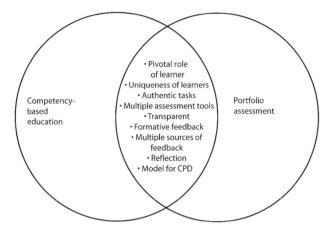

Figure 7-1 Relationship of competency-based education and portfolios. CPD, continuous professional development.

BOX 7-1   Summary of Recent Portfolio Definitions

Reckase MD: Portfolio assessment: A theoretical estimate of score reliability. Educ Measure 1995;14:12–31.

This purposeful collection of student work exhibits to the student (and others) the student's efforts, progress, or achievement in (a) given area(s). The collection must include student participation in selection of portfolio content; the criteria for selection; the criteria for judging merit; and evidence of student reflection.

Martin-Kneip GO: Becoming a Better Teacher: Eight Innovations That Work. Alexandria, VA, Association for Supervision and Curriculum Development, 2000.

This collection of student work exhibits the student's efforts, progress, and achievements in one or more areas. This collection represents a personal investment on the part of the student that is evident through the student's participation in the selection of the contents, the criteria for selection, the criteria for judging the merit of the collection, and the student's self-reflection.

Davis MH, Friedman BDM, Harden RM, et al: Portfolio assessment in medical students' final examinations. Med Teach 2001;23:357–366.

This portfolio is a collection of papers and other forms of evidence that learning has taken place, annotated by the student's reflections on what has been learned in terms of the learning outcomes.

Wilkinson TJ, Challis M, Hobma SO, et al: The use of portfolios for assessment of the competence and performance of doctors in practice. Med Educ 2002;36(10):918–924.

This dossier of evidence collected over time demonstrates a physician's education and practice achievements.

portfolio experience in training may better prepare them for lifelong professional development and maintenance of competence.[13] Portfolios provide the framework for such activity, and some continuing education programs have embraced this concept.[14–16] In training programs, the responsibility for the contents of the portfolio is shared between the program director and the trainees as the latter engage in active learning and self-assessment. This shared responsibility for portfolios is well aligned with the construct of competency-based education, whereby the teacher acts as a guide and facilitator for the self-directed learner.

Second, portfolios are more "authentic," meaning that the contents of the portfolio reflect a comprehensive collection of evidence of what trainees actually do, not just what they could do. This authenticity enhances the face and predictive validity of the portfolio, that is, the link between current trainee performance and what they will be capable of doing later in real world practice. Archibald and Newmann defined authenticity as "the extent to which the outcomes measured represent appropriate, meaningful, significant and worthwhile forms of human accomplishments."[17] Third, and unlike other evaluation methods, portfolios are longitudinal collections of evidence over time and thus capable of demonstrating professional development and progression.

Friedman and colleagues also provided a nice framework to describe the key assessment features of a portfolio that contribute to meaningful evaluation[1]:

1. There are both formative and summative components.
2. Portfolios combine both qualitative and quantitative judgment. The qualitative component is one of the unique aspects of the portfolio, and when it has been integrated with the quantitative component, the combination allows for a more comprehensive assessment of trainees.
3. Portfolios are personalized. The challenge is to balance this personalized assessment with the need for more standardization required for evaluation, especially since the personalized components of the portfolio will be more difficult to evaluate using psychometric methods.
4. Structured portfolios lend a defensible degree of standardization. By using a structured portfolio approach, some components of the portfolio can be standardized for all trainees. By standardizing the evaluation methods, educators can better define the tasks and criteria for evaluation for both teaching faculty and the trainees, and set predetermined pass-fail policies. The outcomes provide the framework for standardization.

Purpose of the Portfolio

In medical education, the portfolio approach can be used for formative and summative assessment. Each program will need to determine what the main purpose(s) of the portfolio will be in their educational program. Educators can use a portfolio in the traditional, formative approach by having the trainees collect examples of their "best" work with narrative reflections about each contribution. Trainees could be given majority control of the contents, with varying degrees of guidance on the types of material entered into the portfolio. Such material might include a particularly excellent write-up of a patient when they made a difficult diagnosis, a videotape encounter with

---

BOX 7-2   Summary of Ten Portfolio Advantages

1. Critical learning skills such as self-assessment, reflection, self-directed learning, and professionalism can be evaluated.
2. Evidence can be collected longitudinally over time.
3. Educators can assess trainee progress toward acquiring the desired learning outcomes and goals.
4. Portfolios can be used for both formative and summative assessment.
5. Portfolios provide a method for trainees to receive continuous feedback *and* to document their feelings and reactions to that feedback for continuous professional development.
6. Trainees have the important opportunity to contribute evidence of their choosing to the overall assessment process.
7. Portfolios can facilitate better communication between educators and trainees.
8. Portfolios help to encourage trainees to learn and remind them that assessment is an interactive two-way process between them and their educators.
9. Portfolios can potentially stimulate reflective skills, which are critical to all physicians' lifelong learning and assessment.
10. Portfolios facilitate a more integrative approach to both individual assessment and actual medical practice.

Adapted from Friedman BDM, Davis MH, Harden RM, et al: AAME Educational Guide 24: Portfolios as a method of student assessment. Med Teach 2001;23:1–23.

---

a standardized patient, a research presentation, journal club write-up, etc. One valuable attribute of the purely formative, learner-driven portfolio is to help faculty gain insight into what the trainee believes he did well (thus potentially providing some window into insight ability), and a measure of the trainee's reflective capabilities. From our perspective, the formative approach is quite reasonable if the primary goal of the portfolio is the development of self-assessment and reflection skills. The difficulty with formative portfolios is that many trainees may not be willing to undertake the amount of work involved in building a portfolio unless it "counts" (i.e., is summative).

If the primary goal of the portfolio is to determine if competence has been achieved (e.g., summative plus formative assessment), faculty will need to address a host of additional important considerations. The most important consideration will be determination of pass/fail criteria for the trainee's portfolio. Traditionally, educators have examined the quality of an evaluation method or tool based on psychometric criteria. However, applying traditional psychometric principles to evaluate a composite, holistic method like portfolios presents some unique challenges. Let's examine some of those challenges.

Challenges in the Evaluation of Portfolios

Several important issues are considered when designing a method to evaluate the quality of a trainee portfolio.

Traditionally, we have applied the psychometric principles of reliability and validity when judging the quality of an evaluation tool. However, using only psychometric methods to portfolio evaluation may be limiting. Recall some of the major strengths of the portfolio process: the collection of *descriptive* evaluation materials, *written* trainee self-assessment and reflection, and the *holistic, composite* nature of a portfolio. Despite these challenges, there is still value to evaluating portfolios using a psychometric framework, and recent work suggests it is also valuable to apply principles from qualitative research methodology to evaluate a portfolio. It is important to remember that each evaluation method (e.g., OSCEs, medical record audits) can be assessed separately as discussed throughout this book. Regardless, methods to evaluate the sum, or "whole," of portfolios continue to evolve, and we expect that more robust, combined psychometric (quantitative) and descriptive (qualitative) approaches will appear soon.

Psychometric Approach to Portfolio Evaluation

The reliability and validity of a portfolio are dependent on two main components. The first component is the psychometric characteristics of the evaluation methods used in the portfolio process. The evaluative component of the portfolio can only be as good as the evaluation methods contained in the portfolio. Second, the process to judge the portfolio needs to possess minimal psychometric characteristics. This process, which by definition includes rating activities by another human, must be able to reliably determine if the portfolio as a whole demonstrates the trainee has achieved the educational end points, especially for summative assessments. This should include a process to judge the reflective activities of the trainee, especially important for gauging the impact of the formative assessment aspect of the portfolio process. One of the strengths of the portfolio process is the ability to use the portfolio contents for *both* formative and summative assessment.

With this background, what are the psychometric issues when programs choose to use the portfolio as the measure of achievement of competency?

Portfolio Content

Many educators do not consider "quantitative" assessments, such as objective structured clinical examinations (OSCEs), results of a medical record audit, and in-training examinations, to be part of the portfolio. However, these evaluation methods are often used for formative purposes and provide a rich opportunity for feedback and subsequent reflection by the trainee. The trainee can also potentially use some of these tools (e.g., a self-audit of medical records) as part of the self-assessment content for the portfolio.[18] Therefore, using evaluation tools that possess solid psychometric properties can enhance the overall reliability and validity of the portfolio. The descriptive content of the portfolio, such as the trainee reflections and narratives, should still be guided by some basic criteria and structure. For example, a program may ask the trainee to answer a series of questions about a particular experience.[18] This descriptive information should also undergo some level of systematic analysis. For example, the summary of a verbal evaluation session with multiple members of the team about students on a medicine clerkship provided valuable information about the students' professionalism.[19] The reflective statements entered by the trainee can be evaluated, but programs will need to develop criteria about how to rate the content and quality of these types of entries.

Standardization

Standardization of portfolio contents can help to improve the reliability of the portfolio assessment process. However, this standardization must be balanced with the trainee's opportunities to determine what they wish to enter into the portfolio as part of their own professional development. Box 7-3 provides some guidance on standardization.

If a program incorporates an oral defense of the portfolio by the trainee, the program needs to carefully consider how it will address several potential factors. These factors include subjectivity of the evaluators, lack of standardized criteria for conducting the oral defense, differences among examiners in their interpretation of trainee responses to questions or portfolio contents, and unequal expectations between evaluators.[20] The suggestions provided in Box 7-3 can help to mitigate these factors. A more realistic expectation may be for the learner to "present" rather than defend the portfolio. Expectations for the presentation, such as up-to-date completion of all work products and review of all evaluations, should be transparent to the learner. The oral defense of the portfolio should enable the examiner to confirm or refute a prejudgment of the student's body of work (the portfolio) in terms of a summative assessment or grade for each outcome, based on the number of assessed documents and materials in the portfolio.

Decision and Evaluator Consistency

Portfolios require judgment by faculty. Thus, faculty raters become a source of error that threatens the "generalizability" of trainee performance. Specific faculty rating issues include the stability of their ratings over time, stability of ratings between different faculty raters, and the reproducibility of pass/fail decisions.[1] One of the biggest concerns about using portfolios for summative purposes in medical education is the lack of several studies demonstrating reasonable reliability, including intra- and inter-rater agreement.[21–24]

BOX 7-3   Suggestions to Improve Evaluation of Portfolios

1. Some assessments or units of the portfolio are assigned to all trainees.
2. The portfolio should contain a minimum amount of standard assessment methods and activities with known reliability and validity characteristics (e.g., objective structured clinical examination or mini-CEX).
3. The criteria and processes for assessment are clearly defined and transparent to the trainees.
4. All portfolios should have clear guidelines and instructions for the trainees and faculty.
5. Evaluation of the portfolio, especially the qualitative components, must follow standard and agreed-upon guidelines by the reviewers. This crucially requires training of the evaluators, including use of techniques such as performance dimension and frame of reference training (see Chapter 8, Direct Observation).
6. The oral defense of the portfolio (if utilized by the program) must also follow a standard protocol with preparation prior to the defense.
7. Summative decisions follow a predetermined and agreed-upon policy and protocol, including policy for how disagreements between evaluators will be handled.

From Friedman BDM, Davis MH, Harden RM, et al: AAME Educational Guide 24: Portfolios as a method of student assessment. Med Teach 2001;23:1–23.

As with any evaluation method, reliability can always be improved by using multiple raters. However, this can be very resource-intensive and time-consuming. Standardization of criteria is an important first step. Koretz argued that high levels of agreement depend on clear criteria, adequately communicating those criteria to the students, robust student orientation materials, a shared faculty understanding of the assessment purpose, and adequate examiner training.[6] A common error in all evaluation is failure to adequately train the faculty who provide the ratings and judgment. Faculty training in portfolio assessment is essential.

It is noteworthy that for several of the early studies showing poor reliability in medical education portfolios little information was provided about faculty training.[21–23] One of the few studies of portfolios to demonstrate good reliability and some evidence for validity involved a full day of rater training at the beginning of the project, followed by retraining with the scoring rubrics prior to actual portfolio review.[25,26] O'Sullivan and colleagues, using this faculty training approach for a portfolio in a psychiatry residency, found that sufficient reliability for relative decisions could be achieved with only two raters, and a generalizability coefficient of 0.7 could be achieved with only one additional rater.[25]

The University of Dundee medical student portfolio contains a broad sampling of the student's work and achievements, including multiple patient and care presentations, log of procedures, special study modules, clinical rotation evaluations, learning contracts, and structured reflection reports. Dundee's evaluation system provides a substantial amount of structure to the portfolio process with clear criteria and expectations for the students.[9] The University of Dundee has experienced results similar to O'Sullivan's; 98% agreement of pass/fail decisions was achieved using two-rater pairs. The Dundee program, like the O'Sullivan program, incorporated substantial rater training.[9]

Validity of Portfolios

Little is known about the validity of the portfolio process. Certainly, the portfolio has a high degree of face validity. O'Sullivan and colleagues performed a validity analysis of their psychiatry portfolio.[25] They found a modest correlation between in-training examination scores and some evidence of increasing portfolio scores with each increasing year of training. One of the main goals of the portfolio process, and one of its greatest strengths, is the promotion of self-directed learning and reflection. O'Sullivan interviewed the residents about their experience and learned that many, but not all, of the residents found the process to be useful personally. Other residents viewed the portfolio as simply a research project. Research is urgently needed to determine whether portfolios can be a robust catalyst for self-directed, lifelong learning.[25]

Qualitative Assessment of Portfolios: The Next Frontier

Given the challenges in using psychometric methods for evaluating portfolios, are there potentially other approaches? We have emphasized throughout this chapter the need to collect both quantitative and qualitative data for the portfolio. Some limited success applying psychometric scales to the qualitative, descriptive aspects of the portfolio has been reported. However, some researchers are beginning to explore new approaches to analyzing portfolios. Recently, Driessen and colleagues developed a new assessment procedure to judge first-year medical student portfolios using qualitative research criteria.[27] They used the qualitative methodological criteria of credibility (e.g., internal validity) and dependability (e.g., reliability). Box 7-4 describes the qualitative methodological strategies they used to ensure credibility and dependability in judging a portfolio.

The Driessen protocol can be viewed in Figure 7-2. Using this protocol, 96% of the portfolios were graded without review by the full committee. This early study suggests that complementary, qualitative approaches are possible for assessment of portfolios, and clearly others will need to replicate Driessen's findings with more advanced trainees. This approach potentially allows educators to "sample through" bias and inter-rater variation by continuing to sample until a stable judgment can be attained. The importance of sampling cannot be overstated. Much of assessment also depends on the context in which the assessment occurs. The greater the sampling, the more likely the program will gather a more robust picture of trainee

---

BOX 7-4 Qualitative Methodological Strategies

Credibility
1. Triangulation: The use of information from different sources about the same construct
2. Prolonged engagement: Sufficient interaction, over time, from the faculty mentor or others
3. Member checking: "Test" the data with the member (e.g., trainee) of the group

Dependability
4. Audit trail: Documentation of the assessment process (over time) to enable external review
5. Dependability audit: Quality assessment procedures performed by an external auditor

---

competency over multiple domains *and* contexts. This is one of the major potential advantages of portfolio assessment.

Self-Assessment and Portfolios

We have emphasized throughout this chapter that a portfolio isn't a portfolio unless it contains substantial evidence of self-assessment and reflection on the part of the trainee. This core requirement begs two critical questions: (1) How good are trainee skills in self-assessment and reflection? (2) Does a portfolio effectively facilitate trainee self-assessment and reflection? The answer to the first question at the present time is troubling. In a recent systematic review of admittedly a modest number of studies of only limited quality, Davis and colleagues found a poor relationship between physician self-ratings of performance and the ratings provided by external raters.[28] Even more worrisome was the finding that inaccuracy in self-rating appears to be worse for the least competent physicians who tend to substantially overestimate their competence.[28-31]

Davis and his colleagues focused on the ability of physicians to perform "self-rating" or use "self-audit" to generate summary judgments of their performance in order to determine their own learning needs and find resources to meet them. When assessment results are judged against an acceptable or passing performance level, the process becomes an "evaluation." Therefore, most of the research into self-assessment has focused more on self-evaluation when a physician had to develop a judgment about his or her "grade" or level of performance.[28]

The work of Eva and Regehr helps to shift the focus of self-assessment away from accuracy by explaining it as a phenomenon that encompasses a number of complex cognitive components such as self-efficacy (focus on consequences), metacognitive theory (using peripheral cues to make inferences about one's own abilities), and social cognitive theory (using others' reactions to one's own behaviors).[31] Thus, they argue the process of self-assessment should be the end point rather than an accurate outcome. They also suggest that the focus in the

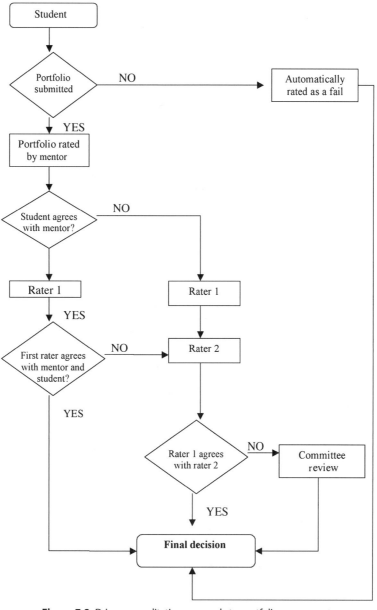

Figure 7-2 Driessen qualitative approach to portfolio assessment.

self-assessment literature is reflection-on-practice as a post-experience reflection, which has detracted from the true essence of self-assessment, which should involve more reflection-in-action or knowing when to ask for help in the act of doing.[31]

True self-assessment should also include guided self-audit. Self-audit refers to the activities trainees can personally perform to assess their level of competence. Self-audit is an active process of looking systematically at the product of one's work (as in chart reviews) or clinical judgments (as in answering multiple-choice questions) in contrast to a potentially more passive process of self-rating performance on a clinical examination or solution of a clinical problem (reflection-on-action). Therefore, portfolios should be an ideal method to foster more effective self-assessment by combining reflection

in-action and on-action.[32] Because portfolios can also be a collaborative process, portfolios could be a powerful tool for *guided* self-assessment and reflection.

Uncovering a gap in knowledge or in clinical performance motivates self-directed professionals to take action to close the gap. When the gap is discovered through self-assessment or self-audit, it seems to have more salience, as well as being more professionally rewarding, than one exposed by someone else. Our personal experience with residents and physicians completing a self-audit of medical records to determine personal performance on standard, validated quality of care measures in two separate studies supports the value of guided self-audit.[33,34] When physicians receive the results of their self-audit as structured feedback, they often experience a surprise or "a-ha" moment.

When trainees and physicians receive credible feedback about their true performance, they may experience what we call "knowledge-performance" discordance. This occurs in situations in which knowledge about the right thing to do is high, and the trainee believes he is doing it, but when the trainee receives feedback about actual performance he gains a more accurate assessment of reality. Additionally, the trainee appropriately experiences emotional discomfort with this discordance that, if handled supportively, provides the necessary energy to motivate change to align actual performance with desired performance. Thus a well-designed portfolio process incorporating this principle of guided self-audit and assessment can be a powerful tool for change.

Why might trainees not be good at recognizing their deficiencies? One reason is they often confuse confidence with competence.[35] Self-assessment of confidence in a particular performance is an area of considerable concern. Confidence is a quality of self-efficacy which tends to correlate in empiric studies with persistence in the face of obstacles and higher achievement.[36] Ratings of confidence can provide a baseline for guiding the structure of feedback provided to novice learners. However, the discordance between the overconfidence of the novice ("fools rush in where angels fear to tread") and the underconfidence of those achieving competence ("once burned, twice cautious") makes the unguided use of confidence measures particularly risky in medicine. The medical culture of "see one, do one, teach one" overemphasizes confidence to the detriment of acquiring true competence if it leads to the erroneous conclusion that actual performance data are not needed unless confidence is threatened.[36]

When it comes to self-evaluation, however, applying personally determined standards for acceptable performance is risky and undesirable. This is particularly so in light of the knowledge that the least competent physicians, as judged by reliable external standards, tend to overrate their abilities. We are just not very good at knowing what we don't know or estimating how well we do. Our experience and the observations of Davis, Eva, and others reinforce the notion that an accurate judgment of performance cannot be made without standard measures based on credible data.[31] Self-evaluation in the absence of credible data is unlikely to be of much value. Guided self-assessment should be incorporated at the earliest stages of medical training as an essential professional skill. Thus, the research around self-assessment lends support for the importance of some level of standardization, reflection with a mentor instead of in isolation, and clear evaluation criteria for portfolios. Tables 7-1 and 7-2 provide a summary of tools that can be used to assess reflective ability in undergraduate and postgraduate trainees. Faculty and mentors may want to consider using these tools with their trainees at the beginning of and during a learning cycle or throughout the portfolio process.

The Structured Portfolio

As you have probably noted by now, most portfolios currently in use by medical educators possess more structure than the traditional learning portfolio. There are important reasons for more structure. First, as described earlier, is the need for a defensible degree of standardization to ensure an acceptable level of reliability if the portfolio is used for more summative decisions. Second, medical educators are required to document whether a trainee has truly attained competence in specific knowledge, skills, and attitudes. One aspect often neglected in the portfolio literature is summative assessment for public accountability. Thus, a portfolio used for summative assessment must not only meet psychometric and qualitative research standards, it must be credible and defensible to the public.

Therefore, we propose using the term "structured portfolio" to denote the contents that are determined by both the training program and trainee to maximize outcomes-based evaluation. Although all portfolios possess some structure, portfolios in medical education must be able to provide sufficient evidence a trainee has attained the desired level of competence and performance. Therefore, medical educators will need to define many of the evaluation tools used in the portfolio, contingent upon local needs and resources.

To date, limited work has been done with residency-based portfolios, especially based on the new Accreditation Council for Graduate Medical Education (ACGME) competencies introduced in Chapter 1.

We present an example in Table 7-3 that lists the potential evaluation tools a residency or fellowship training program might use for a structured portfolio, based on the ACGME general competencies. In all domains, it is important to define the developmental benchmarks for trainees. As noted throughout this book, defining the benchmarks helps to improve the reliability, validity, accuracy, and utility of evaluation.

Table 7-3 demonstrates that a broadly defined portfolio does not function as a single evaluation "tool" but represents a framework and process for collecting, analyzing, and documenting the successful acquisition of competence and performance. Also note that in this framework, other evaluations are considered part of the portfolio, not just those self-assessment activities by the trainee. Reflecting on evaluations provided through other methods can be a valuable learning tool. Furthermore, incorporating actual evaluations into the portfolio, along with trainee reflection, places appropriately greater responsibility on faculty to improve the quality of those evaluations.

Characteristics of a Structured Portfolio

We believe there are six principal characteristics for a structured portfolio:

1. The process must utilize a multifaceted approach to evaluation. Research has shown repeatedly

Table 7-1 **Reflective Ability in Undergraduates**

	Professional Development of Reflective Ability[*]	**Script Concordance Test**[†]	**Reflective Portfolio**[‡]	**Reflection-evoking Case Vignettes**[§]	**Structured Worksheet**[‖]
Institution	University of Dundee	Laval University Medical School, Quebec	University of Nottingham	Free University, Amsterdam	University of London
Course	Professional and personal development	Clerkship in surgery	Communication skills	Clinical ethics	Clinical experience
Year	Years 4 and 5	Medical students	Year 2	Year 4	Dental therapy students
Assessment type	Summative	Formative	Summative	Summative	Formative?
Content	The 12 outcome summary sheets	38 clinical vignettes in four surgical topics: breast lump; gastro-intestinal bleeding; acute abdominal pain; and lump in the thyroid gland	800-word reflective commentary Practical evidence over 6 practicals 6 personal reflection forms 3 peer observation forms 3 teacher observation forms	Semi-structured questionnaire with 4 case vignettes. What are your feelings? What should be the appropriate professional behavior in the case concerned?	What happened? Describe your feelings. Why do you consider this worthy of reflection? What strengths in your clinical practice did this demonstrate? What learning did this reveal? Which one learning need do you address as a priority? Decide exactly what you would like to achieve. Complete "target testing."
Structure	Semistructured	Structured	Flexible	Semistructured	Structured
Assessment criteria	Standardized rubric: based on the ability to identify, evaluate and monitor personal progress		Standardized rubric	Standardized rubric Overall reflection: 10-point scale Perspectives series: 0–2 scale	Qualitative assessment Johns' questions Hatton and Smith's criteria
Psychometric evaluation	Supports construct validity	Acceptable predictive validity Moderate reliability	Supports construct validity and 0.8 inter-rater reliability	Supports construct validity and inter-rater reliability	Good inter-judge agreement especially for Hatton and Smith's criteria
Student attitude	Positive		Neutral	Not mentioned	Positive

[*]Ker JS, Friedman BDM, Pippard MJ, Davis MH: Determining the construct validity of a tool to assess the reflective ability of final year medical students using portfolio evidence. Members' abstracts, Association for the Study of Medical Education (ASME), Annual Scientific Meeting, 2003, pp 20–21.

[†]Brailovsky C, Charlin B, Beausoleil S, et al: Measurement of clinical reflective capacity early in training as a predictor of clinical reasoning performance at the end of residency: An experimental study on the script concordance test. Med Educ 2001;35:430–436.

[‡]Rees C, Sheard C: Undergraduate medical students' views about a reflective portfolio assessment of their communications skills learning. Med Educ 2004;38:125–128.

[§]Boenink AD, Oderwald AK, De Jonge P, et al: Assessing students reflection in medical practice: The development of an observer-rated instrument: Reliability, validity and initial experiences. Med Educ 2004;38:368–377.

[‖]Pee B, Woodman T, Fry H, Davenport ES: Appraising and assessing reflection in students' writing on a structured worksheet. Med Educ 2002;36:575–585.

This table was prepared courtesy of Dr. Gominda Ponnamperuma, University of Dundee, Dundee, Scotland.

Table 7-2 **Assessing Reflective Ability in Postgraduates**

	Reflective Personal Development Plans (PDP)[*]	Pediatric SpR Portfolio Assessment[†]
Institution	Postgraduate deaneries in the United Kingdom	Royal College of Paediatrics and Child Health (RCPCH)
Course year	General practice Continuing professional development	Pediatrics Year 1 to 5 in postgraduate training
Assessment type	Earlier formative, later summative	Summative
Content	Patient focused critical incidents, audits, critical reading, patient and peer feedback	Clinical letters and reports, presentation handouts, ethical submissions and parent information leaflets, feedback educational sessions, thank you letters, course attendance certificates, reports on MSc/MMedSci assignments, group achievements
Structure	Semistructured	Unstructured
Assessment criteria	Identification of learning needs, learning plan, assessment plan, understanding, performance	Global and domain specific rating on an unsatisfactory-fair-good-excellent rating scale. Domains: clinical, communication, ethics-attitudes, self-learning-teaching, evaluation-creation of evidence, management
Psychometric evaluation	Acceptable content and construct validity; reliability of 0.8 with 7 raters and 0.7 with 3–4 raters	Reliability of 0.8 with 4 raters

*Roberts C, Cromarty I, Crossley J, Jolly B: The reliability and validity of a matrix to assess the completed reflective personal development plans of general practitioners. Med Educ 2006;40:363–370.
†Melville C, Rees M, Brookfield D, Anderson J: Portfolio for assessment of paediatric specialist registrars. Med Educ 2004;38:1117–1125.
This table was prepared courtesy of Dr. Gominda Ponnamperuma, University of Dundee, Dundee, Scotland.

Table 7-3 **Examples of Portfolio Evaluation Tools by ACGME Domain of Competence for Residency Training**

Domain of Competence	Assessment Tools
Patient care	Rotation—specific evaluation forms (checklists, global rating scales) Direct observed history, physical examination, and communication Critical incidents Patient and procedure logs Case log of "best" workups and patient interactions as determined by the trainee
Medical knowledge	Shelf examinations (medical school) or specialty in-training examinations Critically appraised topic Evidence-based medical journal log Clinical question log (generated by the trainee) Chart-stimulated recall
Interpersonal and communication skills	Direct observed history and patient communication Multisource evaluations and surveys Trainee reflections on peer and patient feedback Narrative of interview with peer or nursing staff
Professionalism	Multisource evaluations and surveys Critical incidents and praise cards
Practice-based learning and improvement	Individualized learning plan Quality improvement project including self-audit of practice Clinical question logs Self-assessment and reflection Web log dialogue and feedback with advisor
Systems-based practice	Project on navigating the health care system from the perspective of the patient Project on system error, including critical incident analysis Microsystem redesign project Assessment of teamwork skills

*Adapted from Carraccio C, Englander R: Evaluating competence using a portfolio: A literature review and web-based application to the ACGME competencies. Teach Learn Med 2004;16:381–387.

that an evaluation system that only uses global faculty evaluations overestimates resident competency.[37-39] Multiple evaluation approaches are required to truly define the level of competence for trainees,[37,40,41] and as a general rule, each domain of competency should be evaluated by more than one evaluation method.

2. The evaluation program should use the principle of "triangulation." We refer to triangulation in two respects. First, evaluation methods, if used effectively and properly, can be used to evaluate more than one domain of competence. For example, the mini-clinical evaluation exercise can capture skill in both patient care and interpersonal communication.[42] Second, building on the work of Davis, Driessen, and others, the assessment of the portfolio itself should involve more than the perspective of a single evaluator.[9,27]

3. The structured portfolio must be longitudinal and comprehensive in scope and truly represent a composite of a trainee's competence and performance. The trainee, faculty, and mentor should interact on a regular basis over a period of time. This approach can enhance the validity of the process.

4. The process must include evidence of trainee self-assessment and reflection. Without self-assessment and reflection a portfolio cannot exist, and the structured portfolio becomes nothing more than a comprehensive evaluation file. Some aspect of the portfolio must include self-assessment tools and content determined by the trainee. Pitts and colleagues cautioned against too much standardization as a threat to the strengths of the portfolio to drive self-directed learning.[22,23] Allowing the trainee to determine some of the content *and* the evaluation tools used in self-assessment helps to prevent the portfolio from becoming a "glorified" evaluation file. Finally, the portfolio must contain a mechanism to collect and analyze all this important information. Qualitative methods may hold promise in evaluating the "descriptive" aspects of the portfolio.[27]

5. Learners must contribute meaningful work products demonstrating evidence of professional growth and performance to the structured portfolio beyond just evaluations and self-assessment.[43-45] For example, trainees could use research projects and volunteer activities as important contributions to the portfolio. Snadden and Thomas listed a number of items trainees could provide, such as critical incidents of patient events, reflective journal or diary, written descriptions of typical clinical experiences, video recordings of patient care interactions and experiences, clinical care audits, articles reviewed critically using evidenced-based medicine principles, self-selected materials that the trainee believes demonstrate proficiency, and any materials the trainee wishes to keep as a resource for future learning.[44]

6. The portfolio process must be transparent to trainees, and they must have as much access as possible to all contents of the portfolio. In fact, the trainee should "own" the portfolio with agreement between the trainee and the program director regarding the latter's ability to access parts of the portfolio necessary for evaluation. This is part of our obligation as educators and is consistent with the construct of honesty as part of medical professionalism.[46]

In the United States, the ACGME competencies should be the organizing principle for the portfolio. For other educational systems, such as those in Canada and the United Kingdom, the Canadian Medical Education Directions for Specialists (CanMEDS) and Good Medical Practice competencies, respectively, should guide the evaluations.[47,48]

Evaluation Tools for Inclusion in the Portfolio

The minimal evaluation components for a structured portfolio would include at least one method of evaluation from each of the following five broad evaluation methodologies, regardless of what competency framework you may use:

1. Foundational evaluations: At a minimum these should include longitudinal global ratings and monthly evaluations by faculty. These evaluations can and should represent a robust composite of multiple assessments by faculty (see Chapter 3).

2. Direct observations: Observation of the trainee's clinical, communication and interpersonal skills (see Chapters 8 and 9).

3. Practice and data-based learning: Active application by the trainee of personal performance data and system information to improve their practice. One example would be a medical record audit of patients accompanied by self-assessment, reflection, and a quality improvement plan (see Chapters 5 and 11).

4. Multisource evaluations: The perspective of patients and nonphysician health care providers should be included as part of the portfolio (see Chapter 6).

5. Self-assessment and reflection: These methodologies will take two forms. The first will be mostly narrative descriptions of what they have learned, why they have made changes, what they plan to do to improve, and how the portfolio process has changed them. The second should be logs of self-assessment activities such as self-audit of medical records, the results of answering clinical questions, and specific learning plans.

The "foundation" would be the global rating scales/monthly evaluation forms completed by faculty. Despite known problems with such forms, they can provide invaluable information if used properly by faculty. As demonstrated elsewhere in this book, what

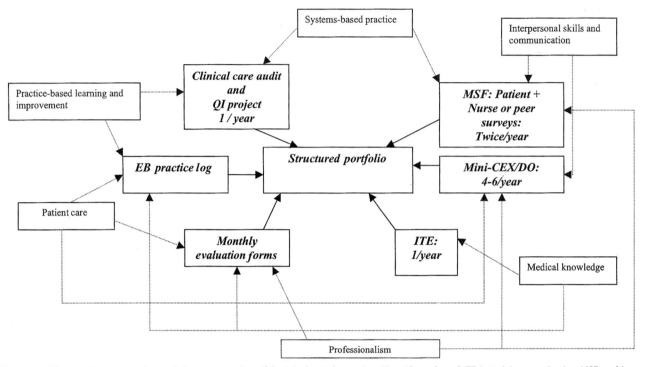

Figure 7-3 Triangulation of evaluation tools for a structured portfolio. DO, direct observation; EB, evidence-based; ITE, in-training examination; MSF, multisource feedback; QI, quality improvement.

is needed is better training of faculty in evaluation and clearly defined descriptions or anchors of each rating on the scale, not new evaluation forms.[37,41,49] With this foundation, programs can implement various tools from the other three components that are feasible and effective for their training setting.

To further illustrate the evaluation components of the structured portfolio framework, we provide an example. Figure 7-3 shows a basic approach for how a program using existing, multifaceted evaluation methods could meet minimum requirements to evaluate the six U.S. ACGME general competencies. Note how one tool can be used to evaluate more than one competency. The figure shows how the use of existing tools, namely monthly evaluation forms, mini-CEX (direct observation), patient and nursing surveys (multisource feedback/360-degree evaluations), the yearly in-training examination (global evaluation of medical knowledge), a medical record audit, and a log of clinical questions using evidenced-based medicine (practice and data-based learning) could address each general competency in multiple ways.

This basic example starts with the monthly global evaluation forms that are best suited to evaluate patient care, medical knowledge, and professionalism. The in-training examination (ITE), given just once a year, is an evidenced-based, effective method to measure a trainee's global medical knowledge[50] (see Chapter 4). For example, the ITE has good predictive validity for the ABIM internal medicine certification examination.

The mini-CEX is a validated, reliable tool for assessing clinical skills through direct observation.[42,51] If programs have faculty perform just four mini-CEXs in

the ambulatory clinic plus one for each inpatient rotation, the majority of trainees would receive over 10 observations per year. Research suggests that 10 to 12 mini-CEXs provide a high degree of reliability; just four will provide sufficient reliability for "pass-fail" determinations.[42] However, other research again highlights the need to train faculty to be more accurate, rigorous observers of clinical skills.[52]

A patient survey and assessment by the nursing staff on selected locations or rotations (360-degree evaluation or multisource feedback evaluation) is an efficient and effective way to include the patient and nonphysician perspective in the trainee's evaluations (see Chapter 6). Multisource evaluations often provide important, different perspectives on the competencies of a trainee[52–54] (see Chapter 6). For example, peers and nurses are often in a better position to judge work ethic, professionalism and interpersonal communication skills.[55] Patient surveys can provide meaningful formative evaluation around communication skills.

Development of competence in practice-based learning and systems-based practice can be substantially facilitated by self-directed activities. For example, residents can perform a medical record audit of their practice as an excellent way to teach practice-based learning and improvement and systems-based practice[56,57] (see Chapter 5). Resident self-audit of practice, combined with a structured curriculum, has been shown to improve patient care and change resident behavior.[33] Other studies have shown how residents can be involved in quality improvement activities and skill building[58–60] (see Chapter 11). Residents can also keep logs of clinical questions and the resources they

Change	Level of motivation to make this change					Anticipated difficulty in making this change				
	Not at all motivated			Highly motivated		Not at all difficult			Extremely difficult	
1.	1	2	3	4	5	1	2	3	4	5
2.	1	2	3	4	5	1	2	3	4	5
3.	1	2	3	4	5	1	2	3	4	5
4.	1	2	3	4	5	1	2	3	4	5
5.	1	2	3	4	5	1	2	3	4	5

Figure 7-4 Commitment to change form.

used to answer them as another effective technique to teach evidenced-based medicine and evaluate practice-based learning and improvement[61] (see Chapter 10).

The Trainee's Contribution

What about the trainee? As noted by others, the trainee must make a meaningful contribution to the portfolio. This can occur in multiple ways. First, the trainee should add evidence of self-directed learning and growth to the portfolio. Examples include the results of answering clinical questions for patient care with reflection on what they learned; results of self-assessment of the clinical practice through chart audit or patient surveys; and research and quality improvement projects. Another example would be written reactions (reflections) to feedback from a mentor, followed by a commitment to change note in the portfolio. Any product, such as a research abstract, poster, or conference presentation, should be included in the portfolio.[44] However, to be most useful trainees must also provide some evidence about the impact and value of the experience on their development.

One feasible and valuable approach to capturing reflection and action is "commitment to change" (CTC) statements.[62–66] In the CTC approach, the learner puts in writing the plan, or "commitment," after a review of his or her performance or an educational experience. This simple process has been shown to increase the likelihood the individuals will actually change their behavior. One example is the American Academy of Pediatrics' online resource for practitioners, called PediLink, to document questions that arise in clinical practice, search resources for answers, and document the "commitment to change" statements that address changes in practice based on new learning.[67]

This approach was successfully used in an internal medicine residency quality improvement curriculum.[18] The documentation of "commitments" also enables follow-up to see if the trainee was successful in making the change. Figures 7-4 and 7-5 demonstrate the CTC baseline and follow-up forms used in the quality improvement study. The CTC statements can become part of the portfolio. A second method simply is to use an open-ended written summary. In the same quality improvement study, the residents were asked at the end of a 4-week block to write a single page reflecting on the following questions:

1. What did I learn about myself as a result of this experience?
2. What did I learn about the systems of care in which I see and care for patients?
3. What recommendations do you have about the rotation and clinic to make things better?

Second, the trainee should provide documentation of his or her reaction to the results of evaluations, along with the action plan or "next steps." Ultimately, the trainee needs to own the evaluation. This reaction can be done on paper at the bottom of the evaluation forms or at the end of a Web-based evaluation entry. This approach has the advantage that it will require the faculty member to complete the evaluation, and the trainee to review and react to it.

Name: _____

At the end of your *<insert name>* rotation during block _____ (/ / to / /), you made the "commitments to change" listed below. For each, please indicate if you have implemented the change in your clinical practice fully, partially, or not at all. For the changes that you have not implemented fully, indicate the primary barrier that prevented your implementation.

1. Practice Change: _____

Which describes the action you have taken? (*circle one*)	Fully implemented change	Partially implemented change	Did not implement change
If only partially or not at all, what was the primary barrier to implementation? (*check one*)	❑ "I have not had enough time to implement this change" ❑ "I need to improve my knowledge / skills before I can implement this change" ❑ "Systems or logistical barriers in my practice prevented me" ❑ "This change is not important enough to my clinical practice" ❑ Other: _____		

2. Practice Change: _____

Which describes the action you have taken? (*circle one*)	Fully implemented change	Partially implemented change	Did not implement change
If only partially or not at all, what was the primary barrier to implementation? (*check one*)	❑ "I have not had enough time to implement this change" ❑ "I need to improve my knowledge / skills before I can implement this change" ❑ "Systems or logistical barriers in my practice prevented me" ❑ "This change is not important enough to my clinical practice" ❑ Other: _____		

Figure 7-5 Commitment to change follow-up form.

When the program director looks at the sum total of the evaluations and the trainee input into the portfolio, she or he must be able to determine if the trainee has attained, at a minimum, competence in the domains of interest by the end of training. Equally important, the trainee must also demonstrate through the reflective input of the portfolio that she or he has assumed the responsibility and accountability for performance and continuous professional development.

Figure 7-6 demonstrates how program directors and training programs could effectively utilize a structured portfolio as the "hub" of an effective evaluation system. Note that active trainee involvement and reflection are vital, essential components of the evaluation system and structured portfolio. As Figure 7-6 demonstrates, the trainee should interact and contribute to the portfolio on an ongoing basis. This will promote trainees taking personal responsibility for their own professional growth. All arrows in the diagram are bidirectional.

The use of the structured portfolio is in its infancy in postgraduate medical training. The most successful examples are found at the medical school level.[1,2,9] However, portfolio use at the residency level is beginning to be reported.[3,25,26,68–70] Although the various components of the portfolio are grounded in empiric educational and evaluation science, future research is needed to determine the optimal approach to implementing and operating a portfolio-based evaluation system at the residency program level. One of the important issues will be how to best operationalize the collection of the data from the various evaluation tools and the residents' interactions with their own portfolios. Web-based technology should enable this process.[64,71–76]

Current vendor-based evaluation products already allow for programs to customize the evaluations used in the program, the types of reports generated, and how the information can be shared among users.

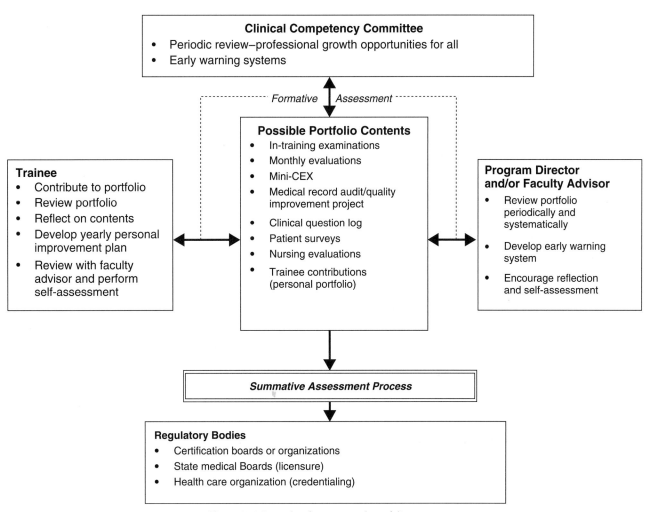

Figure 7-6 Example of a structured portfolio system.

These existing systems could be further modified to allow greater resident interaction and input into these electronic evaluation systems. The ACGME is currently developing a Web-based learning portfolio prototype for pilot testing in 2008 in the United States (ACGME, personal communication) with plans for widespread dissemination in 2009. For portfolios to be feasible in residency programs, a Web-based interface will most likely be needed. As Web-based portfolios are implemented by training programs, the educational community should collaborate to investigate best practices around effectiveness and efficiency, starting with lessons learned in medical schools. Regardless, the portfolio approach holds significant promise to improve assessment in undergraduate and graduate medical education worldwide.

ANNOTATED BIBLIOGRAPHY

1. Friedman BDM, Davis MH, Harden RM, et al: AAME Educational Guide 24: Portfolios as a method of student assessment. Med Teach 2001;23:1–23.

   This comprehensive article provides an in-depth discussion of portfolio assessment and describes in detail the University of Dundee medical student portfolio process. Nice flowcharts about the Dundee process are provided, showing a more structured portfolio assessment system. Despite major concerns about using a psychometric approach, this article does an excellent job of describing the major psychometric issues in portfolio assessment. Finally, important considerations in portfolio implementation are well described.

2. Carraccio C, Englander R: Evaluating competence using a portfolio: A literature review and Web-based application to the ACGME competencies. Teach Learn Med 2004;16:381–387.

   This review is a good compilation of 35 articles published between 1996 and 2002 on portfolios used in medical school, resident training, and continuing medical education. The authors highlight the importance of reflection in professional development and the central role the learners must play in a portfolio-based assessment system. The article also describes a Web-based portfolio used in a residency program based on the six ACGME general competencies. The authors argue that a portfolio needs to balance the trainee's reflective contributions with structured evaluation components. Some of the evaluation tools included in the structured portion of the portfolio included global assessments (e.g., global rating scales), direct observation of history and physical examination skills using a tool based on the mini-CEX, a multi-source evaluation instrument, projects in a quality improvement (e.g., practice-based learning and improvement), and systems-based practice and patient and procedure logs.

3. Davis DA, Mazmanian PE, Fordis M, et al: Accuracy of physician self-assessment compared to observed measures of competence: A systematic review. JAMA 2006;296(9):1094–1102.

   This article nicely summarizes the literature on self-assessment and self-evaluation. Davis and colleagues performed a systematic review of

17 articles that included 20 total comparisons between self- and other assessments. They found that 13 (65%) of the comparisons showed little, no, or an inverse relationship between measures of self-assessment and other indicators. Only seven comparisons demonstrated a positive relationship. Davis and colleagues argued more effort should be directed at the development of feedback processes and tools to help better guide physicians in identifying and selecting opportunities for improvement in performance and self-directed learning.

4. Driessen E, van der Vleuten CPM, Schuwirth L, et al: The use of qualitative research criteria for portfolio assessment as an alternative to reliability evaluation: A case study. Med Educ 2005;39: 214–220.

This important study is one of the first to demonstrate how systematic, qualitative research methods can be used to evaluate the portfolios. The authors focused on the qualitative criteria of credibility and dependability, using the qualitative techniques of triangulation, prolonged engagement, member checking, audit trail, and dependability audit. This approach led to a high degree of agreement between mentors and students, with only a small proportion of portfolio evaluations requiring adjudication by a full committee (9 of 233 portfolios). Figure 7-2 displays the evaluation flow-chart for this study. The key conceptual difference with this approach was the use of adding information during the process to inform judgment until ''information saturation'' was achieved (qualitative methodology) instead of looking for consistency across repeated measurements (traditional psychometric/quantitative methodology). Information saturation simply refers to the process of examining information until no further themes are identified and the judgment no longer changes with the addition of more evaluation information. This approach to portfolio evaluation represents a major shift in the assessment of competence. A word of caution, however, is in order. This study examined portfolios of students early in their training; whether qualitative methods can be used to evaluate competence during later stages of clinical training should be the subject of future studies.

5. Snadden D, Thomas M: The use of portfolio learning in medical education. Med Teach 1998;20(3):192–199.

This well-written article provides some of the history of portfolios and provides guidance on how to develop a portfolio that facilitates the professional development process. Specifically, the authors provide a three-step outline on using portfolios for formative learning. Challenges in using portfolios for summative assessment are described, with the two authors suggesting that portfolios are well suited for high-stakes assessment. Finally, the authors provide helpful suggestions on how to implement and sustain the portfolio process, and they also provide suggestions on workshops to inform and train both faculty and trainees in using portfolios.

6. O'Sullivan PS, Reckase MD, McClain T, et al: Demonstration of portfolios to assess competency of residents. Adv Health Sci Educ 2004;9:309–323.

Despite weaknesses identified here, this is currently one of the few studies to systematically examine the reliability and validity characteristics of a portfolio. The article describes the results of a study involving 18 psychiatry residents over a 4-year period. An important component of O'Sullivan's approach was the training of the portfolio raters. Generalizability analysis found that five entries and two raters were sufficient for normative-based decisions. To reach sufficient reliability for criterion, or absolute decisions, six entries or adding a third rater would be required. Despite the encouraging results on the reliability analysis, the authors still commented they believed the rubric used for scoring the portfolios was somewhat weak, and overall the validity evidence presented was not robust. Regarding validity, the authors did find that portfolio scores improved with increasing years of training, but did not correlate to clinical performance. This latter finding is somewhat disappointing given that an identified strength of portfolios is their authenticity. However, the authors did find that the portfolios provided valuable information on areas of weakness in the curriculum.

REFERENCES

1. Friedman BDM, Davis MH, Harden RM, et al: AAME Educational Guide 24: Portfolios as a method of student assessment. Med Teach 2001;23:1–23.
2. Challis M: AMEE medical education guide no. 11 (revised): Portfolio-based learning and assessment in medical education. Med Teach 1999;4:370–386.
3. Carraccio C, Englander R: Evaluating competence using a portfolio: A literature review and Web-based application to the ACGME competencies. Teach Learn Med 2004;16:381–387.
4. McMullan M, Endacott R, Gray MA, et al: Portfolios and assessment of competence: A review of the literature. J Adv Nurs 2003;41(3):283–294.
5. Smith K, Tillema H: Clarifying different types of portfolio use. Assess Eval Higher Educ 2003;28(6):625–648.
6. Koretz D: Large-scale portfolio assessment in the US: Evidence pertaining to the quality of measurement. Assess Educ 1998;5(3):309–334.
7. Duque G, Finkelstein A, Roberts A: Learning while evaluating: the use of an electronic evaluation portfolio in a geriatric medicine clerkship. BMC Med Educ 2006;6:4.
8. Duque G: Web-based evaluation of medical clerkships: New approach to immediacy and efficacy of feedback and assessment. Med Teach 2003;25:510–514.
9. Davis MH, Friedman BDM, Harden RM, et al: Portfolio assessment in medical students' final examinations. Med Teach 2001;23:357–366.
10. Reckase MD: Portfolio assessment: A theoretical estimate of score reliability. Educ Measure 1995;14:12–31.
11. Martin-Kneip GO: Becoming a Better Teacher: Eight Innovations That Work. Alexandria, VA, Association for Supervision and Curriculum Development, 2000.
12. Wilkinson TJ, Challis M, Hobma SO, et al: The use of portfolios for assessment of the competence and performance of doctors in practice. Med Educ 2002;36(10):918–924.
13. Choudry N, Fletcher R, Soumeral S: Systematic review: The relationship between clinical experience and quality of health care. Ann Intern Med 2005;142:260–273.
14. Campbell C, Parboosingh J, Gondocz T, et al: Study of the factors influencing the stimulus to learning recorded by physicians keeping a learning portfolio. J Cont Educ Health Prof 1999;19(1): 16–24.
15. Campbell CM, Parboosingh JT, Gondocz ST, et al: Study of physicians' use of a software program to create a portfolio of their self-directed learning. Acad Med 1996;71:S49–S51.
16. Holmboe ES, Meehan TP, Lynn L, et al: The ABIM Diabetes Practice Improvement Module: A new method for self assessment. J Cont Educ Health Prof 2006;26:109–119.
17. Archibald DA, Newmann FM: Beyond standardized testing: Assessing authentic academic achievement in the secondary school. Reston, VA, National Association of Secondary School Principals, 1988.
18. Holmboe ES, Prince L, Green ML: Teaching and improving quality of care in a residency clinic. Acad Med 2005;80:571–577.
19. Hemmer P, Hawkins R, Jackson J, Pangaro L: Assessing how well three evaluation methods detect deficiencies in medical students' professionalism in two settings of an internal medicine clerkship. Acad Med 2000;75:167–173.
20. Munger BS: Oral examinations. In Mancall EL, Bashook PG (eds): Recertification: New Evaluation Methods and Strategies. Evanston, IL, American Board of Medical Specialties, 1994.
21. Pitts J, Coles C, Thomas P: Educational portfolios in the assessment of general practice trainers: Reliability of assessors. Med Educ 1999;33:515–520.
22. Pitts J, Coles C, Thomas P: Enhancing reliability in portfolio assessment: ''Shaping'' the portfolio. Med Teach 2001;23(4): 351–356.
23. Pitts J, Coles C, Thomas P, Smith F: Enhancing reliability in portfolio assessment: Discussion between assessors. Med Teach 2002;24(2):197–201.
24. McMullan M, Endacott R, Gray MA, et al: Portfolios and assessment of competence: A review of the literature. J Adv Nurs 2003;41:283–294.
25. O'Sullivan PS, Reckase MD, McClain T, et al: Demonstration of portfolios to assess competency of residents. Adv Health Sci Educ 2004;9:309–323.
26. O'Sullivan PS, Cogbill K, McClain T, et al: Portfolios as a novel approach for residency evaluations. Acad Psychol 2002;26:173–179.
27. Driessen E, van der, Vleuten CPM, Schuwirth L, et al: The use of qualitative research criteria for portfolio assessment as an

alternative to reliability evaluation: A case study. Med Educ 2005;39:214–220.

28. Davis DA, Mazmanian PE, Fordis M, et al: Accuracy of physician self-assessment compared to observed measures of competence: A systematic review. JAMA 2006;296(9):1094–1102.

29. Kruger J, Dunning D: Unskilled and unaware of it: How difficulties in recognizing one's own incompetence lead to inflated self-assessments. J Personality Soc Psychol 1999;77:1121–1134.

30. Kruger J, Dunning D: Unskilled and unaware—But why? A reply to Krueger and Mueller. J Personality Soc Psychol 2002;82:182–192.

31. Eva KW, Regehr G: Self-assessments in the health professions: A reformulation and research agenda. Acad Med 2005;80: S46–S54.

32. Schon DA: The Reflective Practitioner: How Professionals Think in Action. New York, Basic Books, 1983.

33. Holmboe ES, Prince L, Green ML: Teaching and improving quality of care in a residency clinic. Acad Med 2005;80:571–577.

34. Holmboe ES, Meehan TP, Lynn L, et al: The ABIM Diabetes Practice Improvement Module: A new method for self assessment. J Cont Educ Health Prof 2006;26:109–119.

35. Barnsley L, Lyon LM, Ralston SJ, et al: Clinical skill in junior medical officers: A comparison of self-reported confidence and observed competence. Med Educ 2004;38:358–367.

36. Debowski S, Wood RE, Bandura A: Impact of guided exploration and enactive exploration on self-regulatory mechanisms and information acquisition through electronic search. J Appl Psychol 2001(86):1129–1141.

37. Turnbull J, Gray J, MacFayden J: Improving in-training evaluation programs. J Gen Intern Med 1998;13:317–323.

38. Silber CG, Nasca TJ, Paskin DL, et al: Do global rating forms enable program directors to assess the ACGME competencies? Acad Med 2004;79:549–556.

39. Schwind CJ, Williams RG, Boehler ML, Dunnington GL: Do individual attendings' post-rotation performance ratings detect residents' clinical performance deficiencies? Acad Med 2004; 79:453–457.

40. Holmboe ES, Hawkins RE: Evaluating the clinical competence of residents: A review. Ann Intern Med 1998;129:42–48.

41. Gray JD: Global rating scales in residency education. Acad Med 1996;71:S55.

42. Norcini JJ, Blank LL, Duffy FD, Fortna GS: The mini-CEX: A method for assessing clinical skills. Ann Intern Med 2003;138:476–481.

43. Smith K, Tillema H: Clarifying different types of portfolio use. Assess Eval Higher Educ 2003;28(6):625–648.

44. Snadden D, Thomas M: The use of portfolio learning in medical education. Med Teach 1998;20(3):192–199.

45. Webb C, Endacott R, Gray M, et al: Models of portfolios. Med Educ 2002;36:897–898.

46. ABIM Foundation, American College of Physicians, and European Federation of Internal Medicine: Medical professionalism in the millennium: A physician charter. Ann Intern Med 2002;136:243–246.

47. Frank JR, Jabbour M, Tugwell P, et al: Skills for the new millenium: Report of the societal needs working group, CanMEDS 2000 Project. Ann R Coll Phys Surg Can 1996;29:206–216.

48. General Medical Council: Good Medical Practice. London, General Medical Council, 2001.

49. Landy FJ, Farr JL: Performance rating. Psychol Bull 1980;87: 72–107.

50. Garibaldi RA, Subhiyah R, Moore ME, Waxman H: The in-training examination in internal medicine: An analysis of resident performance over time. Ann Intern Med 2002;137: 505–510.

51. Holmboe ES, Huot S, Hawkins RE: Construct validity of the mini-clinical evaluation exercise. Acad Med 2003;78:826–830.

52. Holmboe ES: Faculty and the observation of trainees' clinical skills: Problems and opportunities. Acad Med 2004;79:16–22.

53. Violato C, Lockyer J, Fidler H: Multisource feedback: A method of assessing surgical practice. BMJ 2003;326:546–548.

54. Lockyer J: Multisource feedback in the assessment of physician competencies. J Cont Educ Health Prof 2003;23:4–12.

55. Norcini JJ: Peer assessment of competence. Med Educ 2003; 37:539–543.

56. Thomson O'Brien MA, Oxman AD, Davis DA, et al: Audit and feedback: Effects on professional practice and health care outcomes. The Cochrane Library (Oxford) 2003;1:Update Software.

57. Veloski J, Boex JR, Grasberger MJ, et al: Systematic review of the literature on assessment, feedback and physicians' clinical performance: BEME Guide No. 7. Med Teach 2006;28(2):117–128.

58. Ogrinc G, Headrick LA, Mutha S, et al: A framework for teaching medical students and residents about practiced-based learning and improvement, synthesized from a literature review. Acad Med 2003;78:748–756.

59. Djuricich AM, Ciccarelli M, Swigonski N: A continuous quality improvement curriculum for residents: Addressing core competencies, improving systems. Acad Med 2004;79:S65–S67.

60. Ogrinc G, Headrick LA, Morrison LJ, Foster T: Teaching and assessing resident competence in practice-based learning and improvement. J Gen Intern Med 2004;19:496–500.

61. Wong J, Holmboe ES, Huot S: A novel dayfloat rotation to address the 80 hour work restriction. J Gen Intern Med 2004;19(Part 2):519–523.

62. Mazmanian PE, Mazmanian PM: Commitment to change: Theoretical foundations, methods, and outcomes. J Cont Educ Health Prof 1999;19:200–207.

63. Jones DL: Viability of the commitment-for-change evaluation strategy in continuing medical education. Acad Med 1990; 65:S37–S38.

64. Pereles L, Gondocz T, Lockyer JM, et al: Effectiveness of commitment contracts in facilitating change in continuing medical education intervention. J Cont Educ Health Prof 1997;17:27–31.

65. Mazmanian PE, Johnson RE, Zhang A, et al: Effects of a signature on rates of change: A randomized controlled trial involving continuing education and the commitment-to-change model. Acad Med 2001;76:642–646.

66. Mazmanian PE, Daffron SR, Johnson RE, et al: Information about barriers to planned change: A randomized controlled trial involving continuing medical education lectures and commitment to change. Acad Med 1998;73:882–886.

67. PediaLink Learning Center: Accessed at https://www.pedialink.org/index.cfm, Dec. 12, 2006.

68. Melville C, Rees M, Brookfield D, Anderson J: Portfolios for assessment of paediatric specialist registrars. Med Educ 2004;38:1117–1125.

69. Fung MFK, Walker M, Fung KFK, et al: An Internet-based learning portfolio in resident education: The KOALA multicentre programme. Med Educ 2000;34:474–479.

70. O'Sullivan P, Greene C: Portfolios: Possibilities for addressing emergency medicine resident competencies. Acad Emerg Med 2002;9(11):1305–1309.

71. Supiano MA, Fantone JC, Grum C: A Web-based geriatrics portfolio to document medical student's learning outcomes. Acad Med 2002;77(9):398–937.

72. Sandars J: Commentary: Electronic portfolios for general practitioners: The beginning of an exciting future. Educ Primary Care 2005;16:535–539.

73. Dornan T, Lee C, Stopford A: SkillsBase: A Web-based electronic learning portfolio for clinical skills. Acad Med 2001;76:542–543.

74. Dornan T, Carroll C, Parboosingh J: An electronic learning portfolio for reflective continuing professional development. Med Educ 2002;36:767–769.

75. Dornan T, Meredia N, Hosie L, et al: A Web-based presentation of an undergraduate clinical skills curriculum. Med Educ 2003;37:500–508.

76. Dornan T, Lee C, Stopford A, et al: Rapid application design of an electronic clinical skills portfolio for undergraduate medical students. Computer Methods Prog Biomed 2005;78:25–33.

Direct Observation: Standardized Patients

Richard E. Hawkins, MD, and John R. Boulet, PhD

Accurate appraisal of basic clinical skills requires direct observation of the interaction between the patient (or simulated patient) and the physician-in-training. In this chapter, basic clinical skills are defined as those aptitudes and abilities that are exercised during the doctor-patient interaction. These skills include data gathering through the patient interview and physical examination, as well as general communication and interpersonal skills. Also included in the clinical skills domain are the more complex information sharing and interactive skills that underlie effective counseling, informed decision making, and challenges involved in delivering bad news, dealing with the angry patient, and delivering culturally competent care.

Observation may occur within the context of an actual clinical encounter or, as has become more commonplace, via the simulation of a patient by one of a variety of individuals. For example, faculty or peers may role-play a patient for educational or assessment purposes. In medical education and assessment settings, lay individuals may also be called upon to simulate a variety of conditions and situations. These persons have been referred to by a variety of names such as patient-actors, patient-instructors, programmed patients, standardized patients, or simulated patients. A simulated patient is an individual trained to portray a scripted patient role for medical education or assessment purposes. A simulated patient may also be taught to report on examinee actions/behaviors, to teach, to rate communication and interpersonal skills, and to provide feedback. Simulated patients who undergo more extensive training in order to consistently portray a particular case or objectively score examinee performances are appropriately referred to as standardized patients. However, for the purpose of this chapter, as is most often described in the literature, the term standardized patient (SP) will be used from a broader perspective to describe laypersons simulating actual patients for the purpose of medical education and assessment.

The use of performance-based assessments, including evaluations employing SPs and various types of objective structured clinical examinations (OSCEs), is now widespread.[1-4] From their early introduction as formative assessment tools in medical education,[5,6] they have expanded to become part of the certification and licensure process in several countries.[7-10] This expansion was predicated, in part, on the development of standardized training techniques, the testing and improvement of scoring rubrics, the adoption of technological advances in assessment methodology, a host of psychometric validation studies,[11-13] and the desire to be able to evaluate medical students/graduates under comparable conditions. The widespread adoption of these types of performance-based tests was based on the belief that traditional measurement methods could not provide much needed data on what a physician could do, as opposed to what he/she knew. That is, time-honored paper-and-pencil examinations, on their own, were not a valid testing medium for clinical skills. Moreover, at least for summative evaluations, the observation and assessment of individuals with "real" patients, including typical bedside oral examinations, was difficult to standardize and generally yielded evaluation results that were only marginally reliable and often subject to evaluator bias.[14,15]

A relatively broad range of conditions can be modeled by SPs, some of whom may be "real" patients with stable physical findings. For many conditions, however, SPs can be taught to simulate a wide variety of physical findings in a consistent and reproducible manner.[16] Real patients with physical examination findings are ideal for locally administered examinations in which the addition of clinically relevant historical information and laboratory or radiographic data may enrich the educational or assessment experience. Unfortunately, the use of SPs with real physical findings in multiple-site, high-stakes examinations can be problematic. Here, it is often not possible to standardize their findings, potentially compromising the fairness of the assessment.

Components of a Typical Standardized Patient Encounter

Regardless of whether an SP is used within the context of a single encounter or a multiple station assessment, the clinical interaction generally consists of the following elements (Fig. 8-1).

Introduction to the Encounter (Opening Scenario)

To introduce the clinical material and provide instructions to the trainee regarding the required task, a brief description of the encounter is provided, either in writing or verbally. For example, *Mrs. Jones is referred to your clinic for evaluation of a heart murmur. Please obtain the relevant history, perform a focused physical examination, and then counsel Mrs. Jones regarding the need for antibiotic prophylaxis prior to her dental surgery.* Depending upon the goals of the SP exercise, the background information provided may be brief or detailed.

Standardized Patient Encounter

The trainee is expected to interact with the SP as if interviewing or examining a real patient. Depending upon the focus of the encounter, certain aspects of the physical examination may not be included (e.g., sensitive components such as breast, genital, or rectal examinations). Here, if the examinee wants to perform these physical examination elements, the SP may be trained to respond that the examination has already been performed and then describe the findings or provide written results. Additional clinical information or material may be incorporated into the SP encounter to enrich the educational value of the exercise or to allow faculty to adapt the exercise to the level of the learner. For example, the examinee may be asked to review laboratory or radiographic reports or to interpret the actual clinical materials such as a blood smear, a radiograph, or an electrocardiogram. For the same SP case, a student beginning his or her clinical training may be asked to take a history, perform a physical examination, and offer a differential diagnosis; but a postgraduate trainee would be provided with laboratory and radiographic data and be tasked with the additional challenge of prioritizing the differential diagnosis and formulating plans for therapy. Alternatively, the higher level learner may be asked to inform the patient about worrisome test results or to counsel the patient regarding indicated behavioral modification.

Recording or Scoring of the Standardized Patient Encounter

Several methods have been used to record or score trainee performance during the encounter. Recording or scoring actions may occur during or after the SP encounter, live or via videotape, and by a variety of individuals including the performing SP, another observing SP, the trainee, a faculty observer, or a trainee peer. Different methods or instruments may be used to record, score, or rate trainee performance. These scoring options are detailed later in this chapter.

Post-Encounter (or Inter-station) Activities

Post-encounter stations or exercises are often included to enhance the clinical authenticity of the case(s) or to

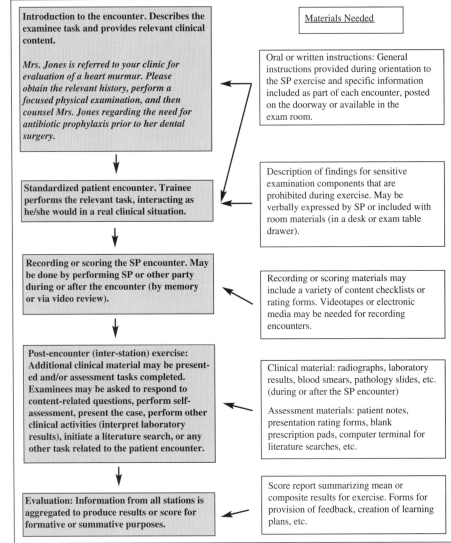

Figure 8-1 Components of a typical standardized patient (SP) encounter.

allow for the expansion of the competence domains being evaluated. For example, after the SP encounter, the examinee may be asked to write a progress note; dispense a prescription for medical, occupational, or physical therapy; or present the case to a consultant or attending physician. In the post-encounter period, examinees may also be asked to complete a series of questions, including multiple-choice, short answer, or other formats. To expand the range of competencies assessed via SP-based methods, trainees might be asked to formulate a question for literature review, seeking evidence to resolve the clinical challenge presented (addressing elements of the *patient care* or *practice-based learning and improvement* competencies) (see Chapter 1 for description of the Accreditation Council for Graduate Medical Education [ACGME]/American Board of Medical Specialties [ABMS] general competencies). Alternatively, within the context of a complex patient presentation, a trainee may be asked to reflect on potential management options that balance the tension between patient advocacy and prudent use of system resources (*systems-based practice* or *professionalism*).

Evaluation

Any or all of the information collected during or after the patient encounter may be used for formative or summative purposes. Case-specific content checklists (i.e., history-taking questions that should be asked, physical examination maneuvers that should be performed) can be used to determine whether the trainee met expected performance standards for data gathering. The same checklist can serve as a discussion template for providing feedback to the trainee regarding his or her success in meeting educational or clinical objectives. Rating scales can be used to provide feedback or to make pass/fail decisions regarding a student or resident's communication and interpersonal skills or humanistic or professional behaviors. Scores from the clinical interview, patient note, case presentation, and multiple choice or other tests associated with individual patient encounters can be combined to obtain a final score that best meets the purpose of the educational or assessment exercise.

Introduction to Reliability and Validity of Standardized Patient–Based Assessment

Although the use of SP-based assessments is now widespread, their utility is contingent on their general purpose (e.g., formative assessment, summative assessment), local health care needs, faculty acceptance, resource availability (e.g., people to be trained as standardized patients, examination rooms, evaluators), available technology, local cultural issues, and, to some extent, psychometric expertise. Historically, SP-based assessments were used primarily for formative purposes and did not demand the level of standardization or psychometric rigor that defines today's performance-based licensure and certification examinations. In general, medical students were observed interacting with an SP, often another medical student, and given immediate feedback regarding their performance. Certain tasks could be repeated until mastery was demonstrated. Typically, scoring was limited to holistic, global impressions, or to the documented completion of a few key (e.g., checklist) items. Post-encounter exercises (e.g., "read an electrocardiogram") were often included to evaluate diagnostic skills. From a practical perspective, students completing these structured exercises were able to get rapid, meaningful feedback concerning their strengths and weaknesses. Although this information may be extremely valuable from a pedagogical perspective, often, little attention was paid to the reliability and validity of the derived ability measures.

Over the past 30 years, however, there has been an expansive list of articles written about the psychometric properties of scores from OSCEs and SP-based assessments.[17–19] In particular, much of the interest in the measurement properties of the scores has been spurred by the introduction of large-scale medical certification and licensure examinations. Research data generated in preparation for these high-stakes examinations, as well as information produced by researchers in medical education settings, provide a sound basis and guidance for the development of SP-based examinations, whether used in certification/licensure or educational programs. It should be noted, however, that regardless of the "stakes" or purpose of the assessment, it is important to gather some evidence to support the psychometric adequacy of the evaluation scores.

In general, the defensibility of any score-based decision (e.g., pass/fail) is dependent on the test's ability to generate reasonably valid and precise measures of ability. To do this, careful attention must be paid to the choice of examination content (e.g., clinical scenarios), the construction of appropriate scoring rubrics, the training of SPs (or other evaluators), the selection and implementation of score equating strategies (if needed), quality assurance, the methods employed to establish performance standards, and, often ignored, the investigation of potential threats to score validity. Thus, the reliability and validity of any SP-based assessment is inextricably linked to examination development and administration processes. For this reason, further discussion of psychometrics is embedded in the broader context of examination development, described in the following section. The steps involved in developing and administering a clinical skills examination are summarized in Figure 8-2.

Development of Standardized Patient–Based Examinations

The specific details on how to set up an OSCE can be found in a number of articles.[20–23] Unfortunately, the generic "how to" publications do not capture the necessary subtleties inherent with local implementations of performance-based evaluation programs. This is especially true for medical schools that do not have an established, well-developed, quantitative competency assessment plan already in place. Although many medical education programs around the world use SPs to evaluate the clinical skills of medical students and, to a lesser extent, residents, how these individuals are employed, where they are recruited from, and how they are trained varies considerably. More important, the use of other personnel (e.g., faculty) in the test development and assessment administration process is not well defined and can certainly differ as a function of the purpose of the assessment, local cultural factors, faculty leadership, and most certainly, available resources.

The test and case development process at many medical schools, albeit less systematic and often idiosyncratic to the culture of the individual institution, is often similar to that employed for high-stakes certification and licensure examinations. For a medical school or residency program, it is important that the faculty member(s) or committee charged with clinical skills assessment-related activities receive training in the case development process or, at the very least, work out a systematic, defendable process that is reproducible over time. Regarding membership, faculty from a variety of medical specialties or subspecialties may need to be recruited to develop individual case scenarios. They should be oriented to the purpose of the assessment, provided with background information on what SPs can and cannot do, and asked for their clinical opinions regarding how the case should play out. Initial scenarios are developed, played out by an SP, and critiqued. Once the case scenario and associated SP portrayal parameters are decided, the history-taking and physical examination checklists can be developed. It should be stressed, however, that case development is an iterative process; until the scenario is acted out, and some pilot administrations undertaken, it is difficult to discern all the potential problems, including those associated with SP portrayal, unanticipated student reactions to the scripted SP responses, and case irregularities (e.g., patient history or physical findings are not consistent with the intended diagnoses) (see Fig. 8-2).

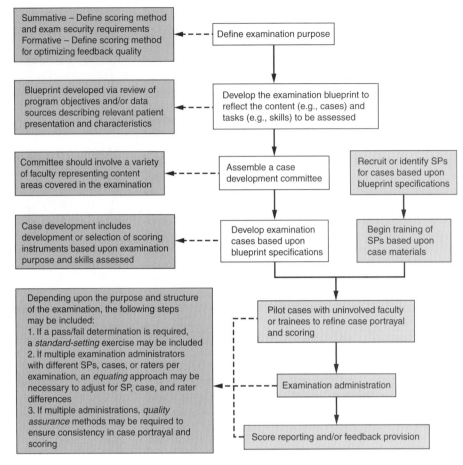

Figure 8-2 Summary of the steps involved in the development and administration of a standardized patient (SP)–based clinical skills examination.

Examination Purpose

When introducing an assessment exercise or program using SPs, it is important to first consider the purpose of such activity. If the purpose is formative in nature, then an important priority should be to determine how assessment results will be compiled and relayed to the examinee as high-quality, individually interpretable feedback. If the purpose is summative in scope, less attention is paid to the quality and nature of the feedback; the focus should be on ensuring adequate reliability and constructing the examination to allow for valid inferences about the clinical skill(s) being assessed. Additionally, if used for making pass/fail or promotion decisions, examination developers will need to consider examination security, especially if cases are to be used in future assessments or across multiple testing sessions.

Examination Content

An essential initial step in examination development is to delineate the general content of the assessment. Regardless of whether its purpose is formative or summative, one must decide what domains (skills) are to be measured and the specific types of clinical encounters that need to be simulated in order to accomplish this. If this is done properly, with particular reference to the

goals of the evaluation, evidence to support the content validity of the assessment will be procured. Delineation of examination content is accomplished via development of a detailed blueprint which maps the skills to be measured (e.g., physical examination) into the specific assessment content (simulated patient presentations, reasons for the patient visiting the doctor) (Fig. 8-3).

The process of developing a blueprint is multifaceted and should involve a review of relevant educational objectives and the curriculum, including textbooks and course outlines. In addition, local, regional, and national healthcare provider statistics can be referenced to ensure that any modeled encounters reflect typical reasons for patient visits to the doctor.[24] Review of educational objectives and materials and the analysis of health care statistics on the frequency of patient presentations are two, often complimentary, approaches for categorizing the clinical material in the blueprint. Categorization per review of health care databases will yield clinical cases that are defined by presenting complaints/reasons for visiting the physician (e.g., leg pain, shortness of breath). Alternatively, review of educational materials or objectives will likely result in a distribution of cases into organ-based or discipline-specific categories. For example, an examination at the end of a medicine clerkship may include cases divided into the common organ-specific subspecialties, one from each of the

	Reason for Visit/ Presenting Complaint				
	Cardiovascular / Respiratory	Gastrointestinal / Genitourinary	Neurology / Psychiatry	General Symptoms	Other: *Skin, nails, and hair; Eyes and ears; Musculoskeletal*
Gender: *at least 3 male 3 female*					
Age: *at least 2 > 64 2 = 45 - 64 2 = 15 – 44*					
Acuity: *at least 2 acute 2 subacute 2 chronic*					
Physical Finding: *at least 2 with findings per form*					

Figure 8-3 Basic blueprint for a multistation standardized patient (SP) assessment. To ensure content validity, the cases are classified according to reasons for visit/presenting complaint (x axis) and patient/case characteristics (y axis). Assuming that a 10-station assessment was being delivered, one could choose two cases from each of the x axis classifications. Although this is fairly straightforward, one must also keep in mind that a mix of patient characteristics (e.g., gender, age) and case representations (e.g., acuity) must also be achieved if accurate representation of a broad clinical population is required. With numerous cases to choose from, as would be the case for a national examination, and reasonable constraints, the process is fairly straightforward. However, if there are relatively few cases, and numerous constraints, it may be very difficult to satisfy any well-meaning test specifications. For a medical school or residency-based assessment, when there are usually limited resources to develop cases, it would be best to develop a general blueprint based on medical content and patient characteristics and then purposefully assemble a limited set of cases that satisfies the necessary constraints.

following areas: cardiology, nephrology, gastroenterology, etc. An end-of-third-year examination may include cases from each of the core clerkships, distributed by specialty or by clerkship duration: one case per clerkship or one case per 6-week interval (thereby allotting more case content to longer clerkships). Regardless of the chosen method of case categorization, one should keep in mind that valid interpretations of examinee performance relate to the extent that examination content reflects important educational goals and objectives, whether it is introduced into a course, clerkship, academic year, or residency program.

A well-developed examination blueprint also serves an important role in optimizing the reliability of the scores produced. Score reliability is dependent on several factors, including heterogeneity of the examinee group, complexity of individual cases, accuracy in SP case portrayal and scoring, the particular skill(s) being tested, and usually most important, the number and type of encounters. Regrettably, while the scoring of SP-based assessments is described in detail in the

literature,[11,13] there is relatively little empirical research available to specifically guide the development and selection of rubrics, the choice and training of evaluators who employ them, or as is often referenced for other testing modalities, optimal test design. However, with respect to performance-based assessments in general, the available literature would suggest that the reliability of the assessment scores is primarily a function of test length (number of encounters) and not the choice of raters. So, in general, if one wants to improve the reliability of assessment scores, it is best to increase the length of the test. In their review of the literature, van der Vleuten and Swanson found that these types of performance-based SP assessments needed to range from 3 to 12 hours in duration to obtain a generalizability coefficient of 0.80.[25] For assessments that are geared toward the formative evaluation of individual trainees or programmatic activities (e.g., determine the adequacy of curriculum content), shorter test lengths may be appropriate. When used for programmatic assessment, compiling aggregate data from individual examinee performances may provide more reliable results, even when one or only a few cases are used.

Because physicians and physicians-in-training demonstrate considerable variability in performance depending upon the clinical content of the case encountered (content or case specificity), the breadth and number of encounters are critical determinants of examination reliability. Content specificity, as mentioned earlier, is the primary variable influencing the reliability of scores from such examinations. Therefore, to obtain a precise measure of an examinee's overall clinical skill, an adequate number of cases of sufficiently broad content should be included in the assessment. Multiple station SP examinations that are designed to sample skills more broadly over the course of the assessment compensate for the psychometric limitations inherent in a single encounter and, in general, lead to more reliable assessment of clinical competence.[26,27]

With respect to the time an examinee must spend with the SP in individual encounters, shorter stations (5 to 10 minutes) are as reliable as longer ones (≥ 20 minutes) and, depending upon resources and total time allotted for testing, may be preferred. For a fixed unit of testing time, they allow inclusion of more cases and the assessment of particular skills over a broader range of content.[28] However, one must be careful to provide sufficient time for the given clinical task; failure to do so may reinforce inappropriate test-taking behaviors (e.g., rapid-fire questioning) that could potentially yield high checklist scores but invalid measures of clinical proficiency. In general, the time allotted to an individual encounter should be appropriate to the task so as to promote behaviors and pace that are relevant to the particular clinical situation.[29]

In terms of the tasks assessed in SP-based examinations, more reliable results are obtained when basic clinical skills (e.g., data gathering) are measured, as opposed to assessment of more complex patient management skills. Stillman found that reliable assessment of data gathering skills required 6 to 10 cases, but 25 or more cases were necessary to reliably assess differential diagnosis ability or the appropriate use of diagnostic studies.[30] Thus, SP-based assessments are most efficiently applied to the assessment of data gathering, communication and interpersonal skills.

Depending upon the assessment goals, in addition to including the relevant skills and clinical cases in the blueprint, it may also be important to consider both the clinical setting and other patient characteristics that reflect the broader population upon which the evaluation is intended to reflect. Related to educational objectives (or perhaps relevant health care statistics), examination developers should decide the proportion of cases that are to represent acute, subacute, and chronic presentations and the setting in which such patients are encountered (inpatient, ambulatory clinic, emergency department, etc). Lastly, depending upon educational goals and health care data, the examination blueprint should also consider relevant patient characteristics such as race, ethnicity, age, and gender. However, as the blueprint becomes increasingly complex and multifactorial, it may be necessary at some point for the examination developer to delimit the critical categories according to curricular objectives and then attempt to reach reasonable proportions for the other areas by careful SP recruiting and case assignment. In many cases it will be helpful to construct a matrix, or examination content outline, to inform case development and allocation (see Fig. 8-3).

Case Development and Standardized Patient Training

One of the assumptions made in writing this chapter is that physicians involved in medical education at the undergraduate or graduate level will have access to a clinical skills center and professional staff, including a standardized patient trainer. Although physician educators may acquire much knowledge and experience in the use of SP-based methods, very few will have either the time or expertise to engage in the many day-to-day activities required to develop and manage SP-based assessment programs. Most of the following information is intended to help physician educators understand their potential contributions to the evaluation process, and to participate effectively and meaningfully in the development and administration of SP-based assessments at their institutions.

Physician educators should understand that SPs comprise a wide variety of individuals with different life and health experiences, educational backgrounds, and occupations. SP trainers and clinical skills center staff apply a variety of implicit or explicit criteria in recruiting and hiring their SPs. They must consider factors such as occupational background (some will likely be actors), intellectual ability, geographic stability, emotional stability, motivation, and availability in general.[20,31] Additionally, in selecting SPs for individual assessments, they need to consider previous health experiences and individual patient characteristics such as age, gender, race, ethnicity, and physical attributes (such as stable or transient physical findings) as they relate to specific clinical case requirements. However, the value of selecting SPs who have prior experience with the medical problem they are supposed to simulate isn't clearly established. Although their previous experience may lead to a more authentic portrayal of the clinical problem, when necessary, they may not be able to disentangle their personal medical history from case simulation requirements.[20,32] As would be expected, people who are hostile or bitter toward the medical profession should not be hired as SPs.

For case development and training, clinician educators play an important role in interacting with SP training staff, and educational or measurement experts.[20] Course, clerkship, and program directors should identify the cases to be included in the assessment or examination. Course directors and faculty can be surveyed to determine which skills need to be measured and how much evaluation emphasis should be placed on each. They should work with the case development team as content experts to create the case materials, either calling upon their own clinical experiences to help develop cases de novo or reviewing existing SP case lists to select those that, with or without modification, will meet assessment goals. Unfortunately, when it comes to developing simulated clinical scenarios, it may be difficult for faculty to provide the most useful case material. Faculty often have a tendency to model initial case scenarios after relatively rare or unnecessarily complex patient presentations. In general, due to the performance demands placed on the standardized patient, these types of cases are difficult to administer and often provide only marginal evaluation data. Nevertheless, with proper case development training, including repeated emphasis on the purpose of the assessment, assembling individual case scenarios can be efficient and productive and, most important, yield valid and meaningful assessment results.

Physician participation in SP training will be valuable in addressing issues that impact portrayal and scoring accuracy. Here, they can help the SP understand the clinical problem that he/she is presenting, provide feedback on affect simulation, and guide individuals in the correct scoring of physical examination maneuvers.[32] Physicians can also provide an important service by performing a thorough screening physical examination on individual SPs. Standardized patients can have unknown or unexpected physical findings that can affect case portrayal and difficulty, causing the examinees to pursue different lines of inquiry than intended by case developers.[33]

Scoring the Assessment/Sources of Measurement Error

Checklists and Rating Scales

Although the number of encounters in an SP-based assessment is the primary determinant of overall score reliability, the choice of assessment instrument can still have an appreciable impact on the psychometric adequacy of the scores. The most common means of evaluating performance during SP examinations involves the use of checklists and rating scales. A content-based checklist is generally used to record whether specific actions are taken by the examinee. These checklists are often used to score history-taking and physical examination performance. Examinee actions are recorded in a categorical fashion (most often, dichotomously) where a check indicates whether the expected history items were asked or specific examination maneuvers were performed (correctly). This is the approach used in the United States Medical Licensing Examination Step 2 Clinical Skills,[34] wherein the SP completes the checklist immediately following the encounter. Another approach to the checklist requires the recorder to indicate whether an examination maneuver was performed incorrectly or correctly, thus allowing for three scoring options. Regardless of how the categorical data are obtained, one can choose to weight specific items based on their clinical relevance. However, given the interdependence among history-taking questions and physical examination maneuvers, and the difficulties inherent with deciding how much more important one action is as opposed to another, the use of weights can be problematic, and may not make much difference in terms of providing meaningful assessment scores.

Most commonly, history and physical examination checklists will be composed during initial case development work and, as a general rule, should be consistent with the goals and objectives of the assessment exercise. Therefore, it is important to decide a priori how checklists will be used. If the intention is to assess the data-gathering abilities of a novice learner in an introductory physical diagnosis course, then it is probably appropriate to include detailed and thorough checklists relevant to the data-gathering task. Such a detailed checklist will allow course or clerkship directors to explicitly define and communicate the learning or clinical objectives related to the skill or clinical task. For higher level learners, or for use in making high-stakes decisions, checklists should reflect the relative importance of specific actions or maneuvers in relation to the presenting complaint(s).

To choose checklist content, the case development team should be attentive to the potential for rewarding thoroughness or inappropriate test-taking behaviors rather than assessing true clinical competence. That is, more capable examinees that arrive at the appropriate diagnostic or management decision via a more efficient, or alternative, data-gathering approach should not be penalized. Clinicians will need to avoid a natural tendency to include too many checklist items. Piloting the case and checklist with more senior trainees or other faculty who are unfamiliar with case details may provide an important "reality check." This process will often serve to reduce the number of unnecessary checklist items and, occasionally, will result in the addition of one or more important items that initial case

developers had not considered. In general, it is a good idea to limit checklist lengths to 10 to 20 items; longer checklists can exceed most SPs' ability to accurately recall specific elements of examinee performance.[35]

It also is important that clinician educators work with SP trainers to ensure individual checklist items represent specific, observable behaviors that are amenable to categorical scoring. Unnecessarily complex checklist items that require SPs to interpret examinee intentions or recall multiple actions can lead to inaccuracies in checklist recording.[35] For example, rather than using "The examinee asked about factors that precipitated my chest pain," separate checklist items should state: "The examinee asked whether physical exertion caused my chest pain;" "The examinee asked if taking a deep breath caused my chest pain;" and "The examinee asked if sitting up caused my chest pain." Checklist items should also reward the kind of communication behaviors, such as use of open-ended questions, emphasized in health communications training. For example, a checklist item on description of pain could be given by the SP for an open-ended question, such as, "Tell me more." This makes the encounter seem more realistic, as opposed to having the SP reply, "What do you want me to tell you, doctor? " When crafting the training materials for the SPs, it is important to provide lists of examples of the kinds of questions examinees may use to receive credit for each item.

Although comprising a large body of information on SP-based methods in general, the academic literature provides little guidance to those developing case-specific checklists.[36] Very few published articles actually describe the process by which checklists were constructed. Nevertheless, it seems prudent to restrict checklist content to those items that are supported by clinical evidence or strong consensus views of faculty. The checklists can then be refined based on pilot administrations of the cases.

Alternative methods for scoring SP-based encounters employ various types of rating scales.[37–39] Rating scales are often used when the skill or behavior being assessed requires some multifaceted judgment of examinee performance that is not amenable to dichotomous scoring. Rating scales are commonly used for measuring communication and interpersonal skills and in assessing humanistic or professional behaviors. Typically, as with global rating scales used by experts in real clinical settings, adequate rater training and the provision of descriptors or anchors within the scale are essential for obtaining a reliable and valid assessment of examinee performance.

For measuring clinical skills, there is, and will probably continue to be, a controversy in the academic literature about the utility of checklists as opposed to global rating scales. Although published data suggest that global ratings may be more valid for discriminating among the clinical skills of more experienced clinicians, the differences described are generally small and probably related (in part) to the fact that both checklists and global ratings have at least some associated measurement error and may be quantifying different performance attributes.[40] Research conducted to date would suggest that, provided the rater training is adequate, the choice of analytic or holistic scales will not have an appreciable impact on score reliability.[41] However, depending on the purpose of the examination, the ability level of the examinees, and the specific construction of the holistic (rating scales) or analytic (checklist) instruments, the validity of the resultant scores could be affected. For example, it has been documented that more experienced physicians may actually score less well on checklists. This is likely due to their ability to take shortcuts, thereby minimizing the amount of information they must collect to formulate a reasonable differential diagnosis. Nevertheless, with careful instrument development or selection and rater training, potential validity problems can be minimized, and the decision whether to use checklists or global ratings can be based primarily upon examination objectives.[18] As mentioned earlier, checklists are better suited for the assessment of whether an examinee asks critical history questions or performs essential physical examination maneuvers for a given case. They are also apropos when specific feedback is being provided to trainees. In contrast, global rating scales are more appropriately applied to the evaluation of multifaceted domains such as communication and interpersonal skills. Here, the SPs or other qualified raters may have a better perspective on what constitutes adequate and inadequate performance. Moreover, the use of checklists (e.g., makes eye contact, introduces self) for constructs such as doctor-patient communication may reward specific actions yet fail to validly capture the essential, and often difficult to quantify, elements of the interaction.

Training the Evaluators

Apart from the choice of scoring rubrics, the evaluators (SPs, peers, faculty observers, or other parties) must be recruited and trained to use the measurement scales consistently and fairly. Even though task sampling variability tends to be high on SP-based assessments, rater variability can still have a measurable impact on score precision, especially when the evaluators are not provided with proper guidance concerning the crediting of correct actions or the assignment of ratings. For the history-taking and physical examination checklists typically employed in SP-based assessments, the SP, or any other person who documents the data-gathering activities, must be trained to understand variations in candidate questioning and discern between correct and incorrect physical examination maneuvers. Physician input into SP training will be helpful in elucidating acceptable and unacceptable variation in clinical approaches to specific cases. For any rating scales employed, the evaluators must be taught to differentiate performance along some relevant continuum. If this training is not done properly, a candidate's score may simply reflect the choice of rater (e.g., "hawk" or "dove") as opposed to his or her true ability.

Fortunately, with proper selection and training, and effective quality assurance procedures, SPs and other evaluators can be trained to provide reasonably reproducible scores. Training often includes role play, review of memorization techniques, and the development and utilization of pilot test exercises involving benchmarked videotapes of modeled clinical encounters. Although both systematic (e.g., bias) and random (e.g., memory) sources of rater error cannot be eliminated entirely, they can be effectively controlled, thus alleviating some potential threats to the validity of the assessment scores. It needs to be emphasized, however, that some individuals (e.g., those with inherent biases against medical practitioners, inadequate memory) will make poor SPs. Likewise, faculty evaluators can have preconceived, and often unrealistic, performance expectations that are not well aligned with learning objectives or, more important, easy to change. Therefore, where possible, it makes sense to screen SPs and other evaluators prior to using them as part of an assessment team.

Score-Equating Strategies

For SP-based assessments, especially those used for high-stakes decisions such as academic promotion or licensure, steps must be taken to ensure that all examinees have a fair and equal opportunity to show their "true" ability. As mentioned in the previous section, regardless of training, some evaluators may be more stringent or lenient than others. Therefore, if examinees are not assessed under identical conditions (i.e., the same evaluators) it is important that score adjustments, where necessary, be made. Otherwise, the fairness of the assessment could be called into question. Similarly, because different cases are often used as part of the same assessment, one must account for their difficulty. If difficulty is ignored, an examinee who encountered a more challenging set of cases would receive a test score that would most certainly underestimate his/her true ability. In contrast, without any adjustments, an examinee who encountered an easier test form (mix of cases) would benefit, potentially compromising the validity of the assessment results.

For many medical school or residency-based SP assessments, especially those whose purpose is primarily formative in nature, there is usually no need for score adjustment. Here, most students will see the same cases and SPs, usually over the course of several assessment sessions. Moreover, the assessment results will be used to provide feedback and perhaps to identify those trainees who are in need of remediation. When the assessment is more summative in nature, as is the case for certification and licensure examinations, or as part of medical school graduation requirements, the application of equating strategies specifically developed for performance-based assessments is relatively straightforward, provided that specific attention is paid to test administration (e.g., selection of cases, SPs) and data collection.[19] Thus, regardless of the difficulty of the test form, or the choice of particular evaluators, all examinees will be treated fairly.

For summative medical school or residency assessments (e.g., those used as a graduation requirement), where the number of examinees encountering a particular case and the number of evaluators employed can be small, it can sometimes be difficult to implement score-equating strategies. This is due to the fact that estimates of case difficulty and rater stringency will be less precise with fewer test takers. However, if some of the same cases are used from year to year, estimates derived from previous student performances can be used to ascertain the difficulty of specific cases and test forms. Provided that the overall student ability from year to year does not fluctuate much, these "common" cases can be used to link assessment forms. For measured traits such as doctor-patient communication, at least for examinations that measure basic clinical skills, one would not expect that the choice of case would overly influence student performance. Assuming that the evaluators, on average, encounter students of relatively equal ability, simply calculating the mean performance, by evaluator, will yield estimates of rater stringency/leniency. These statistics can be used to make adjustments to individual student ratings, thus preserving the fairness of the assessment.

Quality Assurance

Despite efforts to develop high-quality checklist items and limit checklist length, it is likely that recording errors will occur.[42,43] SPs tend to commit more errors of commission than omission, giving examinees credit for action not taken about two or three times more often than failing to record actual examinee actions.[35,44] Nevertheless, efforts to ensure that SPs are optimally prepared for their simulations, including the implementation of quality assurance programs that provide for periodic observation and monitoring of SP portrayal and scoring accuracy can significantly reduce SP errors in these areas.[45]

To ensure the accuracy of examinee scores, specific steps must be taken to document the numerous evaluative processes that take place in an SP-based assessment. First, albeit qualitative in nature, some indication of portrayal fidelity must be secured. If an SP is not performing the case as expected (e.g., affect is not consistent with the case), then the examinee may be less likely to ask certain questions or perform related physical examination maneuvers. As a result, the data-gathering score for the examinee, be it obtained via checklists or more holistic ratings, will be error-prone. Quality assurance through periodic observation, either live or via videotaped encounters, with feedback provided to the SP regarding accuracy in portrayal will likely improve consistency.

Another quality assurance approach can be implemented using a second rater. For any scores that are obtained, some subset should be verified, usually through the use of a second rater, either an SP, a trainer, or a physician evaluator. Although this second score will likely do little to enhance the overall reliability of the assessment currently being conducted, provided that a proper sampling framework is utilized, these data can be used to identify SPs who may not be scoring accurately or other evaluators who are not using the rating scales as intended. It should be noted that if additional SPs are available, and enhanced overall reliability is the goal, it makes more sense to add an extra case rather than provide additional scores for existing cases.[46] Finally, it is extremely important to periodically review case materials, including checklists. The practice of medicine is not static, and the importance of certain interview questions or physical examination maneuvers may change over time.

With respect to who should be doing the scoring, the available research suggests that there is not much difference in accuracy between SP or physician raters for assessing history-taking or physical examination skills; however, if more complex diagnostic or management skills are being evaluated, where expertise and experience are paramount, it is probably necessary to have experienced physicians rate examinee performance.[30,47,48] Research has also shown that when multiple SPs play the same case, appropriate training and feedback lead to accuracy and consistency in case portrayal and checklist recording.[49] Finally, SPs are marginally better in simulating and recording aspects of the history than in portraying affect (severity of pain) or in scoring aspects of the physical examination.[35,44]

Standard Setting

For many SP-based assessment activities, there is little need to develop or apply specific performance standards. If the evaluation is formative in nature, and competency or proficiency decisions are not desired, setting specific performance standards is usually not necessary. Instead, the scores (i.e., specific checklist performance, summary ratings), often tabulated as percentiles, are used to provide normative feedback to the examinees. If, however, the assessment is being used for summative purposes (e.g., course success, graduation), there will be a need to determine the score, or scores, that delimit those who possess adequate skills from those who do not.

Regrettably, unlike traditional multiple-choice tests, the development of standard-setting methodologies for SP-based assessments is relatively immature. Nevertheless, by borrowing from the performance assessment literature, and adapting some common techniques, reasonably efficient and effective methods to set standards for SP-based clinical simulations have been produced.[50,51] The most promising techniques generally involve the recruitment of clinician experts to review performances (e.g., videotapes) or adequate proxies (e.g., completed checklists) and make judgments regarding the competencies of those individuals who are represented in the performances.[52] These judgments are then regressed onto the scores to delimit the point on the score scale that maximally discriminates between those who have the necessary skills and those who do not. For example, a panel of physicians may be shown a series of videotapes of student performances and asked to make summary proficiency judgments regarding the adequacy of doctor-patient communication. For truly poor performance, it is likely that all panelists will agree that proficiency was not evidenced; a similar consensus is likely for excellent performance. However, somewhere along the ability continuum, the panelists will disagree with respect to proficiency. Provided that there is a sufficient number of panelists, and adequate samples of student performances, the judgments can be used to ascertain the point on the score scale that discriminates between proficient and not proficient performance. Mathematical techniques (e.g., linear regression) can easily be used to delimit this specific point.

Regardless of the method chosen to set performance standards, those involved in the process (i.e., physicians) tend to have unrealistically high performance expectations. This is probably related, at least in part, to the fact that some physicians have little insight into the abilities of their trainees, having rarely observed them interacting with patients. Additionally, current checklist development practices are often not adequately informed by clinical evidence, allowing consensus-based approaches to drive a performance standard that may not be consistent with good clinical practice.[53] Therefore, when embarking upon the standard-setting process for SP-based examinations, it is particularly important that the standard-setting panelists (usually physicians) have a common definition of the purpose of the assessment and are intimately aware of the complexities and nuances of the evaluation method. Often, in addition to a thorough orientation, standard-setting panelists are invited to partake in part of the assessment (e.g., be an examinee for a few cases) as a means to align their expectations with reality.

Identifying Threats to Validity

In conjunction with a defined quality assurance plan, it is essential to investigate potential threats to the validity of the assessment, especially for ones that involve human ratings, cover relatively limited content, or are used for high-stakes decisions. This may involve a number of strategies, including the investigation of test administration protocols (e.g., examinees have enough time for certain cases),[29] the identification of biased evaluators,[54,55] the analysis of the relationships between SP-based assessment scores and other markers of ability,[56,57] the examination of test security issues (e.g., students who take the examination later in the cycle benefit from prior information),[58–60] or if cut-scores are used, the validation of the standards.[61] Over time, these research practices will help to ensure that the examinee scores are true reflections of their abilities. Also, provided that the results from these investigations do not identify serious threats to the interpretability of the assessment scores, trainees will be more accepting of the evaluation and less likely to challenge their results.

Standardized Patient–Based Methods for Evaluating the ACGME General Competencies

SP-based assessment methods can be applied to measurement of educational outcomes in each of the ACGME competencies. In particular, SP-based methods

are ideally suited for assessing *interpersonal and communications skills* and the patient-centered elements (eliciting patient information and preferences in making informed decisions, gathering essential and accurate information from patients, and counseling and educating patients) within the *patient care* domain. As highlighted in the previous sections, SP-based assessments can provide reliable and valid measures of basic clinical skills such as history taking, physical examination, communication, and interpersonal skills. Multiple-station SP examinations may be used in measuring educational needs or outcomes before, during, and upon completion of a wide range of educational programs, courses, clerkships, rotations, and academic years. For learning and subsequently evaluating basic and more advanced skills, SPs, as with other simulation methods, provide for the safe transition from the classroom to the clinic.

Although SP-based methods are not efficient when applied to the evaluation of *medical knowledge*, they may be used to measure the application of knowledge in simulated patient care situations. The SP encounter can be supplemented with structured global ratings such as the mini-CEX or, to tap other important skills, combined with a patient note or some form of chart-stimulated recall process. Because these types of evaluation approaches model those currently used in real clinical settings, they are more readily accepted, both by those who are responsible for the assessment and by those who are being assessed. Here, program or clerkship directors may also decide to employ SPs for assessment of knowledge application in important medical cases that are infrequently or inconsistently encountered during clinical rotations.

Standardized patients may be used individually, or as part of multiple-station exercises, to assess behaviors intrinsic to *professionalism*. Although it is apparent that SPs are useful in determining whether students and residents have the capacity to behave in a professional and humanistic manner, demonstration of these skills within the context of an instructional or assessment exercise does not guarantee that the associated behaviors will be manifest in day-to-day performance. Continuous and episodic observation of trainee performance in a variety of clinical contexts, by a diverse group of assessors, is needed to ensure maintenance of professional behaviors (see Chapter 6).

The flexibility of SP-based methods also facilitates development of assessment exercises to measure competence in *practice-based learning and improvement* (PBLI), *systems-based practice* (SBP), and in the patient management aspects (developing and carrying out patient management plans, providing preventive health care services) of the *patient care* competency. Faculty, clerkship, and program directors can work with SP training staff to develop cases to evaluate trainees' abilities to analyze their own patient care experience; to search, appraise, and apply scientific evidence in patient management; to use information technology in managing patient information and online resources; and to provide appropriate care for selected conditions and health maintenance. Similarly, cases can be constructed to measure the capacity to function within a health care team, the cost-effective use of diagnostic and therapeutic modalities for a range of clinical presentations, and the ability to advocate for patients in negotiating system-related complexities and obstacles to effective health care.

The Use of Unannounced Standardized Patients for Assessing Patient Care, PBLI, and SBP

The placement of unannounced SPs into real clinical settings can be an effective method for measuring important educational outcomes. An initial study of physician performance using unannounced SPs may also provide the impetus and evidence for trainee or faculty developed approaches to quality improvement. The utility of this approach spans undergraduate, graduate, and continuing medical education. Published studies describe a variety of applications, ranging from the assessment of quality of care and resource utilization for common conditions to the evaluation of more focused efforts in preventive care or select abilities, such as HIV risk assessment, cancer prevention, screening for domestic violence, interviewing skills, or counseling for behavioral modification.[62–68]

The rationale for using SPs in this manner is related to concerns about conventional measures of clinical performance and quality of care.[66,69,70] Commonly used measures, such as audits of medical records, claims or utilization data, physician self-reports, videotaped patient encounters, or simulation-based approaches in a testing center context, are plagued by an array of methodological and psychometric hurdles. For example, the suboptimal sensitivity and specificity of medical record audits raise questions about their validity for measuring quality of care.[71,72]

The use of unannounced (also referred to as blinded, covert, incognito, undetected, or unidentified) SPs has the potential to circumvent some of the measurement problems and potential biases associated with conventional evaluation methods.[66,69,70] Highly trained SPs portraying realistic clinical scenarios, and using well-developed scoring instruments and appropriate supplemental information, have produced evaluations with acceptable psychometric properties, allowing for valid interpretations of performance related to multiple attributes and health care outcomes.[64,69,73,74] To the extent that they are undetected, unannounced SPs provide for unobtrusive assessment of authentic behaviors in the actual practice setting. Careful case selection and development, coupled with standardized and consistent portrayal and scoring, can negate selection bias and obviate the need for case-mix or complexity adjustments.[75] However, inconsistencies in portrayal or scoring may adversely affect the accuracy of performance assessment, and evaluators should understand that valid interpretations of overall performance may be limited by typical (and appropriate) physician behaviors during single or first patient visits.[44,76] Capturing preventive health care practices or discussions of sensitive issues may require assessment approaches that span more than one visit. When important decisions are made about physician performance using unannounced SPs, ensuring accuracy in scoring through rigorous pretesting and quality assurance practices (such as audio- or videotape monitoring of SP performance) or supplementing SP scoring with other data (medical record audits, test requests) should be considered.[44]

Based on past research, unannounced SPs are able to provide for reliable and valid assessment of clinical performance. Some experts suggest that unannounced SPs are the "gold standard" for assessing quality of health care as well as measuring the effect of education on practice.[53,74] Residents and practicing physicians who have participated in studies using unannounced SPs have been satisfied with their experience, have been agreeable to future participation with this method, and have endorsed the validity and usefulness of the feedback provided and positive effects on patient care.[77] Nevertheless, methodological and logistical demands, including related costs, may limit the practical application of these techniques.[70] In particular, the intensity of SP training requirements and the rigorous attention to detail necessary to avoid exposure limit their deployment for more routine assessment activities.[75] Their use probably should be restricted to obtaining specific and detailed information in focused quality studies, evaluating the performance of groups of physicians, or identifying deficiencies in educational programs.

Strengths and Weaknesses of Standardized Patient–Based Methods for Education and Assessment

Strengths

One of the notable advantages of using SPs for teaching and evaluating clinical skills is the requirement for direct observation of the interaction between the student or resident and the SP. Regardless of whether the observer/rater is a trained SP, faculty member, peer, or other party, the assessment of skills is not inferred from case presentations, preceptor sessions, or review of the medical record. The incorporation of some form of direct observation of students and residents is critical in that there are ample data suggesting that trainees at all levels have deficiencies in basic physical diagnosis skills and often lack adequate training in these areas in medical school.[78–80]

The integration of SPs into educational activities allows the program, course, or clerkship director to exert a degree of control over instructional and assessment activities. Encounters with SPs can be scheduled to coincide with, or complement, other relevant educational or assessment activities in a manner that is consistent with learner needs. This is quite different from education in actual clinical settings where a particular learning experience depends on if and when patients are available. The SP exercise can be manipulated to be consistent with the academic level of the learner or to serve specific individual or programmatic needs. For example, slight modifications in case emphasis or portrayal can change a history-taking task to one requiring counseling or more complex communication skills; adding a patient note as a post-encounter exercise can change the focus of the case from assessment of data gathering to evaluation of diagnostic management and documentation. In addition to modifying SP cases to focus on different aspects of clinical competence, encounters can be manipulated to incorporate a range of clinically relevant phenomena, such as variability in clinical presentation for the same or similar conditions, or the effect of time on clinical processes.

While allowing for flexibility in tailoring instruction and formative assessment to the level and needs of the learner and program, SP-based methods may also be used to promote consistency and standardization of clinical content for the purposes of higher stakes assessment. Examinees are exposed to the same clinical problem presented uniformly, eliminating the need to control for the uncertainties of case complexity and comorbidity, patient preferences, and other complex factors associated with patient care. The ability to standardize clinical content, case portrayal, and scoring allows SP methods to be deployed in multiple station examinations at various junctures in the educational process. As a result, important decisions regarding advancement, promotion, or even graduation, can be made.

From the student and resident perspective, the use of SPs for formative assessment allows them to practice and receive feedback on their clinical skills in an environment that is nonthreatening and poses no risk of harm to real patients. However, depending upon the trainee's ability to suspend disbelief and buy into the simulation, some exposure to SPs may be necessary before he/she feels fully comfortable and is able to obtain maximum pedagogical benefit. Nonetheless, the nonthreatening nature and low risk for such exercises makes the use of SPs an ideal method for teaching and assessment of difficult or sensitive communication or physical examination challenges. In particular, SPs have proved to be a valuable resource for teaching and assessment of an examinee's ability to deliver bad news to a patient, to discuss preferences for end-of-life care, to engage in patient counseling or education, and in teaching and assessing breast, rectal, and genitourinary examinations.[81–83] As the use of SPs allows manipulation of the clinical encounter to focus teaching/assessment on various aspects of clinical competence, simulated encounters can also be manipulated to enhance the quality of feedback provided and offer opportunities for trainees to learn different approaches and develop flexibility in their strategies when encountering various patient problems and presentations. For example, use of the "freeze-frame" or "time-out" technique, where the SP encounter is interrupted in order to provide formative assessment and feedback, allows the trainee to practice those skills or develop alternative approaches to difficult clinical situations.

The use of SPs for formative assessment activities often enhances the quality of feedback provided. Various observers can provide immediate and corrective feedback to examinees, focusing on discrete skills and behaviors. The SPs themselves can also be trained to provide valuable patient perspectives regarding trainee skills and behaviors. Videotaped encounters can be rated by faculty, peers, SPs, or the trainees themselves. Review of videotapes can be accomplished using a stimulated-recall process, allowing evaluators to gather important diagnostic information, including when errors of commission or omission occur. Such techniques will certainly be useful in the evaluation of marginal or problem students or residents.

The use of SPs, either individually or as part of multiple-station clinical skills examinations, not only allows clerkship and program directors to obtain valuable feedback concerning individual trainees but also enables them to determine whether the program as a whole has been successful in achieving important curricular objectives. Using SP-based methods for program evaluation is ideal in that it identifies the patient encounter as a critical event in which learning should occur and on which individual assessment will focus. The well-known influence of assessment on learning will result in renewed interest in clinical medicine and focus attention on developing patient-centered skills. Because a sound educational program is dependent upon the synergistic relationship and interaction between course objectives, curriculum, and evaluation, thinking about how assessment will link to learning objectives and educational experiences will encourage course and program directors to think broadly about educational strategies and how limited resources may be best deployed. For example, patient logs may indicate that certain important clinical experiences are rarely or unpredictably encountered in the course of various clinical rotations. By introducing SPs during or after the educational experience, faculty can ensure that trainees have the relevant experience, better enabling them to develop critical knowledge and skills.

Weaknesses

One of the obvious concerns about the implementation of SP-based teaching and assessment programs is the potential cost. Hiring SP trainers and SPs can be expensive, and depending upon the location of the program, they may be difficult to locate and recruit. Likewise, finding the time and space to conduct SP-based teaching and assessment activities may be difficult for programs that do not have clinical skills centers or are not affiliated with institutions where such centers are located. Faculty development efforts may also be necessary for individuals to participate meaningfully in case and test development, feedback, standard setting, and evaluation activities. Unfortunately, the observation and rating skills that faculty may have obtained in real clinical settings do not automatically transfer when passing through the doors of a simulation center or clinical skills laboratory. Conversely, faculty who lack adequate observation and rating skills probably will not spontaneously acquire them within the confines of a clinical skills center. Faculty development continues to be an important priority for educational leaders, regardless of the content or processes involved in educational or assessment activities.

As a remedy for logistical and cost concerns, there is an increasing trend toward the introduction of clinical skills facilities in academic institutions as well as the continued development of regional consortia focusing on the use of SPs (and other simulation methods) in education and assessment. Programs and institutions combine resources and expertise, minimizing financial and other resource commitments and ensuring the availability of SPs, case material, and trained personnel. Such consortia have already been created in various geographic areas.[84,85]

One marked weakness of SP-based methods is that there is a limit on the number of physical findings that can be demonstrated or simulated. In this respect, it is important to remember that SPs are a supplement to, not a replacement for, real patients. A high volume of "real" patient contact is still required for a trainee to appreciate the diversity of clinical presentations. A recent study also raised concerns regarding the ability to make judgments about overall physical examination skills based upon demonstration of technical proficiency alone. Chalabian and Dunning noted that there was a limited relationship between breast examination skills assessed during an SP encounter and breast lump detection sensitivity and specificity using breast models.[86]

Following on this theme, it is important to remember that the performance of students and residents in assessment environments may not define their capacity to perform in real clinical settings. In fact, data describing the use of SPs in assessing practicing physician competence suggest that there may be a significant difference between demonstrated capacity to perform (competence) and actual performance in practice.[87,88] There is clearly an observation effect (Hawthorne effect) operating under such simulated conditions. Although it is important for educators to require that trainees periodically demonstrate acquisition of the relevant competencies, this should not be taken as absolute evidence that such abilities will be exercised in real clinical settings. Therefore, building evaluation systems that ensure that the relevant knowledge, skills, and behaviors are manifest in the day-to-day activities of future physicians is critical.

Conclusion

Standardized patients are a valuable tool for inclusion in a multifaceted assessment program. They are particularly well suited for measuring basic clinical skills. Deployed covertly into real clinical settings, they provide for precise and accurate assessment of a variety of clinical skills and patient management practices. A particular advantage provided by SP-based methods is their unique malleability. They can be applied to a wide range of assessment objectives and trainee levels, allowing for flexibility in instructional and formative assessment approaches. Amenability to standardization allows SP-based methods to support important summative assessment as well. Regrettably, a significant requirement for capital and expertise limits their broad application and acceptance in the medical education community. As with any other assessment tool, their inclusion in comprehensive educational and evaluation programs will depend upon institutional culture, goals and objectives, and resources.

ACKNOWLEDGMENT

The authors wish to thank Gail Furman, PhD, RN, for her thoughtful review and suggestions for improving this chapter.

ANNOTATED BIBLIOGRAPHY

Assessment and Case Development

1. King AM, Pohl H, Perkowski-Rogers LC: Planning standardized patient programs: Case development, patient training, and costs. Teach Learn Med 1994;6(1):6–14.
2. Stillman P, Swanson D, Regan MB, et al: Assessment of clinical skills of residents utilizing standardized patients. A follow-up study and recommendations for application. Ann Intern Med 1991;114(5):393–401.
3. Olive KE, Elnicki DM, Kelley MJ: A practical approach to developing cases for standardized patients. Adv Health Sci Educ Theory Pract 1997;2:49–60.
4. Stillman PL: Technical issues: Logistics. AAMC Acad Med 1993;68(6):464–468.
   These articles address some of the main issues involved in examination and case development, including SP selection and training.

Quality Assurance

5. Wallace P, Garman K, Heine N, Bartos R: Effect of varying amounts of feedback on standardized patient checklist accuracy in clinical practice examinations. Teach Learn Med 1999;11(3): 148–152.
6. Boulet JR, McKinley DW, Whelan GP, Hambleton RK: Quality assurance methods for performance-based assessments. Adv Health Sci Educ Theory Pract 2003;8(1):27–47.
   These papers describe the need for quality assurance of SP scoring and provide information regarding optimal frequency of feedback.

Psychometrics

7. van der Vleuten C, Swanson DB: Assessment of clinical skills with standardized patients: State of the art. Teach Learn Med 1990;2(2):58–76.
8. Norcini J, Boulet J: Methodological issues in the use of standardized patients for assessment. Teach Learn Med 2003;15(4):293–297.
9. Whelan GP, Boulet JR, McKinley DW, et al: Scoring standardized patient examinations: Lessons learned from the development and administration of the ECFMG Clinical Skills Assessment (CSA). Med Teach 2005;27(3):200–206.
10. Vu NV, Barrows HS: Use of standardized patients in clinical assessments: Recent developments and measurement findings. Educ Res 1994;23(3):23–30.
11. Swanson DB, Clauser BE, Case SM: Clinical skills assessment with standardized patients in high–stakes tests: A framework

for thinking about score precision, equating, and security. Adv Health Sci Educ Theory Pract 1999;4(1):67–106.

12. Boulet JR, De Champlain AF, McKinley DW: Setting defensible performance standards on OSCEs and standardized patient examinations. Med Teach 2003;25(3):245–249.

13. Newble D: Techniques for measuring clinical competence: Objective structured clinical examinations. Med Educ 2004;38(2): 199–203.

14. Colliver JA, Swartz MH, Robbs RS, Cohen DS: Relationship between clinical competence and interpersonal and communication skills in standardized-patient assessment. Acad Med 1999; 74(3):271–274.

15. Wilkinson TJ, Newble DI, Frampton CM: Standard setting in an objective structured clinical examination: Use of global ratings of borderline performance to determine the passing score. Med Educ 2001;35(11):1043–1049..

These articles provide an excellent overview of issues concerning the reliability and validity of scores obtained from SP-based assessments. They also offer a detailed synopsis of score-equating strategies and standard-setting methodologies.

Application of SP-Based Methods in Real-World Settings

16. Gorter SL, Rethans JJ, Scherpbier AJ, et al: How to introduce incognito standardized patients into outpatient clinics of specialists in rheumatology. Med Teach 2001;23(2):138–144.

17. Glassman PA, Luck J, O'Gara EM, Peabody JW: Using standardized patients to measure quality: Evidence from the literature and a prospective study. Jt Comm J Qual Improv 2000; 26(11):644–653.

18. Tamblyn RM, Grad R, Gayton D, et al: McGill Drug Utilization Research Group: Impact of inaccuracies in standardized patient portrayal and reporting on physician performance during blinded clinic visits. Teach Learn Med 1997;9(1):25–38.

These articles describe the benefits and challenges of using unannounced SPs for the assessment of physicians.

SP-Based Examinations within Comprehensive Evaluation Programs

19. Dupras DM, Li JT: Use of an objective structured clinical examination to determine clinical competence. Acad Med 1995; 70(11):1029–1034.

20. Joorabchi B, Devries JM: Evaluation of clinical competence: The gap between expectation and performance. Pediatrics 1996; 97(2):179–184.

21. Hull AL, Hodder S, Berger B, et al: Validity of three clinical performance assessments of internal medicine clerks. Acad Med 1995;70(6):517–522.

22. Schwartz RW, Donnelly MB, Sloan DA, et al: The relationship between faculty ward evaluations, OSCE, and ABSITE as measures of surgical intern performance. Am J Surg 1995; 169(4):414–417.

These articles describe the relationship between SP-based examinations and other assessment modalities used in medical education programs.

General Reading

23. Ferrell BG: Clinical performance assessment using standardized patients: A primer. Fam Med 1995;27(1):14–19.

24. Williams RG: Have standardized patient examinations stood the test of time and experience? Teach Learn Med 2004; 16(2):215–222.

25. Boulet JR, McKinley DW, Norcini JJ, Whelan GP: Assessing the comparability of standardized patient and physician evaluations of clinical skills. Adv Health Sci Educ Theory Pract 2002; 7(2):85–97.

26. De Champlain AF, Schoeneberger J, Boulet JR: Assessing the impact of examinee and standardized patient ethnicity on test scores in a large-scale clinical skills examination: Gathering evidence for the consequential aspect of validity. Acad Med 2004;79(10 Suppl):S12–S14.

27. Hauer KE, Hodgson CS, Kerr KM, et al: A national study of medical student clinical skills assessment. Acad Med 2005;80(10 Suppl):S25–S29.

28. Worth-Dickstein H, Pangaro LN, Macmillan MK, et al: Use of "standardized examinees" to screen for standardized-patient scoring bias in a clinical skills examination. Teach Learn Med 2005;17(1):9–13.

29. Petrusa ER: Taking standardized patient-based examinations to the next level. Teach Learn Med 2004;16(1):98–110.

30. Richards BF, Rupp R, Zaccaro DJ, et al: Use of a standardized-patient-based clinical performance examination as an outcome measure to evaluate medical school curricula. Acad Med 1996;71(1 Suppl):S49–S51.

These articles provide some general information concerning the use of SP-based assessment methods in medical schools and residency programs. They also describe some interesting research findings that can be used to help support the validity of these types of performance-based assessments.

REFERENCES

1. Barzansky B, Etzel SI: Educational programs in US medical schools, 2003–2004. JAMA 2004;292(9):1025–1031.

2. Patil NG, Saing H, Wong J: Role of OSCE in evaluation of practical skills. Med Teach 2003;25(3):271–272.

3. Colliver JA: Status of standardized patient assessment series. Teach Learn Med 2003;15(4):226.

4. Newble D: Techniques for measuring clinical competence: Objective structured clinical examinations. Med Educ 2004;38(2): 199–203.

5. Harden RM, Stevenson M, Downie WW, Wilson GU: Assessment of clinical competence using objective structured examination. Br Med J 1975;1:447–451.

6. Barrows HS, Abrahamson S: The programmed patient: a technique for appraising student performance in clinical neurology. J Med Educ 1964;39:802–805.

7. Whelan G: High-stakes medical performance testing: The clinical skills assessment program. JAMA 2000;283(13):1748.

8. Trewby PN: Assisting international medical graduates applying for their first post in the UK: What should be done? Clin Med 2005;5(2):126–132.

9. Dillon GF, Boulet JR, Hawkins RE, Swanson DB: Simulations in the United States Medical Licensing Examination (USMLE). Qual Saf Health Care 2004;13(Supp. 1):i41–i45.

10. Reznick RK, Blackmore D, Dauphinee WD, et al: Large-scale high-stakes testing with an OSCE: report from the Medical Council of Canada. Acad Med 1996;71(1 Suppl):S19–S21.

11. Norcini JJ, Stillman PL, Sutnick AI: Scoring and standard setting with standardized patients. Eval Health Prof 1993;16(3): 322–332.

12. Vu NV, Barrows HS: Use of standardized patients in clinical assessments: Recent developments and measurement findings. Educ Res 1994;23(3):23–30.

13. Whelan GP, Boulet JR, McKinley DW: Scoring standardized patient examinations: Lessons learned from the development and administration of the ECFMG Clinical Skills Assessment (CSA). Med Teach 2005;27(3):200–206.

14. Burchard KW, Rowland-Morin PA, Coe NP, Garb JL: A surgery oral examination: Interrater agreement and the influence of rater characteristics. Acad Med 1995;70(11):1044–1046.

15. Leichner P, Sisler GC, Harper D: A study of the reliability of the clinical oral examination in psychiatry. Can J Psychiatry 1984;29(5):394–397.

16. Barrows HS: An overview of the uses of standardized patients for teaching and evaluating clinical skills. AAMC Acad Med 1993;68(6):443–451.

17. Newble DI, Swanson DB: Psychometric characteristics of the objective structured clinical examination. Med Educ 1988; 22(4):325–334.

18. Norcini J, Boulet J: Methodological issues in the use of standardized patients for assessment. Teach Learn Med 2003;15(4): 293–297.

19. Swanson DB, Clauser BE, Case SM: Clinical skills assessment with standardized patients in high-stakes tests: A framework for thinking about score precision, equating, and security. Adv Health Sci Educ Theory Pract 1999;4(1):67–106.

20. King AM, Pohl H, Perkowski-Rogers LC: Planning standardized patient programs: Case development, patient training, and costs. Teach Learn Med 1994;6(1):6–14.

21. Olive KE, Elnicki DM, Kelley MJ: A practical approach to developing cases for standardized patients. Adv Health Sci Educ 1997;2:49–60.

22. de Almeida Troncon LE: Clinical skills assessment: limitations to the introduction of an ''OSCE'' (Objective Structured Clinical Examination) in a traditional Brazilian medical school. Sao Paulo Med J 2004;122(1):12–17.

23. Boursicot K, Roberts T: How to set up an OSCE. Clin Teach 2005;2(1):16–20.

24. Boulet JR, Gimpel JR, Errichetti AM, Meoli FG: Using National Medical Care Survey data to validate examination content on a performance-based clinical skills assessment for osteopathic physicians. J Am Osteopath Assoc 2003;103(5):225–231.

25. van der Vleuten C, Swanson DB: Assessment of clinical skills with standardized patients: State of the art. Teach Learn Med 1990;2(2):58–76.

26. Stillman P, Swanson D, Regan MB, et al: Assessment of clinical skills of residents utilizing standardized patients. A follow-up study and recommendations for application. Ann Intern Med 1991;114(5):393–401.

27. Petrusa ER, Blackwell TA, Ainsworth MA: Reliability and validity of an objective structured clinical examination for assessing the clinical performance of residents. Arch Intern Med 1990; 150(3):573–577.

28. Shatzer JH, Darosa D, Colliver JA, Barkmeier L: Station-length requirements for reliable performance-based examination scores. Acad Med 1993;68(3):224–229.

29. Chambers KA, Boulet JR, Gary NE: The management of patient encounter time in a high-stakes assessment using standardized patients. Med Educ 2000;34(10):813–817.

30. Stillman PL, Swanson DB, Smee S, et al: Assessing clinical skills of residents with standardized patients. Ann Intern Med 1986; 105(5):762–771.

31. Stillman PL: Technical issues: Logistics. AAMC Acad Med 1993;68(6):464–468.

32. Tamblyn RM, Klass DK, Schanbl GK, Kopelow ML: Factors associated with the accuracy of standardized patient presentation. Acad Med 1990;65(9 Suppl):S55–S56.

33. Peitzman SJ: Physical diagnosis findings among persons applying to work as standardized patients. Acad Med 2001;76(4):383.

34. Federation of State Medical Boards I, National Board of Medical Examiners: 2004 USMLE Step 2 CS Content Description and General Information Booklet. Philadelphia, FSMB and NBME, 2003.

35. Vu NV, Marcy MM, Colliver JA, et al: Standardized (simulated) patients' accuracy in recording clinical performance check-list items. Med Educ 1992;26(2):99–104.

36. Gorter S, Rethans JJ, Scherpbier A, et al: Developing case-specific checklists for standardized-patient-based assessments in internal medicine: A review of the literature. Acad Med 2000;75(11): 1130–1137.

37. Rothman AI, Blackmore D, Dauphinee WD, Reznick R: The use of global ratings in OSCE station scores. Adv Health Sci Educ 1997;1:215–219.

38. Solomon DJ, Szauter K, Rosebraugh CJ, Callaway MR: Global ratings of student performance in a standardized patient examination: Is the whole more than the sum of the parts? Adv Health Sci Educ 2000;5:131–140.

39. Boulet JR, Ben David MF, Ziv A, et al: Using standardized patients to assess the interpersonal skills of physicians. Acad Med 1998;73(10 Suppl):S94–S96.

40. Reznick RK, Regehr G, Yee G, et al: Process-rating forms versus task-specific checklists in an OSCE for medical licensure. Medical Council of Canada. Acad Med 1998;73(10 Suppl):S97–S99.

41. Boulet JR, McKinley DW, Norcini JJ, Whelan GP: Assessing the comparability of standardized patient and physician evaluations of clinical skills. Adv Health Sci Educ Theory Pract 2002; 7(2):85–97.

42. Boulet JR, McKinley DW, Whelan GP, Hambleton RK: Quality assurance methods for performance-based assessments. Adv Health Sci Educ Theory Pract 2003;8(1):27–47.

43. De Champlain AF, Margolis MJ, King A, Klass DJ, et al: Standardized patients' accuracy in recording examinees' behaviors using checklists. Acad Med 1997;72(10 Supp. 1):S85–S87.

44. Tamblyn RM, Grad R, Gayton D, et al: McGill Drug Utilization Research Group: Impact of inaccuracies in standardized patient portrayal and reporting on physician performance during blinded clinic visits. Teach Learn Med 1997;9(1):25–38.

45. Wallace P, Garman K, Heine N, Bartos R: Effect of varying amounts of feedback on standardized patient checklist accuracy in clinical practice examinations. Teach Learn Med 1999;11(3):148–152.

46. van der Vleuten CP, Norman GR, De Graaff E: Pitfalls in the pursuit of objectivity: Issues of reliability. Med Educ 1991; 25(2):110–118.

47. Martin JA, Reznick RK, Rothman A, et al: Who should rate candidates in an objective structured clinical examination? Acad Med 1996;71(2):170–175.

48. Elliot DL, Hickam DH: Evaluation of physical examination skills. Reliability of faculty observers and patient instructors. JAMA 1987;258(23):3405–3408.

49. Vu NV, Steward DE, Marcy M: An assessment of the consistency and accuracy of standardized patients' simulations. J Med Educ 1987;62(12):1000–1002.

50. Dauphinee WD, Blackmore D, Smee S, et al: Using the judgments of physician examiners in setting the standards for a national multi-center high stakes OSCE. Adv Health Sci Educ 1997; 2:201–211.

51. Boulet JR, De Champlain AF, McKinley DW: Setting defensible performance standards on OSCEs and standardized patient examinations. Med Teach 2003;25(3):245–249.

52. McKinley DW, Boulet JR, Hambleton RK: A work-centered approach for setting passing scores on performance-based assessments. Eval Health Prof 2005;28(3):349–369.

53. Williams RG: Have standardized patient examinations stood the test of time and experience? Teach Learn Med 2004;16(2): 215–222.

54. Chambers KA, Boulet JR, Furman GE: Are interpersonal skills ratings influenced by gender in a clinical skills assessment using standardized patients? Adv Health Sci Educ Theory Pract 2001;6(3):231–241.

55. van Zanten M, Boulet JR, McKinley D, Whelan GP: Evaluating the spoken English proficiency of international medical graduates: Detecting threats to the validity of standardised patient ratings. Med Educ 2003;37(1):69–76.

56. Ayers WR, Boulet JR: Establishing the validity of test score inferences: Performance of 4th-year U.S. medical students on the ECFMG Clinical Skills Assessment. Teach Learn Med 2001;13(4):214–220.

57. Whelan GP, McKinley DW, Boulet JR, et al: Validation of the doctor-patient communication component of the Educational Commission for Foreign Medical Graduates Clinical Skills Assessment. Med Educ 2001;35(8):757–761.

58. De Champlain AF, Macmillan MK, Margolis MJ, et al: Modeling the effects of a test security breach on a large-scale standardized patient examination with a sample of international medical graduates. Acad Med 2000;75(10 Suppl):S109–S111.

59. Niehaus AH, DaRosa DA, Markwell SJ, Folse R: Is test security a concern when OSCE stations are repeated across clerkship rotations? Acad Med 1996;71(3):287–289.

60. Boulet JR, McKinley DW, Whelan GP, Hambleton RK: The effect of task exposure on repeat candidate scores in a high-stakes standardized patient assessment. Teach Learn Med 2003;15(4): 227–232.

61. Kane MT, Crooks TJ, Cohen AS: Designing and evaluating standard-setting procedures for licensure and certification tests. Adv Health Sci Educ 1999;4:195–207.

62. Carney PA, Ward DH: Using unannounced standardized patients to assess the HIV preventive practices of family nurse practitioners and family physicians. Nurse Pract 1998;23(2):56–58.

63. Day RP, Hewson MG, Kindy P Jr, Van KJ: Evaluation of resident performance in an outpatient internal medicine clinic using standardized patients. J Gen Intern Med 1993;8(4):193–198.

64. McLeod PJ, Tamblyn RM, Gayton D, et al: Use of standardized patients to assess between-physician variations in resource utilization. JAMA 1997;278(14):1164–1168.

65. Grad R, Tamblyn R, McLeod PJ: Does knowledge of drug prescribing predict drug management of standardized patients in office practice? Med Educ 1997;31(2):132–137.

66. Grant C, Nicholas R, Moore L, Salisbury C: An observational study comparing quality of care in walk-in centres with general practice and NHS Direct using standardised patients. BMJ 2002;324(7353):1556.

67. Dresselhaus TR, Peabody JW, Lee M, et al: Measuring compliance with preventive care guidelines: Standardized patients, clinical vignettes, and the medical record. J Gen Intern Med 2000; 15(11):782–788.

68. Carney PA, Dietrich AJ, Freeman DH Jr, Mott LA: A standardized-patient assessment of a continuing medical education program to improve physicians' cancer-control clinical skills. Acad Med 1995;70(1):52–58.

69. Beullens J, Rethans JJ, Goedhuys J, Buntinx F: The use of standardized patients in research in general practice. Fam Pract 1997;14(1):58–62.

70. Gorter SL, Rethans JJ, Scherpbier AJ, et al: How to introduce incognito standardized patients into outpatient clinics of specialists in rheumatology. Med Teach 2001;23(2):138–144.

71. Rethans JJ, Martin E, Metsemakers J: To what extent do clinical notes by general practitioners reflect actual medical performance? A study using simulated patients. Br J Gen Pract 1994;44(381):153–156.

72. Luck J, Peabody JW, Dresselhaus TR, et al: How well does chart abstraction measure quality? A prospective comparison of standardized patients with the medical record. Am J Med 2000; 108(8):642–649.

73. Carney PA, Dietrich AJ, Freeman DH Jr, Mott LA: The periodic health examination provided to asymptomatic older women: An assessment using standardized patients. Ann Intern Med 1993;119(2):129–135.

74. Luck J, Peabody JW: Using standardised patients to measure physicians' practice: Validation study using audio recordings. BMJ 2002;325(7366):679.

75. Glassman PA, Luck J, O'Gara EM: Using standardized patients to measure quality: Evidence from the literature and a prospective study. Jt Comm J Qual Improv 2000;26(11):644–653.

76. Tamblyn RM, Abrahamowicz M, Berkson L, et al: First-visit bias in the measurement of clinical competence with standardized patients. Acad Med 1992;67(10 Suppl):S22–S24.

77. Epstein RM, Levenkron JC, Frarey L, et al: Improving physicians' HIV risk-assessment skills using announced and unannounced standardized patients. J Gen Intern Med 2001;16(3):176–180.

78. Stillman PL, Regan MB, Swanson DB, et al: An assessment of the clinical skills of fourth-year students at four New England medical schools. Acad Med 1990;65(5):320–326.

79. Sachdeva AK, Loiacono LA, Amiel GE, et al: Variability in the clinical skills of residents entering training programs in surgery. Surgery 1995;118(2):300–308.

80. Holmboe ES: Faculty and the observation of trainees' clinical skills: problems and opportunities. Acad Med 2004;79(1):16–22.

81. Chalabian J, Garman K, Wallace P, Dunnington G: Clinical breast evaluation skills of house officers and students. Am Surg 1996;62(10):840–845.

82. Colletti L, Gruppen L, Barclay M, Stern D: Teaching students to break bad news. Am J Surg 2001;182(1):20–23.

83. Foley KL, George G, Crandall SJ, et al: Training and evaluating tobacco-specific standardized patient instructors. Fam Med 2006;38(1):28–37.

84. Morrison LJ, Barrows HS: Developing consortia for clinical practice examinations: The macy project. Teach Learn Med 1994;6(1):23–27.

85. Pangaro LN, Worth-Dickstein H, Macmillan MK: Performance of "standardized examinees" in a standardized-patient examination of clinical skills. Acad Med 1997;72(11):1008–1011.

86. Chalabian J, Dunnington G: Do our current assessments assure competency in clinical breast evaluation skills? Am J Surg 1998;175(6):497–502.

87. Rethans JJ, Sturmans F, Drop R, et al: Does competence of general practitioners predict their performance? Comparison between examination setting and actual practice. BMJ 1991;303(6814):1377–1380.

88. Kopelow ML, Schnabl GK, Hassard TH, et al: Assessing practicing physicians in two settings using standardized patients. Acad Med 1992;67(10 Suppl):S19–S21.

Direct Observation by Faculty

Eric S. Holmboe, MD

Medical educators have a major responsibility to evaluate the clinical skills of trainees and to provide them with timely, useful feedback to ensure continued progress and correction of deficiencies. Despite tremendous advances in technology, the basic clinical skills of interviewing, physical examination, and counseling remain essential to the successful care of patients. The Association of American Medical Colleges (AAMC), Accreditation Council for Graduate Medical Education (ACGME), and American Board of Medical Specialties (ABMS) strongly endorse the evaluation of students, residents, and fellows in these clinical skills.[1-3] The Institute of Medicine has placed *patient-centered care* at the heart of its five core competencies for all physicians (Fig. 9-1).[4]

The direct observation of trainees performing a medical interview, physical examination, or counseling is mandatory for the reliable and valid assessment of these skills.

As highlighted in Chapter 8, the use of standardized patients (SPs) to evaluate and teach clinical skills is a valuable methodology in medical education and assessment. The development of standardized patients to evaluate clinical skills is unquestionably a major advance in competency assessment as rigorous SP training and scoring methods support the security and reliability requirements of high-stakes examinations.[5-10] There are limitations, however, in the application of SP-based methods for teaching and evaluation along the continuum of education and practice. Standardized patients are optimally applied in clinical skills teaching and assessment as a supplement to similar activities in the real clinical setting; they cannot replace the observation of trainees by physicians on an ongoing basis with actual patients.[11-16] Standardized patients may also have less validity with more advanced trainees because assessment instruments used for SP exercises, depending upon case development and standard setting approaches, may favor completeness over efficiency.[14-19]

Therefore, clinician-educators need to embrace their professional responsibility for evaluating these skills through direct observation of trainees in real clinical settings. George Miller's assessment pyramid best captures the important role of faculty of evaluating what the trainee actually "does" (e.g., a trainee's performance) with patients, despite the possibility the act of observation may change the level of performance[20] (Fig. 9-2).

Stop for a moment and imagine the triangle now as a spear. At the tip of the spear is the patient, meaning that the behaviors and actions of the trainee directly affect the well-being of the patient. Unfortunately, this obvious fact has too often not resulted in effective observation and supervision of trainees in the clinical setting,[21] despite the fact many trainees actually want better supervision![22] Exacerbating this situation is the sobering research demonstrating many faculty members are ill prepared to accurately observe and provide

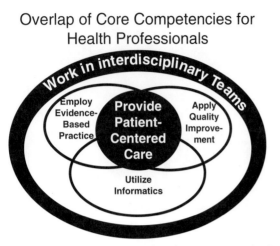

Figure 9-1 Institute of Medicine's clinical competencies for health professionals.

effective corrective feedback about clinical skills.[21] The good news is that observation is a skill that can be acquired by faculty, but faculty members must acknowledge that direct observation is important, is a professional obligation of a teacher, and requires training like any other skill. Being a good clinician and teacher does not equate to skill in observing trainees' clinical skills. In this chapter we will first explore problems in trainees' clinical skills and the challenges faced by faculty performing direct observation. The purpose of this background is to give educational leaders "ammunition" to highlight the importance of clinical skills and the need to teach and observe them. We will then outline some practical methods to help you improve observation skills among your faculty. Some useful tools faculty can use when performing observations will also be highlighted.

Reasons for and Challenges of Direct Observation

It has long been recognized that students and residents have substantial deficiencies in the basic clinical skills of

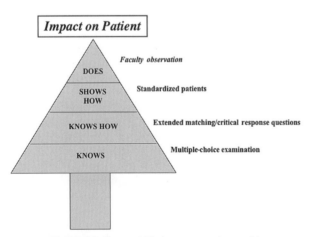

Figure 9-2 George Miller's assessment pyramid.

medical interviewing, physical examination, and counseling. Numerous studies have documented serious deficiencies in medical interviewing that have persisted over time and in the views of some, history-taking skills may have actually declined.[23–27] Furthermore, communication skills do not appear to improve after completion of training. In a study using unannounced standardized patients, Ramsey found that a group of primary care physicians only asked 59% of essential history items.[28] Braddock found that among 1057 counseling sessions involving primary care physicians and surgeons, only 9% of encounters met basic criteria for effective informed decision making.[29] Other studies have shown that physicians fail to elicit over half of patient complaints and that many of the public's complaints about physicians relate to communication problems.[30–34] Effective communication has been shown to improve patient outcomes and adherence, and most patients want an active role in the decision-making processes.[35–38] Errors are also common in physical examination skills.[40–48] For example, deficiencies in auscultatory skills among trainees were noted over 40 years ago[41,42] and poor cardiac and pulmonary physical examination skills continue to plague U.S. students and residents today.[43,44]

These findings are relevant because we know that despite advances in technology, accurate data collection during the medical interview and the physical examination remains the most potent diagnostic tool available to physicians.[49–51] Two important studies showed that the medical interview alone produced the correct diagnosis in nearly 80% of patients presenting to an ambulatory care clinic with a previously undiagnosed condition.[47,48] Bordage recently noted that errors in data collection are one of the principal factors in diagnostic errors committed by physicians.[52]

The preceding findings have resulted in a significant push to re-emphasize both the training and evaluation of clinical skills.[53–57] Without accurate evaluation of clinical skills, which must be accomplished by direct observation, improvement in the clinical skills of our trainees is highly unlikely. First, trainees have to know *how* to perform a skill before they can acquire experience through practice with actual patients. Second, physicians in general are poor at self-assessment in the absence of guidance and data.[58,59] For clinical skills, the guidance and data to drive assessment is direct observation by faculty.

Lack of Direct Observation by Faculty

Perhaps the biggest problem in the evaluation of clinical skills is simply getting faculty to observe trainees. For decades faculty members have taken at face value the veracity of the history and physical examination presented on inpatient and outpatient rounds without ever watching the trainee actually perform any of these skills. Two of the most prominent physician-scientists and educators of the twentieth century, the late Alvan Feinstein and George Engel, strongly advocated direct observation of the history and physical examination skills of trainees over 30 years ago.[60,61] Dr. George Engel commented in a 1976 editorial,

> Evidently it is not deemed necessary to assay students' (and residents) clinical performance once they have entered the clinical years. Nor do clinical instructors more than occasionally show how they themselves elicit and check the reliability of clinical data. To a degree that is often at variance with their own professed scientific standards, attending staff all too often accept and use as the basis for discussion, if not recommendations, findings reported by students and housestaff without ever evaluating the reporter's mastery of the clinical methods utilized or the reliability of the data obtained.[62]

The AAMC found that among 97 medical schools it visited between 1993 and 1998, faculty members rarely observed student interactions with patients, noting that the majority of a student's evaluation was based on faculty and resident recollections of student presentation skills and knowledge.[63] Observation of residents and fellows by faculty is even less frequent. There is little evidence even today of greater faculty involvement in teaching and observing clinical skills.[21]

Quality of Faculty Observation

Although several studies show that four to seven observations produce sufficient reliability in the evaluation of clinical skills for "pass-fail" determinations, little is known about the validity of faculty ratings. Noel and Herbers, in two important studies of the American Board of Internal Medicine's (ABIM) traditional "long case" clinical evaluation exercise (CEX), found substantial deficiencies in the accuracy of faculty ratings.[64,65] They demonstrated that faculty failed to detect up to 68% of errors committed by a resident scripted to depict marginal performance on a training videotape. Use of specific checklists prompting faculty to look for certain skills increased accuracy of error detection nearly twofold, but the checklist did not produce more accurate overall ratings of competence. Nearly 70% of faculty members still rated a resident depicting marginal performance as satisfactory or superior overall. A brief informational videotape shown to a group of faculty members about the traditional CEX and its purpose failed to improve ratings.[64]

Kalet examined the reliability and validity of faculty observation skills using videotapes of student performance on an objective structured clinical examination (OSCE) designed to evaluate interviewing skills.[66] She found that faculty were inconsistent in identifying the use of open-ended questions and empathy, and that the positive predictive value of faculty ratings for "adequate" interviewing skills was only 12%. Another study found that faculty members could not reliably evaluate 32% of the physical examination skills assessed and had the most difficulty with examination of the head, neck, and abdomen.[67]

Finally, practicing physicians have also been shown to have significant deficiencies in clinical skills.[28,29,31,34]

A medical educator who possesses deficiencies in his or her clinical skills is obviously less likely to detect those deficiencies among trainees. Let's be honest, if faculty members lack the skill or feel uncomfortable about their own proficiency, it seems pretty unlikely they would be critical of a trainee's performance. Faculty members are very uncomfortable about admitting their own limitations, despite the powerful role modeling such an act engenders. Given the decline in clinical skills of the last 10 to 20 years, a major focus of faculty development will have to be clinical skills training for the faculty as well as the trainees.

Practical Approaches to Training Faculty

Given the essential role of faculty observation in the evaluation of basic clinical skills, medical schools and residency programs must train faculty for this important task. Industry and the field of psychology have grappled with the challenges of rater training in performance appraisal for decades. In 1980, Landry and Farr, pleading for a moratorium on the endless search for the "perfect" evaluation form, highlighted the need to redirect energies on training the evaluator in the most appropriate and effective use of the evaluation form.[68] Yet, over the last 25 years medicine has continued to seek the "holy grail" of evaluation tools and forms. An assessment or evaluation is only as good as the individual performing it. Training approaches do exist that can improve the evaluation of performance in the clinical training setting. Early research in medical education has demonstrated that these training approaches do indeed improve observation skills. The following paragraphs summarize a set of training methods that can be used for faculty development in direct observation.

Behavioral Observation Training

Behavioral observation training (BOT) focuses on improving the detection, perception, and recall of actual performance.[69] Three main strategies are emphasized in BOT. The first strategy is simply to get faculty to increase the number of their observations of their trainees. This helps to improve recall of performance and provides multiple opportunities for skill practice in observation by the faculty, the "practice makes perfect" principle. The second strategy is to provide some form of observational aid that raters can then use to record observations, sometimes referred to as "behavioral diaries" or "aide-de-memoir" devices. Studies show that even something as simple as a 3-inch × 5-inch index card used to record observation notes improves the quality of information provided on evaluation forms.[70]

Simply getting faculty to make notes on a regular basis can help them to be more specific when observing performance. In this electronic age, such notes can be quickly entered into computers or portable personal digital assistants (PDAs). It is important to encourage this activity as a habit in faculty. For example, I always carried a 3 × 5 card for teaching and clinical interactions with my trainees. Every day I strove to write down at least one thing the trainee did well, one thing they could improve, and my plan to help them improve. I took 5 to 10 minutes to enter these notes into a simple word document on my computer. By doing this on a regular basis, I had a rich source of observations I could simply "cut and paste," with a little editing, onto the final evaluation form at the end of the rotation. The mini-CEX form and checklists can also serve as an immediate "behavioral diary" to record an assessment of an observation.

The third important strategy is to help faculty members learn how to *prepare* for an observation. To prepare, faculty members should determine the objectives or goals of the observation before entering the patient's room with the trainee. For example, if you plan to perform an observation of trainee's physical examination skills, what would be the appropriate components of a physical examination for the patient's chief complaint or medical condition? Obviously, you would need to have heard some of the patient's history in order to determine what the critical aspects of the physical examination will be. Although rapidly becoming a lost art, bedside presentations are a valuable and efficient way to hear about the patient's history with the added benefit that patients actually appreciate such presentations.[71]

Other aspects of preparation include the following: How should you position yourself in order to ensure proper technique is used by the trainee? How and when will you confirm (if you deem necessary) the physical findings obtained by the trainee? This preparation helps to maximize the effectiveness of the observation. Positioning is very important because as faculty you want to minimize interference with the trainee-patient interaction whenever possible. Don't become a distraction to both the trainee and patient. Remember, protect the trainee-patient bond whenever possible. Figure 9-3 demonstrates the principle of triangulation that maximizes the ability of the faculty

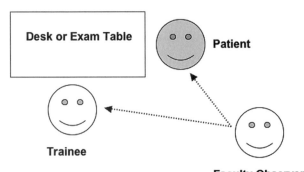

Figure 9-3 Principle of triangulation for direct observation.

member to observe while minimizing interference. Table 9-1 lists some important yet simple rules for performing trainee observation.

Performance Dimension Training

Performance dimension training (PDT) is designed to teach and familiarize the faculty with the appropriate performance dimensions used in their own evaluation system. Although PDT alone probably does not improve rater accuracy, it is a critical structural element for all rater training programs.[72–74] PDT simply starts with a review of the definitions and criteria for each dimension of performance or competency. The goal should be to define all the criteria and trainee behaviors that constitute a superior performance from the perspective of patient outcomes. For residency or fellowship training, the six new general competencies developed by the ACGME would be an appropriate starting point. The next step in PDT is to give faculty the opportunity to "interact" with the definitions to improve their understanding of the definitions and criteria. The overarching goal of PDT is to ensure that the faculty understands the definitions and criteria for the competency of interest to reach a high level of consensus.

This consensus can then facilitate calibrating faculty to utilize these assessment criteria in a more standardized

Table 9-1 Four Simple Rules for Observation

Rule	Description
Correct positioning	As the rater, try to avoid being in the line of sight of either the patient or trainee, especially when they are communicating. Use the principle of triangulation. However, during physical examinations be sure you can view the trainee's techniques accurately.
Minimize external interruptions	Let your staff know you will be with the resident for 5–10 minutes, avoid taking routine calls, etc.
Avoid intrusions	Don't interject or interrupt if at all possible. Once you interject yourself into the resident-patient interaction, the visit is permanently altered. However, there will be often be a point in the visit where you need to interject yourself in order to correct misinformation, etc., from the resident.
Be prepared	Know before you enter the room what your goals are for the observation session. For example, if a physical examination, have the resident present the history first; then you will know what the key elements of the PE should be.

fashion, which in turn will improve the fairness, reliability, and validity of the observation. This simple faculty development technique is seldom used in training programs. Faculty members need frameworks in order to perform evaluation effectively. In Chapter 3, we covered various frameworks for the effective use of global rating scales and longitudinal evaluation forms. Performance dimension training is a validated method to help faculty both understand and then *use* a framework and specific criteria effectively for not only direct observation but other evaluation tools as well. The important message is that faculty training is crucial to effective observation of clinical skills.[21,64,65,75]

Appendix 9-1 provides a very straightforward and useful proactive PDT exercise that can be done with faculty to facilitate interaction with competency in clinical skills. As an example, one simple clinical scenario is a trainee prescribing a medication for a patient with a newly diagnosed medical condition. The clinical skill competency here is counseling and patient education. The question for the PDT exercise would simply be, What should an effective counseling session look like for a patient starting a new medication? The main task for the faculty will be to define the trainee *behaviors* of an effective counseling session. A focus on behaviors is crucial because trainee behaviors are what faculty will observe. I recommend performing PDT exercises in small groups and then having the small groups share their results. Inevitably, differences occur between the groups. These differences, however, lead to productive discussions on what constitute the core elements and criteria of competency in counseling, or other clinical skills. This type of PDT exercise can be done for two clinical skills over approximately 1 hour. Another approach to PDT is reactive: using actual evaluations or videotapes of clinical skills that faculty can react to when performing the PDT exercise. The accompanying DVD (Faculty Guidelines to Training) provides a number of scripted clinical encounters you can use for a PDT exercise.

Frame of Reference Training

Frame of reference training (FORT) specifically targets accuracy in rating.[72,73] Table 9-2 describes the complete FORT process.

As you can see, FORT is really an extension of PDT; the main goal of FORT is achieving consistency (using the result of the consensus process in PDT) among faculty regarding application of the different performance criteria to distinguish *levels* of performance. For FORT, I encourage faculty to focus on defining four levels of performance: unsatisfactory, marginal, satisfactory, and superior. The PDT exercise should define the criteria and definitions for a superior performance from the perspective of optimal patient outcomes. The second step of the exercise, as shown in Appendix 9-1, is to define the minimal criteria for a *satisfactory* performance. These criteria for a satisfactory performance serve as an important anchoring point to define marginal and unsatisfactory performance in step 3. Once the group defines marginal criteria, by default any lesser performance is unsatisfactory. This important technique helps faculty members to distinguish levels of performance and to provide more specific feedback to the trainee.

Evidenced-based standards for many of the clinical skills provide an excellent foundation and resource to help faculty reach consensus on performance standards for basic clinical skills. For example, use of open-ended questions at the beginning of history taking is more likely to yield more complete and accurate information from the patient.[76,77] Other examples include the Calgary-Cambridge and SEGUE models for medical interviewing and the informed decision-making model for counseling.[29,78,79] Several resources now exist on the evidence for the utility of a number of clinical skills, including skills from the surgical disciplines.[75,80–83] I recommend that these types of resources be available when possible as a guide for PDT and FORT exercises.

Table 9-2 **Steps for Frame of Reference Training**

Step	Description of Task
1	Performance dimension training (PDT). Faculty observers are given descriptions for each dimension of competence followed by a discussion of what they believe the qualifications are for each dimension.
2	Faculty observers define what constitutes superior (the most effective criteria and behaviors) performance from the perspective of optimal patient outcomes.
3	Next, faculty members define and reach consensus on the minimal criteria for satisfactory performance. Once the satisfactory criteria are set, marginal criteria are defined. Everything else by default is unsatisfactory performance.
4	Participants are given clinical vignettes describing critical incidents of performance from unsatisfactory to average to outstanding (frame of reference). For clinical skills, videotaped encounters are the best method.
5	Participants use the vignettes to provide ratings on a behaviorally anchored rating scale.
6	Session trainer/facilitator provides feedback on what the "true" ratings should be along with an explanation for each rating.
7	Training session wraps up with an important discussion on the discrepancies between the participants' ratings and the "true" ratings.

Direct Observation of Competence Training

Using the evidence from BOT, PDT, FORT, and SP training methods (Chapter 8) my colleagues and I developed a new approach called direct observation of competence (DOC) training. DOC training is a multifaceted approach that incorporates the key elements of these previously validated rater training methods but adds relevant, practical exercises in direct observation.

DOC training can be delivered in multiple formats ranging from 1.5- to 2-hour to full-day workshop formats. Each workshop typically begins with a scripted videotape (provided on the accompanying DVD) that portrays a standardized resident performing either a history, physical examination, or counseling session with a standardized patient who has a common medical problem. Three tapes were developed for each basic skill depicting different levels of performance that vary in the quality and quantity of errors committed by the resident. Typically a tape demonstrating "satisfactory" performance is shown to start the workshop and the participants are asked to rate the resident using a standard evaluation form and to write down what they saw the resident do well and any specific deficiencies they noted on the tape. Workshop participants are then given a 30-minute interactive presentation reviewing the problems with resident clinical skills and direct observation by faculty. Participants then break into small groups to work on PDT exercises for the clinical skill of interest.

The workshop leader next facilitates a group discussion to reach some preliminary consensus about what constitutes an effective clinical skill. Whenever possible, the participants should compare their PDT checklist against an evidenced-based standard. For example, after a PDT exercise focused on counseling/informed decision-making skills, we introduce the informed decision-making criteria of Braddock and colleagues.[29] This helps to further standardize and calibrate the faculty on the criteria they will use in the observations. At the completion of this discussion, the participants view the same videotape encounter again but using the criteria they have developed to evaluate the performance on the tape. Finally, each participant shares the scores they gave the resident from the opening tape and how this evaluation compares with their second rating of the tape. Feedback is provided by the session trainer on the errors committed by the resident on the tape. The other two tapes, depicting different levels of performance, are shown followed by discussion and feedback to provide the "frame of reference." A checklist is also provided to participants for use in evaluating the specific clinical skill covered in the training. This aspect of DOC training can be done as an abridged workshop, without showing the additional tapes, in 1.5 to 2 hours. If you wish to include the behavioral observation techniques and the additional tapes, give yourself about 3 to 3.5 hours to complete.

The second workshop session involves actual practice with live standardized residents and patients. The first part of this live training focuses on the principles of behavioral observation training discussed earlier in the chapter. Each participant is given an opportunity to sit in the examination room observing the standardized resident and patient in a simulated clinical encounter. The resident is instructed to perform at different levels of competence for each faculty participant. At the end of the encounter the faculty member provides his/her evaluation with feedback to the standardized resident. The standardized resident is also trained to respond to the feedback in different ways.

The other faculty members observe both the clinical encounter and the evaluation/feedback session. Once the participant finishes the evaluation/feedback session, the group shares their evaluation of the resident and provides feedback to the faculty observer of their evaluation and feedback to the resident. If desired, the standardized resident and patient can also provide feedback to the faculty observer. The session trainer facilitates the feedback and points out errors made and provides suggestions for improving the observation and feedback. In total, the second session is designed to allow each faculty participant to perform two observations among the three clinical skills depicted. This is a very valuable approach if you have access to standardized patients. Chief residents and junior faculty are excellent sources for standardized residents and can be easily trained using scripts depicting varying levels of performance skill. The steps for DOC training are provided in Table 9-3. DOC training could be completed over the course of a single day, or the live standardized patient/resident session could be performed on a different day. A randomized controlled trial of DOC training demonstrated that this method of faculty development leads to meaningful changes in faculty evaluation.[84]

Useful Tools to Guide Observation

The Mini-Clinical Evaluation Exercise

The mini-CEX is designed to evaluate residents in a setting reflective of day-to-day practice. Faculty observe a resident performing a *focused* history, physical examination, or counseling session during routine care experiences on the inpatient wards, intensive care units, outpatient clinics, and the emergency department. Unlike the traditional long case that can require several hours to complete, mini-CEX observation lasts from 5 to 30 minutes depending on the goals of the observation. Faculty complete a 9-point rating scale at the end of the exercise evaluating specific skills and overall competency and provide immediate feedback to the resident. The mini-CEX facilitates multiple observations over time by different faculty members. This improves both the reliability and validity of the evaluations. This longitudinal nature of the mini-CEX is one

Table 9-3 **Direct Observation of Competence (DOC) Training**

Workshop Element	Approximate Time
Half-Day Workshop*	
Introduction: Viewing and rating of clinical skills: videotape	15 min
Current state of clinical skills and direct observation skills: lecture	30 min
Performance dimension training (PDT): small group exercise	20 min
Review of PDT exercise results: large group exercise	15 min
Review of ratings of initial videotape: large group exercise	15 min
Review of second clinical skills: videotape/ frame of reference training (FORT): large group exercise	15 min
Behavioral observation training: lecture	10 min
Conclusions: large group discussion	15 min
Full-Day Workshop (Afternoon Session)	
Live observation/feedback training with standardized patient and resident: small groups	2.5–3 hr

*Breaks not included.

of its most important strengths as an evaluation tool and method.

In the first large study of the mini-CEX, Norcini and colleagues[85] reported on the results of 388 mini-CEX evaluations for 88 residents at five different residency programs. Over half of the encounters occurred in the inpatient setting. In this initial study, most of the participating residents were in the PGY-1 year, and each resident underwent a mean of 4.4 observations (range 2 to 10). The mean ratings for each category were significantly correlated with scores for overall competence. Higher resident ratings were noted for longer CEX interactions. The authors noted that between 12 and 14 encounters would be necessary to reach a reproducibility of 0.80, sufficient for high-stakes determinations, but the standard error noted for just four mini-CEXs per resident was acceptable for pass-fail determinations. Trainees reported high satisfaction ratings for the mini-CEX format, and interestingly, there was a modest correlation between faculty satisfaction ratings and resident performance.

In a more recent study of the mini-CEX involving a more diverse set of residency programs, several new findings were noted. First, the scores on the mini-CEX suggested that interns displayed growth in clinical skills over the course of the year, with the biggest gains occurring in the dimensions of clinical judgment and organization/efficiency. Finally, the authors concluded that the mini-CEX had higher fidelity and was less expensive than the long case CEX.[86] In a separate report, Norcini also found that ratings did not differ by the setting of the exercise, specific institution, or type of patient. Norcini concluded that it may be possible to compare ratings from different clinical settings because examiners do not appear to rate residents differently based on the setting. There is also evidence related to the validity of the mini-CEX. My colleagues and I, using scripted videotapes, found that the mini-CEX evaluation form does possess construct validity.[87] However, we were not able to conclude if this occurs with actual observations of resident performance, and the ratings on each tape had a wide range among a group of 40 faculty members.

Feedback and the Mini-CEX

An essential component of the mini-CEX, as with any evaluation, is feedback. A recent study investigated the feedback generated from the mini-CEX observation by audiotaping the attending/resident feedback session, with a particular focus on interactive feedback.[88] Interactive feedback was defined as any feedback that provided a recommendation plus self-assessment, allowing the learner to react to the feedback, and development of an action plan. The study showed that 80% of the feedback sessions included at least one recommendation for improvement for the resident, and on average each feedback session contained two recommendations. The majority of recommendations, as might be expected, involved the clinical skills of medical interviewing, physical examination, and counseling. However, despite the large number of recommendations, few concluded with a specific action plan from the faculty member on how to carry out the recommendation or improve.[81] This is a very important aspect of feedback: including an action plan to enable the learner to act on the recommendations provided.

Checklists

The mini-CEX is an example of a global rating scale for which faculty training (described in the previous section) is crucial to the effective use of the mini-CEX form (Fig 9-4). Checklists targeting specific skills are another tool that can improve the quality of faculty observation. In one of the original studies of the long case CEX the use of a checklist doubled the detection of errors committed on a scripted videotape. As described in Chapter 8, checklists are the foundation for standardized patient assessments. However, because the purpose of faculty direct observation is to assess performance of actual clinical practice, it is not feasible to develop highly detailed checklists for every patient encounter. Some degree of faculty interpretation of behavior and skills will be required when working in actual clinical settings. A number of checklists for assessment of interviewing skills have been developed

Mini Clinical Evaluation Form

Evaluator: _____   Date: _____

Complexity: ☐ Low   ☐ Moderate   ☐ High

Focus: ☐ Data gathering   ☐ Diagnosis   ☐ Therapy   ☐ Counseling

1. **Medical interviewing** (☐ Not observed)

    1   2   3   4   5   6   7   8   9
    UNSATISFACTORY   SATISFACTORY   SUPERIOR

2. **Physical Examination Skills** (☐ Not observed)

    1   2   3   4   5   6   7   8   9
    UNSATISFACTORY   SATISFACTORY   SUPERIOR

3. **Humanistic Qualities/Professionalism** (☐ Not observed)

    1   2   3   4   5   6   7   8   9
    UNSATISFACTORY   SATISFACTORY   SUPERIOR

4. **Clinical judgment** (☐ Not observed)

    1   2   3   4   5   6   7   8   9
    UNSATISFACTORY   SATISFACTORY   SUPERIOR

5. **Counseling Skills** (☐ Not observed)

    1   2   3   4   5   6   7   8   9
    UNSATISFACTORY   SATISFACTORY   SUPERIOR

6. **Organization/Efficiency** (☐ Not observed)

    1   2   3   4   5   6   7   8   9
    UNSATISFACTORY   SATISFACTORY   SUPERIOR

7. **Overall Clinical Competence** (☐ Not observed)

    1   2   3   4   5   6   7   8   9
    UNSATISFACTORY   SATISFACTORY   SUPERIOR

Comments:

Figure 9-4 Mini-clinical evaluation form.

and tested for reliability. Both the SEGUE and Calgary-Cambridge checklists are useful tools to guide the evaluation of process and general content of medical interviewing.[78,79]

The choice of instruments depends primarily on the objectives of the teaching or assessment exercise. Drawing upon the standardized patient literature, the use of checklists may increase the reliability of observation compared to less structured global ratings in the hands of physician observers.[12] On the other hand, concerns have been raised about the validity of such a highly structured approach.[14–18] However, the differences between global ratings and checklist scores in these studies were relatively small and it may be that the different approaches were measuring different constructs.[88,89] At the present time, it seems reasonable to conclude that checklists may provide a reliable means of assessing whether critical data-gathering actions are completed and facilitate the provision of explicit feedback to trainees. Identification of essential examinee actions for a particular patient encounter may reduce the propensity of such instruments to over-reward thoroughness. The use of global ratings supports the valid assessment of communication and interpersonal skills and allows faculty to gauge various aspects of examinee performance against an internal or professional standard (see Chapter 8). Faculty development activities that include the above-mentioned training approaches will serve to instill a

common standard among raters and therefore optimize the reliability and validity of assessment.

Creating an Observation System

There are three simple steps in creating a faculty observation system. First, determine what your faculty is doing in regard to observation. If no observation is occurring, you will probably have to create a "need" for observation through culture change. You can start by highlighting with your faculty the substantial documented deficiencies in trainees' clinical skills to reinforce the need to perform observation.

Second, if you have the resources and access, consider an OSCE or other standardized patient baseline assessment with your trainees. Lypson and colleagues discovered in an entry OSCE that brand-new interns lacked basic skills faculty believed they should have on day 1.[90] This type of information, especially if accompanied by videotape for review by the faculty, can be a powerful motivator. My own experience with an OSCE for early fourth-year medical students was similar and productively led to a revision of the curriculum for teaching physical examination skills (once the depression among the teaching faculty had lifted).

Third, start small and get the faculty to simply perform observation of their trainees. Invariably at some point a faculty member will observe these deficiencies and experience the powerful "you will not believe what I saw today" moment. Once that happens, it becomes very difficult for your faculty to argue they no longer need to observe trainees, especially from a patient-centered perspective.

The next step is to improve faculty skill in observation, and depending on your educational climate, this can be done concurrently with creating the need for observation. We recommend you start with performance dimension and behavioral observation training. This can be done in a series of brief workshops as described earlier in the chapter, and can then be reinforced in small aliquots of time at competency committee or other scheduled faculty meetings. Once your group feels comfortable with the definitions and criteria for the clinical skills competencies, you can then move on to frame of reference training and direct observation of competence training to further improve faculty accuracy and ability to distinguish between levels of competence.

Conclusion

The successful practice of medicine requires the effective application of medical interviewing, physical examination, and counseling skills. Studies continue to document significant deficiencies in all three of these clinical skills areas among students, residents, and practicing physicians. Despite the advances in clinical skills evaluation afforded by standardized patients and potentially computer simulation, direct observation by medical faculty remains an essential method to assess core basic clinical skills with actual patients.

Furthermore, faculty observers are in the best position to assess a trainee's acquisition and refinement of clinical skills longitudinally over time. Several practical approaches, described in this chapter, exist to help improve faculty skills in observation.

ANNOTATED BIBLIOGRAPHY

1. Noel GL, Herbers JE, Callow MP, et al: How well do internal medicine faculty members evaluate the clinical skills of residents? Ann Intern Med 1992;117:757–765.

   This was one of the first studies to systematically evaluate problems in faculty observation skills. Although the tool used for the study (the "traditional" long-case clinical evaluation exercise [CEX]) is infrequently used today, the lessons from the study about the importance of training faculty remain valuable.

2. Norcini JJ, Blank LL, Arnold GK, Kimball HR: The mini-CEX (clinical evaluation exercise): A preliminary investigation. Ann Intern Med 1995;123:795–799.

3. Norcini JJ, Blank LL, Duffy FD, Fortna GS: The mini-CEX: A method for assessing clinical skills. Ann Intern Med 2003;138:476–481.

   These two articles report on the feasibility and reliability characteristics of the mini-clinical evaluation tool (mini-CEX). These two studies combined involved over 30 internal medicine programs in the United States.

4. Holmboe ES, Hawkins RE, Huot SJ: Direct observation of competence training: A randomized controlled trial. Ann Intern Med 2004;140:874–881.

   This is one of the few controlled trials of a faculty development intervention to attempt to improve observation skills. Faculty in the intervention group who underwent direct observation of competence training reported improved comfort in observation, and an efficacy analysis showed the training changed their rating behavior at follow-up 8 months later compared to the control group.

5. Holmboe ES: The importance of faculty observation of trainees' clinical skills. Acad Med 2004;79:16–22.

   This article offers a basic review of the importance of clinical skills and the continued need for faculty to observe and evaluate trainees while caring for actual patients.

REFERENCES

1. Accreditation Council for Graduate Medical Education: The General Competencies. Accessed July 16, 2007 at www.acgme.org.

2. American Board of Internal Medicine: Portfolio for internal medicine residency programs. Philadelphia, American Board of Internal Medicine, 2001.

3. American Association of Medical Colleges: AAMC Educational Outcomes Project. Accessed July 16, 2007 at www.aamc.org.

4. Institute of Medicine: Health Professions Education: A Bridge to Quality. Washington, DC, National Academy Press, 2003.

5. Richards BF, Rupp R, Zaccaro DJ, et al: Use of a standardized patient based clinical performance examination as an outcome measure to evaluate medical school curricula. Acad Med 1996;71:S49–S51.

6. Anderson MB, Stillman PL, Wang Y: Growing use of standardized patients in teaching and evaluation in medical education. Teach Learn Med 1994;6:15–22.

7. Scoles PV: An evaluation of clinical skills in the United States Medical Licensing Examination: A report from the National Board of Medical Examiners. J Med Licensure Discipline 2002;88:66–69.

8. Sloan DA, Donnelly MB, Schwartz RW, Strodel WE: The objective structured clinical examination: The new gold standard for evaluating postgraduate clinical performance. Ann Surg 1995;222:735–742.

9. Stillman PL, Swanson D, Regan MB, et al: Assessment of clinical skills of residents utilizing standardized patients. A follow-up study and recommendations for application. Ann Intern Med 1991;114:393–401.

10. Barrows HS: An overview of the uses of standardized patients for teaching and evaluating clinical skills. Acad Med 1993;6:443–453.

11. Brailovsky CA, Grand'Maison P, Lescop J: Construct validity of the Quebec licensing examination SP-based OSCE. Teach Learn Med 1997;9:44–50.

12. Van der Vleuten CPM, Swanson DB: Assessment of clinical skills with standardized patients: State of the art. Teach Learn Med 1990;2:58–76.

13. King AM, Perkowski-Rogers LC, Polh HS: Planning standardized patient programs: Case development, patient training and costs. Teach Learn Med 1994;6:6–14.

14. Ram P, van der Vleuten C, Rethans JJ, et al: Assessment of family physicians: Comparison of observation in a multiple-station examination using standardized patients with observation of consultations in daily practice. Acad Med 1999;74:62–69.

15. Kopelow ML, Schnabl GK, Hassard TH, et al: Assessment of performance in the office setting with standardized patients: Assessing practicing physicians in two settings using standardized patients. Acad Med 1992;10:S19–S21.

16. Rethans JJ, Sturmans F, Drop R, et al: Does competence of general practitioners predict their performance? Comparison between examination setting and actual practice. BMJ 1991;303:1377–1380.

17. Hodges B, Regehr G, McNaughton N, et al: OSCE checklists do not capture increasing levels of expertise. Acad Med 1999;74:1129–1134.

18. Regehr G, MacRae H, Reznick RK, Szalay D: Comparing the psychometric properties of checklists and global rating scales for assessing performance on an OSCE-format examination. Acad Med 1998;73:993–997.

19. Hawkins R, MacKrell Gaglione M, LaDuca T, et al: Assessment of patient management skills and clinical skills of practising doctors using computer-based case simulations and standardised patients. Med Educ 2004;38(9):958–968.

20. Miller G: The assessment of clinical skills/competence/performance. Acad Med 1990;65(Suppl):S63–S67.

21. Holmboe ES: The importance of faculty observation of trainees' clinical skills. Acad Med 2004;79:16–22.

22. Kilminster SM, Jolly BC: Effective supervision in clinical practice settings: A literature review. Med Educ 2000;34:827–840.

23. Platt FW, McMath JC: Clinical hypocompetence: The interview. Ann Intern Med 1979;91:898–902.

24. Meuleman JR, Caranasos GJ: Evaluating the interview performance of internal medicine interns. Acad Med 1989;64:277–279.

25. Beaumier A, Bordage G, Saucier D, Turgeon J: Nature of the clinical difficulties of first year family medicine residents under direct observation. Can Med Assoc J 1992;146:489–497.

26. Sachdeva AK, Loiacono LA, Amiel GE: Variability in the clinical skills of residents entering training programs in surgery. Surgery 1995;118:300–309.

27. Pfeiffer C, Madray H, Ardolino A, Willms J: The rise and fall of student's skill in obtaining a medical history. Med Educ 1998;32:283–288.

28. Ramsey PG, Curtis R, Paauw DS, et al: History-taking and preventive medicine skills among primary care physicians: An assessment using standardized patients. Am J Med 1998;104:152–158.

29. Braddock CH, Edwards KA, Hasenberg NM: Informed decision making in outpatient practice. Time to get back to basics. JAMA 1999;282:2313–2320.

30. Stewart MA, McWhinney IR, Buck CW: The doctor-patient relationship and its effect upon outcome. J R Coll Gen Pract 1979;29:77–82.

31. Richards T: Chasms in communication. BMJ 1990;301:1407–1408.

32. Katz J: The Silent World of Doctor and Patient. New York, Free Press, 1984.

33. Simpson M, Buckman R, Stewart M, et al: Doctor-patient communication: The Toronto consensus statement. BMJ 1991;303:1385–1387.

34. Shapiro RS, Simpson DE, Lawrence SL, et al: A survey of sued and nonsued physicians and suing patients. Arch Intern Med 1989;149:2190–2196.

35. Novack DH: Therapeutic aspects of the clinical encounter. J Gen Intern Med 1987;2:346–355.

36. Assessing the effects of physician-patient interactions on the outcomes of chronic disease. Med Care 1989;27(Suppl 3): S110–S127.

37. Deber RB, Kraetschmer N, Irvine J: What role do patients wish to play in treatment decision making? Arch Intern Med 1996;156: 1414–1420.

38. Institute of Medicine: Crossing the Quality Chasm. A New Health System for the 21st Century. Washington, DC, National Academy Press, 2001.

39. Weiner S, Nathanson M: Physical examination. Frequently observed errors. JAMA 1976;236:852–855.

40. Wray NP, Friedland JA: Detection and correction of house staff error in physical diagnosis. JAMA 1983;249:1035–1037.

41. Butterworth JS, Reppert EH: Auscultatory acumen in the general medical population. JAMA 1960;174:32–34.

42. Raferty EB, Holland WW: Examination of the heart, an investigation into variation. Am J Epidemiol 1967;85:438–444.

43. Mangione S, Nieman LZ: Cardiac auscultatory skills of internal medicine and family practice trainees. A comparison of diagnostic proficiency. JAMA 1997;278:717–722.

44. Mangione S, Burdick WP, Peitzman SJ: Physical diagnosis skills of physicians in training: A focused assessment. Acad Emerg Med 1995;2:622–629.

45. Li JTC: Assessment of basic examination skills of internal medicine residents. Acad Med 1994;69:296–299.

46. Johnson JE, Carpenter JL: Medical house staff performance in physical examination. Arch Intern Med 1986;146:937–941.

47. Fox RA, Clark CLI, Scotland AD, Dacre JE: A study of pre-registration house officers' clinical skills. Med Educ 2000;34: 1007–1012.

48. Todd IK: A thorough pulmonary exam and other myths. Acad Med 2000;75:50–51.

49. Peterson MC, Holbrook JH, Hales DV: Contributions of the history, physical examination, and laboratory investigation in making medical diagnoses. West J Med 1992;156:163–165.

50. Kirch W, Schaffi C: Misdiagnosis at a university hospital in 4 medical areas: Report on 400 cases. Medicine 1996;75:29–40.

51. Hampton JR, Harrison MJG, Mitchell JRA, et al: Relative contributions of history-taking, physical examination, and laboratory investigation to diagnosis and management of medical outpatients. BMJ 1975;2:486–489.

52. Bordage G: Why did I miss the diagnosis? Some cognitive explanations and educational implications. Acad Med 1999;74: S138–S143.

53. Turnbull J, Gray J, MacFacyen J: Improving in-training evaluation programs. J Gen Intern Med 1998;13:317–323.

54. Duffy DF: Dialogue: The core clinical skill. Ann Intern Med 1998;128:139–141.

55. Johnson BT, Boohan M: Basic clinical skills: Don't leave teaching to the teaching hospitals. Med Educ 2000;34:692–699.

56. Cunnington JPW, Hanna E, Turnbull J, et al: Defensible assessment of the competency of the practicing physician. Acad Med 1997;72:9–12.

57. Long DM: Competency-based residency training: The next advance in graduate medical education. Acad Med 2000; 75:1178–1183.

58. Davis DA, Mazmanian PE, Fordis M, et al: Accuracy of physician self-assessment compared to observed measures of competence: A systematic review. JAMA 2006;296:1094–1102.

59. Duffy FD, Holmboe ES: Self-assessment in lifelong learning and improving performance in practice: Physician know thyself. JAMA 2006;296(9):1137–1139.

60. Feinstein AR: Clinical Judgment. Baltimore, Williams & Wilkins, 1967, pp 1–71, 291-349.

61. Engel GL: The deficiencies of the case presentation as a method of teaching: Another approach. N Engl J Med 1971;284:20–24.

62. Engel GL: Are medical schools neglecting clinical skills? JAMA 1976;236:861–863.

63. Scenes P: The role of faculty observation in assessing students' clinical skills. Contemp Issues Med Educ 1997;1:1–2.

64. Noel GL, Herbers JE, Callow MP: How well do internal medicine faculty members evaluate the clinical skills of residents? Ann Intern Med 1992;117:757–765.

65. Herbers JE, Noel GL, Cooper GS: How accurate are faculty evaluations of clinical competence? J Gen Intern Med 1989;4:202–208.

66. Kalet A, Ear JA, Kilowatts V: How well do faculty evaluate the interviewing skills of medical students? J Gen Intern Med 1992;97:179–184.

67. Elliot DL, Hickam DH: Evaluation of physical examination skills. Reliability of faculty observers and patient instructors. JAMA 1987;3405–3408.

68. Lindy FJ, Farr JL: Performance rating. Psychol Bull 1980;87: 72–107.

69. Heinemann RL, Wesley KN: The effects of delay in rating and amount of information observed on performance rating accuracy. Acad Management J 1983;26:677–686.

70. Holmboe ES, Fiebach NF, Galaty L, Huot S: The effectiveness of a focused educational intervention on resident evaluations from faculty: A randomized controlled trial. J Gen Intern Med 2001;16:1–6.

71. Ludmerer KM: Time to Heal: American Education from the Turn of the Century to the Era of Managed Care. Oxford, Oxford University Press, 1999.

72. Woehr DJ, Huffcutt AI: Rater training for performance appraisal: A quantitative review. J Occup Org Psychol 1994;67:189–205.

73. Hauenstein NMA: Training raters to increase the accuracy of appraisals and the usefulness of feedback. In Smither JW (ed): Performance Appraisal. San Francisco, Jossey-Bass, 1998, pp 404–442.

74. Stamoulis DT, Hauenstein NMA: Rater training and rating accuracy: Training for dimensional accuracy versus training for rater differentiation. J Appl Psychol 1993;78:994–1003.

75. Beard JD: Setting standards for the assessment of operative competence. Eur J Endovas Surg 2005;30:215–218.

76. Lipkin M, Quill TE, Napadano RJ: The medical interview: A core curriculum for residencies in internal medicine. Ann Intern Med 1984;100:277–284.

77. Smith RC, Hoppe RB: The patient's story: Integrating the patient and physician centered approaches to interviewing. Ann Intern Med 1991;115:470–477.

78. MacKoul G: The SEGUE framework for teaching and assessing communication skills. Patient Educ Counsel 2001;45:23–34.

79. Cegala DJ, Broz SL: Physician communication skills training: A review of the theoretical backgrounds, objectives, and skills. Med Educ 2002;36:1004–1016.

80. McGee S: Evidenced-Based Physical Diagnosis. Philadelphia, WB Saunders, 2001.

81. Sackett DL, Rennie D: The science of the art of the clinical examination. JAMA 1992;267:2650–2652.

82. Sackett DL, Rennie D: A primer on the precision and accuracy of the clinical examination. JAMA 1992;267:2638–2644.

83. Golnik KC, Goldenhar L: The ophthalmic clinical evaluation exercise. Reliability determination. Ophthalmology 2005;112: 1649–1654.

84. Holmboe ES, Hawkins RE, Huot SJ: Direct observation of competence training: A randomized controlled trial. Ann Intern Med 2004;140:874–881.

85. Norcini JJ, Blank LL, Arnold GK, Kimball HR: The mini-CEX (clinical evaluation exercise): A preliminary investigation. Ann Intern Med 1995;123:795–799.

86. Norcini JJ, Blank LL, Duffy FD, Fortna GS: The mini-CEX: A method for assessing clinical skills. Ann Intern Med 2003;138:476–481.

87. Holmboe ES, Huot S, Hawkins RE: Construct validity of the mini-clinical evaluation exercise. Acad Med 2003;78: 826–830.

88. Holmboe ES, Williams F, Yepes M, Huot S: Feedback and the mini-CEX. J Gen Intern Med 2004;19(part 2):558–561.

89. Norcini J, Boulet J: Methodological issues in the use of standardized patients for assessment. Teach Learn Med 2003;15:293–297.
90. Lypson ML, Frohna JG, Gruppen LD, Wolliscroft JO: Assessing residents' competencies at baseline: Identifying the gaps. Acad Med 2004;79:564–570.
91. Reznick RK, Regehr G, Yee G, et al: Process-rating forms versus task-specific checklists in an OSCE for medical licensure. Acad Med 1998;10:S97–S99.

APPENDIX 9-1
Sample Performance Dimension Training and Frame of Reference Exercise

The purpose of this group exercise is to develop specific criteria for a dimension of clinical competency. The dimension we will focus on today is counseling. Counseling is a core component of the new ACGME general competency of patient care.

Situation: A resident is seeing a patient who has been diagnosed with a new medical condition. The resident now needs to start a new medication for this patient. What are the criteria for a superior, highly effective counseling and patient education session? In other words, what criteria will you use to judge the counseling and patient education performance of this resident? Once you have defined all the criteria, check off those criteria a resident would have to perform in order to receive a *satisfactory* rating.

With your group: Define the components/criteria of *effective* patient counseling and education, based on the knowledge, skills, attitudes (KSA) model (Box 9-1). Be sure your criteria are ''behavioral''; remember that you are developing these elements in the context of faculty observation.

BOX 9-1	Knowledge, Skills, Attitudes (KSA) Model

Knowledge
What questions and "content" should the resident ask the patient?

Skills
How should the resident conduct the interview? Ask questions?

Attitudes
Define behaviors that would signal to an attending a resident was displaying a compassionate, interested, professional attitude.

Evaluating Evidence-Based Practice

Michael L. Green, MD, MSc

Evidence-based practice (EBP) has emerged as a national priority in efforts to improve health care quality.[1] EBP may be defined as the integration of the best research evidence with patients' values and clinical circumstances in clinical decision making.[2] In a recent consensus statement, authors preferred the term "evidence-based practice" over "evidence-based medicine" to "reflect the benefits of the entire health care teams and organizations adopting a shared evidence-based approach."[3] This ideal, however, remains far from realization. Physicians leave the majority of their clinical questions unanswered,[4,5] often consult non-evidence-based sources of information, witness their up-to-date medical knowledge and practice performance deteriorate over the years following their training,[6] and often

fail to implement clinical maneuvers with established efficacy.[7,8] And traditional didactic-based continuing medical education (CME) remains of limited utility as a remedy.[9,10]

In response, professional organizations have called for increased EBP training at all levels of medical education.[11-14] The Accreditation Council for Graduate Medical Education (ACGME) emphasized EBP in its "outcomes project,"[13] which shifted the currency of accreditation from structure and process to educational outcomes corresponding to six competencies. EBP is represented most prominently in the "patient care" and "practice-based learning and improvement (PBLI)" general competencies. Similarly, the Institute of Medicine includes "employ evidence-based practice" and "utilize informatics" among five essential competencies for all health professions.[11] In short, program directors must now document that trainees "investigate and evaluate their patient care practices, appraise and assimilate scientific evidence, and improve their scientific practices."[13]

In my thinking, reflective physicians encounter two distinct types of deficits as they "investigate and evaluate" their practices and undertake two different "improvements" accordingly. Let's take a clinical example, which I will return to throughout the chapter:

A 70-year-old man visits his physician for a periodic health examination. His only new complaint is a 3-month history of a mild intermittent nonproductive cough. His medical history includes benign prostatic hypertrophy, osteoarthritis, and isolated systolic hypertension. In the past he smoked about one pack per day but stopped at age 60. He has received all the routinely recommended preventive health care, including a normal colonoscopy, a pneumococcal polysaccharide vaccine (Pneumovax), and yearly influenza vaccines. Near the end of the visit he tells you that his bocci partner was recently hospitalized emergently for a ruptured abdominal aortic aneurysm (AAA). He asks, "Can you check me for that, doc?"

Unaware of recent studies and recommendations, this physician encounters a knowledge deficit. In descriptive studies of how physicians (or other professionals) learn, these deficits have been variously called "breakdowns,"[15] "problems,"[16] or "surprises."[17] We call them "clinical questions," in the parlance of evidence-based practice. The physician must then *ask* the question in an answerable format, *acquire* the best evidence, *appraise* the evidence for its validity and usefulness, *apply* the evidence to the decision making or counseling for this individual patient, and *assess* her performance. If she then reflects on the process, this new information will become part of her working knowledge and can be applied in future scenarios, almost reflexively, without a "surprise." She is, I might say, "knowing (from) what she does" in this evidence-based practice moment. In this chapter, I review the psychometric properties of instruments and strategies to evaluate this aspect of PBLI and offer recommendations for current educational practice and future research. In addition, I provide a list of resources in Appendix 10-1.

Alternatively, in the preceding scenario, the physician may already know that, based on a meta-analysis of screening trials, the United States Preventive Services Task Force (USPSTF) now recommends one screening abdominal ultrasound for men 65 years of age or older with a history of smoking.[18] In retrospectively investigating her practice via a record audit, she might discover that only 60% of her elderly male patients with a smoking history have been screened for AAA. This discovery would trigger a quality improvement initiative, which might include examining physician, patient, and office microsystem barriers to screening; a practice intervention such as a reminder system; and an evaluation of its effect on screening rates. The physician is, in this case, "doing what she knows." This aspect of PBLI is covered in Chapter 11.

General Issues in Evaluation in Medical Education

In analyzing EBP evaluation instruments, I defer to the classification developed by the Joint Committee on Standards for Educational and Psychological Testing of the American Educational Research Association, American Psychological Association, and National Council on Measurement in Education[19] and Downing's recent methodologic treatises[20-25] (Table 10-1).

Recent scholars have rejected the use of "construct validity" to describe a particular type of validity evidence.[20] Rather, all validity is construct validity, as it represents evidence that the instrument is accurately approximating an intangible psychological "construct" that cannot be measured directly. This is certainly true for knowledge, skills, and attitudes. Behaviors, on the other hand, can be directly observed. However, because resource and time constraints often make such observations impractical, investigators resort to surrogate measures. In this case, evidence for validity should demonstrate that the surrogate measures approximate the actual behaviors.

Finally, there is no single hierarchy for preferred types of validity evidence. Rather, appropriate analyses should be dictated by the intended evaluation uses of the instrument. For example, responsive validity may be more critical for an instrument to evaluate the programmatic effectiveness of an EBP curriculum, whereas instruments with established discriminative validity may be more appropriate to assess individual learners. Higher stakes evaluations, such as certification or promotion, require more robust validity (multiple types of evidence from strong scientific studies) than formative evaluation used for corrective feedback.

EBP Evaluation Domains

Table 10-2 lists several EBP evaluation domains, drawing from previously published conceptual frameworks for EBP evaluation.[26-28] An evidence-based practitioner must have the *knowledge and skills* to perform the five steps, alliteratively phrased as the five "A's." First, she must recognize emerging information needs and *ask* answerable clinical questions. Clinical questions can be classified as *background* (general) or *foreground* (specific, patient-based)[29] and associated with particular *clinical tasks*, such as therapy, diagnosis, or prognosis.[30] Furthermore, foreground questions can be constructed in the PICO format, explicitly identifying characteristics of the patient, intervention, comparison, and outcome.[31] For the clinical scenario described earlier in the chapter, we might ask, "In a 70-year-old patient with a history of hypertension and smoking, will screening for AAA with abdominal ultrasound result in a decreased risk of death from AAA rupture?" Asking such questions may help in selecting information resources, choosing search terms, knowing when to stop searching, applying the evidence in decision making, and communicating with other providers.[32-35]

Table 10-1 **Classification and Terminology for Types of Validity Evidence**

Sources of Validity Evidence	Description	Analysis*
Based on test content	Analysis of the relationship between the instrument's content and the construct it is intended to measure. Content refers to the themes, wording, and format of the items, tasks, or questions on a test as well as the procedures for administration and scoring.	Often determined by external review by experts (*content validity*)
Based on response processes	Data collected on the "processes" that examinees use in completing or that observers use in rating the instrument.	
Based on internal structure	The degree to which the relationships among the test items and test components conform to the construct on which the proposed test core interpretations are based.	Detection, among the items, of a unified latent construct or, if specified in advance, discrete subthemes, often determined with factor analysis (*dimensionality*)
		Relationship between items within either the entire instrument or within a prespecified section of the instrument, often measured with Cronbach's Alpha Coefficient (*internal consistency*)
Based on relationship to other variables	Analysis of the relationship of test scores to external variables (criteria) hypothesized to measure or represent the same constructs. Two designs may be distinguished. A *predictive* study indicates how accurately test data can predict criterion scores obtained in the future. A *concurrent* study obtains predictor and criterion information at the same time.	Correlation with scores on another test with established psychometric properties (*criterion validity*) Comparison of scores between groups assumed to have different levels of expertise (*discriminative validity*) Comparison of pre versus post scores with respect to an educational intervention (*responsive validity*)

Descriptive labels in italics in Analysis column represent terms in common use but are not taken from this source.
*Classification proposed by Joint Committee on Standards for Educational and Psychological Testing of the American Educational Research Association; the American Psychological Association; and the National Council on Measurement in Education: Standards for Educational and Psychological Testing. Washington, DC, American Educational Research Association, 1999.

However, the findings of one recent study of clinical questions have challenged some of these hypotheses.[36]

In performing the steps in which they *acquire* and *appraise*, clinicians practice in one of three EBP "modes,"[28,37] depending on the nature of the encountered condition, time constraints, level of EBP expertise, and personal preference. For frequently encountered conditions and with minimal time constraints, we may operate in the "doing" mode, seeking and critically appraising original clinical research reports. For less common conditions or for more rushed clinical situations, we might eliminate the critical appraisal step and operate in the "user" mode, conserving our time by restricting our search to rigorously pre-appraised resources. Editors of these evidence-based secondary information resources search, select, appraise, and summarize evidence from original research in the form of "syntheses" (systematic reviews) and "synopses" of studies and systematic reviews, adhering to accepted explicit methodologic criteria.[38,39] In our case, operating in the "user" mode, we might turn to a rigorous systematic review supporting new recommendations for screening for AAA.[18] Finally, in the "replicator" mode we trust and directly follow the recommendations of respected EBP consultants (abandoning at least the search for evidence and its detailed appraisal).

Doctors may practice in any of these modes at various times, but their activity will probably fall predominantly into one category. In a survey of U.K. general practitioners, 72% reported practicing at least part of their time in the "user mode," using evidence-based summaries generated by others.[40] On the other hand, fewer claimed to understand the "appraising" tools of number needed to treat (35%) and confidence intervals (20%). Finally, only 5% believed that "learning the skills of evidence-based medicine" (all five steps) was the most appropriate method for "moving from opinion-based medicine to evidence-based medicine."

In any of the modes, the clinician must then *apply* the evidence to the decision making for an individual patient. In this, she relies on her clinical expertise to integrate the evidence, the patient's particular clinical circumstances, and the patient's preferences.[2] Finally, the clinician *assesses* her performance in the entire EBP process.

Attitude domains include points of view about the appropriateness, effectiveness, feasibility, practice preferences, advantages, "untoward consequences," and perceived barriers to EBP. In addition, as a strategy for lifelong learning, EBP requires "readiness" or "inclination" for self-directed learning, a related construct borrowed from educational psychology.

Table 10-2 **EBP Evaluation Domains**

Psychometric Domain	Description
Knowledge and skills: EBP steps	
Ask	Identifying emerging information needs
	Discriminating between "background" and "foreground" questions
	Recognizing the "clinical task" associated with the clinical question
	Phrasing foreground questions in PICO format
Acquire	General computer/Internet skills[27]
	Recognizing and choosing between different EBP modes (doer, user, replicator)[28]
	Doer: Searching databases of original research (e.g., Medline) *User*: Appraising secondary databases of evidence-based summaries 　　Searching secondary databases of evidence-based summaries (e.g., Cochrane Library) *Replicator*: Knowing EBP performance of consultants
Appraise	*Doer*: Primarily appraising study design and conduct *User*: Understanding and appreciating a critical appraisal done by others
Apply	Individualizing measures of effect*
	Considering patient's particular clinical state and circumstances
	Considering patient's preferences
Assess	Assessing one's performance of EBP
Attitudes	Attitudes toward EBP
	Self-directed learning "readiness"
Behaviors	Performing EBP steps in practice
	Performing evidence-based clinical maneuvers in practice
	Affecting desirable patient outcomes
Global ratings	Global rating of EBP competence

*For example, recasting number needed to treat based on patient's baseline risk or determining posttest probability of disease using patient's pretest probability and likelihood ratio of diagnostic test.

We can consider EBP behaviors at two levels. First, we can ask: "Does a trainee perform the five EBP steps in her actual practice?" Alternatively, we can look further downstream and examine her clinical practice directly, asking, "Does she perform evidence-based clinical maneuvers in her practice?" And finally, we can examine patient outcomes as a desired "result" of EBP.

EBP Evaluation Instruments

A systematic review of EBP curricula in 1999 found that only a minority of published reports of EBP curricula included an evaluation.[41] Among these, evaluation instruments focused on critical appraisal to the exclusion of other EBP steps, measured EBP knowledge and skills but did not objectively document behaviors in actual practice, and often lacked established validity and reliability. Similarly, a national survey of internal medicine residency programs found that, among the 37% offering an EBM curriculum, only one third evaluated their curricula.[42] And very few of these attempted to objectively measure resident skills. Editorialists at the time lamented[43]:

Despite the widespread teaching of EBM, however, most of what is known about the outcomes of EBM curricula relies on observational data. Although evaluation of the quality of research evidence is a core competency of EBM, the quantity and quality of the evidence for effectively teaching EBM are poor. Ironically, if one were to develop guidelines for how to teach EBM based on these results, they would be based on the lowest level of evidence.

Fortunately, the last few years have witnessed the development of a wider range of EBP evaluation instruments, some of which are supported by robust psychometric testing. A recent systematic review, covering all health professions education, summarized the development, formats, learner levels, EBP domains, feasibility, and psychometric properties of 104 EBP evaluation instruments.[44] Although, as before, the instruments most commonly evaluated skills in critically appraising evidence, several new instruments have emerged to evaluate the *ask*, *acquire*, and *apply* steps. Within the *acquire* step, however, most of the instruments assess Medline searching and do not evaluate the appraisal, selection, and searching of resources containing preappraised summaries. Similarly, most of the Apply instruments are limited to consideration of research evidence in decision-making, neglecting skills in integrating clinical circumstances and patient preferences. Regarding EBP behaviors, the systematic review identified several new objective approaches to document the performance of EBP steps in practice and a few instruments that assess the performance of evidence-based clinical maneuvers.

Among the 104 instruments in the review, 53% were supported by at least one type of validity evidence but only 10% were supported by three or more types of validity evidence. In the following sections, I describe the more psychometrically robust instruments and suggest their suitability for different EBP evaluation purposes.

EBP Knowledge and Skills

Instruments with the Multiple Types of Evidence for Validity, Including Discriminative Validity

Table 10-3 summarizes the specific domains, formats and psychometric properties of the instruments supported by established inter-rater reliability (if applicable), objective (non-self reported) outcome measures, and multiple (3 or more) types of established validity evidence, including at least *discriminative validity*. Given their ability to distinguish between different levels of expertise, these instruments should be suitable to evaluate the EBP competence of individual trainees. Furthermore, the robust psychometric properties in general should support their use in formative or summative evaluations. However, in the absence of well-defined "passing standards" for different learner levels, they should not yet be used for very high stakes evaluations, like academic promotion or certification.

Among the instruments in Table 10-3, the Fresno Test[45] and Berlin Test[46] represent the only ones that evaluate all four EBP steps. In taking the primarily free text Fresno Test, trainees perform realistic EBP tasks, exposing their underlying thinking process as they demonstrate their applied knowledge and skills. However, this same feature requires more time and expertise to grade this instrument (although the authors do not offer feasibility data). The Fresno Test and grading template are available on the Internet (see Appendix 10-1). The multiple choice format of the Berlin Test restricts assessment to EBP applied knowledge but also makes it easier to implement. The other instruments in Table 10-3 evaluate a narrower range of EBP steps as indicated.

Instruments with "Strong Evidence" for Responsive Validity

In addition to four of the instruments in Table 10-3,[46–49] six additional instruments fulfill criteria for "strong evidence" of responsive validity (Table 10-4). These instruments are supported by (1) established inter-rater reliability (if applicable), (2) a randomized

controlled trial or pre-post controlled trial design, and (3) an objective (non-self-reported) outcome measure. Generally, these instruments have less robust psychometric properties than those in Table 10-3, which enjoy support from multiple types of validity evidence. However, given their ability to detect knowledge and skill changes after an educational intervention, these instruments should be suitable to determine the programmatic level impact of EBP curricula. For this type of evaluation, the Society of General Internal Medicine EBP Task Force recommends tailoring evaluation strategies to the learners (including their level and particular needs), the intervention (including the curriculum objectives, intensity, delivery method, and targeted EBP steps), and the outcomes (including knowledge, skills, attitudes, behaviors, or patient level outcomes).[28]

Among the instruments in Table 10-4, only Smith's EBP examination[50] measures all four EBP steps. Residents articulated clinical questions, conducted MEDLINE searches, performed calculations, and answered free text questions about critical appraisal and application of the evidence. In this study, gains in skills persisted on retesting at 6 months, indicating both concurrent and predictive responsive validity. The instrument described by Green and Ellis[51] required free text responses about the appraisal of a redacted journal article and application of the results to a patient. The three multiple choice tests[52–54] detected improvements in trainees' EBP knowledge. However, in two of the studies, this gain did not translate into improvements in critical appraisal skills as measured with a test article[53] or the incorporation of literature into admission notes.[52] Finally, in Villanueva's study,[55] librarians identified elements of the Patient-Intervention-Comparison (PICO) format[31] in clinical question requests, awarding one point for each of four elements included. This instrument detected improvements in a randomized controlled trial (RCT) of providing instructions and clinical question examples as part of an "evidence search and critical appraisal service."

Additional EBP Knowledge and Skill Instruments

The following instruments, in spite of their more limited psychometric testing, are worthy of mention because of either an innovative evaluation strategy or an assessment of EBP steps other than "appraise." (As noted previously, many older EBP evaluation instruments measured critical appraisal knowledge and skills, to the exclusion of the other EBP steps.)

Objective Structured Clinical Examinations

Objective structured clinical examinations (OSCEs) measure knowledge and skills as applied in a realistic clinical setting ("shows how" level in Miller's classification;[56] see Chapter 1). Investigators have reported EBP OSCEs using standardized patients,[57,58] computer stations,[59,60] and written cases.[61,62] In Berner's study, students at a medical school with a "mature informatics curriculum" scored significantly higher on 4 of the 11 tasks than students (with higher MCATs and USMLE II scores) at another school that offered "no formal instruction."[59]

Evaluating Ask: Articulating Clinical Questions

In addition to the one instrument in Table 10-4,[55] two additional investigators developed approaches to evaluate clinical questions formulation, using 4-point[63] and 2-point[64] scales corresponding to inclusion of PICO elements.

Evaluating Acquire: Searching for Evidence

In several studies, librarians rated trainees' Medline search strategies according to predetermined criteria, usually developed by consensus.[65–69] Search strategy criteria often include the efficient use of boolean operators, Medical Subject Headings (MeSH), "explode" function, and methodologic (or publication type) filters. Three studies demonstrated evidence of responsive validity,[66,68,69] one provided evidence of criterion validity,[69] but none of the studies examined the interrater reliability or discriminative validity of these Medline search strategy ratings. As described in Haynes' studies[70–72] in Table 10-3, we can reliably assess searching skills by examining looking beyond the intermediate outcome of the search strategy to the captured articles.

It is notable that nearly all the evaluation approaches for the *acquire* step exclusively assess Medline searching skills. Of four instruments that include secondary preappraised evidence-based medical information resources, only the Fresno Test[45] (see Table 10-3) assesses skills, and only a few of the others[40,63,73] include a few survey questions about "awareness of" or "preference for" these resources.

Evaluating Apply: Applying Evidence to Decision Making

Evaluating this EBP step remains largely unexplored. Some of the general EBP instruments include one or two questions relating to applying evidence to an individual patient, but none comprehensively assess skills in "individualizing" evidence and integrating it with the patient's particular clinical context, preferences, and potential actions. Some promising approaches to this type of evaluation include having standardized patients rate students' explanations of therapeutic decisions after reviewing research evidence,[57,58] scoring of residents' free text justification of applying results of a study to "paper case,"[51] and documenting decision making before and after access to a research abstract[61,62] or Medline searching.[74]

EBP Attitudes and "Readiness"

Although many EBP instruments include a few questions about attitudes, few explore this domain in depth.[40,75–77] McAlister's survey assessed EBP attitudes, perceived barriers to EBP, preferred sources of information, and self-reported confidence in EBP skills.[75] The study reported correlations between some scales within the instrument, such as self-reported use of EBM and preference for primary research articles, as evidence for validity. In the attitude section of McColl's survey, respondents report their attitudes toward EBP, awareness of medical information resources, ability to access information databases, understanding of EBP terms, perceived barriers to EBP, and views on how to "move from opinion-based to evidence-based medicine."[40] In a subsequent RCT, EBP academic detailing did not influence general practitioners' attitudes (but did improve their scores on the multiple-choice knowledge section) as measured with this instrument.[78] Young's survey addressed views of EBP, understanding of technical terms in EBP, barriers to EBP, preferred strategies to support EBP, and familiarity with information databases.[77] In Baum's uncontrolled study, residents' attitudes improved after an EBP workshop.[76] In addition to these quantitative surveys, investigators have employed qualitative techniques to analyze the responses of focus groups and structured interviews.[79–86]

Some EBP attitude domains, such as the inclination to seek information to answer clinical questions emerging in practice, seem closely related to the educational psychology construct of self-directed learning (SDL) "readiness," which has been defined as "the degree [to which] the individual possesses the attitudes, abilities, and personality characteristics necessary for SDL."[87] The Self-Directed Learning Readiness Scale (SDLRS)[88] is the most widely used instrument for assessing SDL "readiness." This instrument includes 58 statements with Likert-style responses ranging from 1 (almost never true of me; I hardly ever feel this way) to 5 (almost always true of me; there are very few times when I don't feel this way). Subjects receive a single score, ranging from 58 (indicating a low level of readiness to direct one's learning) to 290. The national norm for general adult learners is 214.

Factor analyses in different populations, not surprisingly, have found different factor structures,[89–92] but most seem similar to the themes determined in the original developmental studies. In higher education studies, the SDLRS showed excellent interitem consistency and test-retest reliability. Several studies have confirmed criterion validity, documenting correlations with adult learning (measured with the Student's Orientation Questionnaire),[93] preference for structure (inverse),[94] and learning projects, SDL time, and SDL behaviors.[95]

There is limited experience with the SDLRS in health professions education. In Harvey's cross-sectional study at a single medical school, there was no increase in SDLRS score by curriculum year.[96] Shokar administered the SDLRS to beginning third-year students after completing 2 years of a PBL curriculum.[97] Their SDLRS scores correlated with their final grade and all of its components in two clerkships, but only the association with the faculty preceptor evaluation achieved statistical significance. In the only GME experience with the SDLRS, obstetrics-gynecology residents using an Internet-based learning portfolio for a longer period of time scored higher than residents with a shorter exposure.[98]

Table 10-3 EBP Knowledge and Skill Instruments with Multiple Types of Validity Evidence, Including Discriminative Validity

Knowledge and Skill Domains	Description	Experience	Inter-rater Reliability*	Validity
Instrument: Berlin Questionnaire[46,134]				
Knowledge about interpreting evidence Skills to relate a clinical problem to a clinical question Best design to answer a question Use quantitative information from research to solve specific patient problems	2 separate sets of 15 MCQs built around "typical" clinical scenarios	43 "experts," 20 third-year students, 203 participants in EBM course in development study[46] 49 internal medicine residents in controlled trial of EBM curriculum[134]	N/A	Content Internal consistency Discriminative Responsive
Instrument: Taylor[†,48,135-137]				
Knowledge of critical appraisal Knowledge of MEDLINE searching	Sets of 6 MCQs with 3 potential answers, each requiring a true, false, or don't know response Best score on each set = 18	152 health care professionals in development study[48] Modified and "revalidated" instrument on 55 delegates at international EBP conferences[135] 175 students in RCT of self-directed versus workshop-based EBP curricula[136] 145 general practitioners, hospital physicians, allied health professionals, and health care managers in RCT of critical appraisal training[137]	N/A	Content Internal consistency Discriminative Responsive
Fresno Test[†,45,138]				
Formulate a focused question Identify appropriate research design for answering the question Show knowledge of electronic database searching (including secondary sources) Identify issues important for the relevance and validity of an article Discuss the magnitude and importance of research findings	Short-answer free text questions and calculations relating to 2 pediatric clinical scenarios. Scored by using a standardized grading rubric.	53 "experts" and 43 family practice residents and faculty in development study[45] 114 occupational therapists in pre/post uncontrolled trial of 2-day EBP workshop combined with outreach support[138]	Yes	Content Internal consistency Discriminative Responsive
Instrument: MacRae[†,49,139]				
Critical appraisal skills	55 short-answer questions and 7-point methodologic ratings related to 3 articles	44 surgery residents in development study[49] 55 surgeons in RCT of Internet-based EBP curriculum[139]	Yes	Internal consistency Discriminative Responsive

Instrument	Description	Sample	Reliability*	Validity
Instrument: Weberschock[140]				
EBP knowledge and skills (specific skills not specified)	5 sets of 20 MCQs (5 "easy," 10 "average," and 5 "difficult") linked to clinical scenarios and pertaining to data from published research articles	132 third-year medical students and 11 students with advanced training in "EBM working group" in development and pre/post uncontrolled study of peer teaching EBP curriculum[140]	N/A	Internal consistency Discriminative Responsive Criterion
Instrument: Bennett[47]				
Critical appraisal skills	Set of case-based problems that require a diagnostic or treatment decision matched with an article advocating the test or treatment; students have to "take a stand" and "defend" it in writing; graded on preset criteria	79 medical students on various clerkships in pre/post controlled trial.[47]	Yes‡	Content Discriminative Responsive
Instrument: Haynes[†,70-72]				
Medline searching skills	Search output scored by comparison to searches (for same clinical questions) by an expert end-user physician and a librarian; "relative recall" calculated as number of relevant citations from a given search divided by number of relevant citations from the 3 searches (subject, expert physician, and librarian); "precision" calculated as the number of relevant citations retrieved in a search divided by the total citations retrieved in that search; article "relevance" rated reliably on a 7-point scale	158 clinicians (novice users), 13 "expert end searcher" clinicians (expert end users), and 3 librarians[70,71] 308 physicians and physicians-in-training in RCT of one-on-one precepting and searching feedback[72]	Yes‡	Content Discriminative Responsive

*Reliability testing was deemed "not applicable" for instruments, such as multiple-choice tests, that required no rater judgment to score.

†Demonstrated both inter-rater and intrarater reliability.

‡Instruments evaluated in more than one study. Results from all of the studies were used to determine number of trainees, reliability, and validity.

MCQ, multiple-choice question; RCT, randomized controlled trial.

Adapted from Shaneyfelt T, Baum KD, Bell D, et al: Instruments for evaluating education in evidence-based practice: A systematic review. JAMA 2006;296(9):1116-1127.

Table 10-4 **EBP Knowledge and Skill Instruments Supported by "Strong Evidence" of Responsive Validity***

Instrument	Knowledge and Skill Domains	Description	Study Settings/ Participants	Inter-rater Reliability[†]	Validity
Landry[‡52]	Research design and critical appraisal knowledge	10-item test	146 medical students in controlled trial of two 90-minute seminars[52]	NA	Content Responsive
	Skills in applying medical literature to clinical decision making	Blinded review of patient "write-ups" looking for literature citations		No	None
Linzer[‡53]	Epidemiology and biostatistics knowledge	MCQ test (knowledge); 15 questions chosen so that perfect score would allow access to 81% of medical literature (1983)[141]	44 medical residents in RCT of journal club curriculum[53]	NA	Content Responsive
	Skills in critical appraisal	Free text critical appraisal of text article; scoring based on "gold standard" criteria developed by consensus of faculty		Yes	Content Discriminative
Green[51]	Skills in critical appraisal Skills in applying evidence to individual patient decision making	9-question test (requiring free text response) relating to a case presentation and a redacted journal article	34 residents in controlled trial of a 7-session EBP curriculum[51]	Yes	Content Responsive
Stevermer[105]	EBP behavior (performance of EBP steps in practice)	Test of awareness and recall of recently published articles reporting "important findings about common primary care problems" (selected by faculty physicians)	59 family practice residents in RCT of EBP "academic detailing"[105]	NA	Responsive
Smith[50]	Skills in formulating clinical questions Skills in Medline searching Skills in critical appraisal Skills in applying evidence to individual patient decision making Knowledge of quantitative aspects of diagnosis and treatment studies	Test including sets of questions (format not specified) relating to 5 clinical cases	55 medical residents in pre/post controlled cross-over trial of 7-week EBP curriculum, which included interactive sessions and computer lab training[50]	Yes	Responsive[¶]
Villanueva[55]	Skills in formulating clinical questions	Librarians identified elements of the patient-intervention-comparison (PICO) format in clinical question requests; one point awarded for each of 4 elements included	39 health care professional participants in a library "evidence search and critical appraisal service" in an RCT of providing instructions and clinical question examples[55]	Yes	Responsive

Table 10-4 **EBP Knowledge and Skill Instruments Supported by "Strong Evidence" of Responsive Validity*** *(Continued)*

Instrument	Knowledge and Skill Domains	Description	Study Settings/ Participants	Inter-rater Reliability[†]	Validity
Ross[54]	EBP knowledge (specific steps not specified)	50-item "open book" MCQ test	48 family practice residents in controlled trial of 10-session EBP workshop (control residents in different program)[54]	NA	Content Responsive
	EBP behavior (enacting EBP steps in practice)	Analysis of audiotapes of resident-faculty interactions, looking for phrases related to literature searching, clinical epidemiology, or critical appraisal		No	Content Responsive

*To qualify for "strong evidence," instruments must demonstrate inter-rater reliability (if applicable) and responsive validity must be established by studies with a randomized controlled trial or pre/post controlled trial design and an objective (non-self-reported) outcome measure. Four instruments from Table 10–3 also showed "strong evidence" of responsive validity.[46–49]

[†]Reliability testing was deemed "not applicable for instruments, such as MCQ tests, that required no rater judgment to score.

[‡]Met "strong evidence" criteria for the EBP knowledge portion of overall instrument, not for the EBP skill portion.

[¶]Gains in skills persisted after 6 months, indicating both concurrent and predictive (responsive) validity.

EBP, evidence-based practice; MCQ, multiple-choice question; RCT, randomized controlled trial.

Adapted from Shaneyfelt T, Baum KD, Bell D, et al: Instruments for evaluating education in evidence-based practice: A systematic review. JAMA 2006; 296(9):1116–1127.

The Jefferson Scale of Physician Lifelong Learning (JSPLL), which includes 19 items answered on a 4-point Likert scale, measures physicians' "orientation" toward lifelong learning.[99] Psychometric testing demonstrated excellent internal consistency (coefficient alpha 0.89) and the test-retest reliability. In a survey of 444 physicians, factor analysis yielded 4 subscales entitled "professional learning beliefs and motivation," "scholarly activities," "attention to learning opportunities," and "technical skills in seeking information," which are consistent with recognized features of lifelong learning.[100] The criterion validity of the scale and its subscales was supported by significant correlations with responses to additional questions about respondents' professional activities that presumably require continuous learning.

EBP Behaviors (Performance)

EBP behavior remains the most challenging domain for evaluators. Nonetheless, we must ensure that trainees implement their EBP skills in actual practice.[101] The range of evaluation strategies is summarized in Table 10-5.

Evaluating the Performance of EBP Steps in Practice

Regarding EBP steps, we can simply ask a trainee if she, for example, consistently searches for the evidence to answer her clinical questions. However, retrospective self-reports of EBP behaviors remain extremely biased, as physicians tend to underestimate their information needs and overestimate their pursuit of them.[4] At the opposite extreme of rigor, we can shadow a trainee in the course of her patient encounters, document her emerging clinical questions, and follow up

later to see if she has acquired, appraised, and applied the evidence. The question collection might involve passive "anthropological" observation[102] or active debriefing.[4,5,103] Although this direct observation yields more valid data, it is generally not feasible outside the research setting. Thus, educators have looked for intermediate approaches to evaluating EBP performance.

In two studies, investigators analyzed audiotapes of resident-faculty interactions, looking for phrases related to literature searching, clinical epidemiology, or critical appraisal.[54,104] Family practice residents'

Table 10-5 **Strategies for Evaluating Physician EBP Behaviors and Patient Outcomes***

Performing EBP steps in practice
Retrospective self-reports of performing EBP steps
Frequency of EBP terminology in analysis of recorded teaching interactions
Recall and knowledge or recent articles important to particular practice and specialty
Electronic capture of searching behavior, including number of "log-ons," searching volume, abstracts or articles viewed, and time spent searching
EBP learning portfolios
Direct observation and debriefing
Performing evidence-based clinical maneuvers in practice and affecting desirable patient outcomes
Record audit for primary diagnosis and therapy and determination of level of supporting evidence
Record audit for quality performance indicators or patient outcomes
Clinical vignettes

*See text for further discussion.

"EBP utterances" increased from 0.21 per hour to 2.9 per hour after an educational intervention.[54] In my view, however, this outcome lacks face validity as a suitable surrogate for EBP performance. Taking a different approach, investigators questioned residents about their awareness and knowledge of findings in recent journal articles deemed relevant to primary care practice.[105] In this pre-post RCT, residents exposed to "academic detailing" recalled more articles and correctly answered more questions about them.

Educators can also electronically capture trainees' searching behaviors, including number of "log-ons," searching volume, abstracts or articles viewed, and time spent searching.[72,106] In an RCT, Cabell demonstrated that these measures were responsive to an intervention including a 1-hour didactic session, the use of well-built clinical question cards, and practical sessions in clinical question building.[106] In Haynes' RCT, physicians receiving additional help from a personal clinical preceptor and feedback from a librarian did not search more often than controls receiving a 2-hour training session alone.[72] Although this approach is quite feasible, the crude measure of searching "volume" fails to capture the pursuit and application of information in response to particular clinical questions.

Another approach is to have trainees catalogue their EBP learning activities in "learning portfolios," which represent "a purposeful collection of student work that exhibits to the student (and/or others) the student's efforts, progress, or achievement in (a) given area(s)."[107] EBP portfolios might include "educational prescriptions," which faculty members "dispense" when a moment of uncertainty arises in the course of patient care.[108–112] A typical educational prescription describes the clinical problem, states the question, specifies who is responsible for answering it, and reminds the trainee and faculty of a follow-up time. Some variations have the trainee articulate foreground questions in the PICO format, document the information resources searched, grade the level of evidence, or summarize what she learned. (See Appendix 10-2 for examples.)

EBP learning portfolios can be maintained in sophisticated Internet-based databases.[98,113–115] Educators implemented a Computerized Obstetrics and Gynecology Automated Learning Analysis (KOALA) at several residency programs.[98] This portfolio allowed residents to record their clinical encounters; directly link to information resources; and document "critical learning incidents." During a 4-month pilot period at four programs, 41 residents recorded 7049 patient encounters and 1460 critical learning incidents. Residents at one of the programs, which had a prior 1-year experience with KOALA, demonstrated higher "self-directed learning readiness" (measured with a validated instrument[88]). In another program, internal medicine residents entered their clinical questions, accompanied by Medline reference links and article summaries, into a similar Internet-based compendium.[113] The EBP exercises produced "useful information" for 82% and altered patient management for 39% of 625 clinical questions over 10 months.

Evaluating the Performance of Evidence-Based Clinical Maneuvers and Affecting Patient Outcomes

Ellis devised a reliable method for determining the primary therapeutic intervention chosen by a practitioner and classifying the quality of evidence supporting it.[116] In this scheme, interventions are (1) supported by individual or systematic reviews of randomized controlled trials, (2) supported by "convincing non-experimental evidence," or (3) lacking substantial evidence. This method has been employed in descriptive studies in inpatient medicine,[116,117] general outpatient practice,[118] emergency ophthalmology,[119] dermatology,[120] anesthesiology,[121] general surgery,[122] pediatric surgery,[123] and inpatient psychiatry[124] settings. Straus's pre-post study of a multifaceted EBP educational intervention provides initial evidence of the "responsive" validity of this evaluation strategy.[125] Patients admitted after the intervention were more likely to receive therapies proved to be beneficial in RCTs (62% versus 49%; $p = 0.016$). Of these trial-proved therapies, those offered after the EBM intervention were more likely to be based on high-quality randomized controlled trials (95% versus 87%; $p = 0.023$).

Lucas's study showed that this method of classifying the quality of supporting evidence may not be sensitive to clinicians' selections among evidence-based therapies.[126] On an inpatient medical service, 86% of inpatients of 33 providers received "evidence-based treatments" (level 1 or 2 of Ellis classification) at baseline. After then receiving a standardized literature search related to the primary diagnosis, the practitioners altered their treatment for 23 (18%) of the patients. However, the proportion of patients classified as receiving "evidence-based treatments" did not significantly change (86% to 87%). The Ellis "protocol" appears most suited to evaluate changes in EBP performance after an educational intervention or simply just over time. To use it to document some absolute threshold of performance, one would have to know, for every trainee's set of patients, the "denominator" of evidence-based therapeutic options, making it impractical on a programmatic scale.

We can also document the provision of evidence-based care by auditing records for adherence to evidence-based guidelines or quality indicators. Hardly a new development, this type of audit is commonly performed as part of internal quality initiatives or by third-party payers or regulatory agencies. Langham used a quality audit to evaluate the impact of an EBP curriculum, documenting, in an RCT, improvements in practicing physicians' documentation, clinical interventions, and patient outcomes relating to cardiovascular risk factors.[127] Epling showed improvements in residents' performance of recommended diabetes mellitus care measures after they participated in a curriculum that involved the development of a practice guideline.[128]

Clinical vignettes may represent a more feasible, yet valid, alternative for measuring the quality of clinical practice.[129]

Finally, patient level outcomes remain the most elusive to evaluators, remaining subject to myriad influences apart from physician performance. Nonetheless, investigators have documented changes in patient outcomes, albeit intermediate outcomes such as blood pressure, glycemic control, and serum lipids, following EBP educational interventions.[127,128,130]

Which Level of EBP Behaviors Should We Measure?

One could argue that trainees' enactment of EBP steps, however measured, represents an intermediate behavioral outcome. That is, we assume that physicians who consistently perform EBP steps will provide more evidence-based care, which, in turn, will lead to more evidence-based practice actions and better patient outcomes. But our clinical experience reminds us that intermediate outcomes may fail to guarantee the ultimate outcomes of interest. Should educators, then, "cast their line" beyond EBP steps to measures of evidence-based practice performance and, if possible, clinical outcomes in patients?

I believe we should document *both* types of EBP behavior outcomes. Although practice performance measures represent the ultimate outcome, they remain, by virtue of their "downstream" vantage, blunt instruments. A physician's performance, for instance, in screening her elderly male patients for abdominal aortic aneurysm represents the end result of myriad inputs, some of which remain outside her control. Would a record audit "detect" that the patient did not adhere with her recommendation to undergo screening because of denied insurance coverage? Or perhaps the physician did *not* recommend screening but her decision reflected a careful consideration of the patient's particular clinical circumstances and preferences,[2,83] rather than a failure to consider the new guidelines supported by a systematic review of the evidence. Perhaps, for example, a chest radiograph revealed a pulmonary nodule, and she deferred screening until lung cancer was excluded. Finally, we should ensure trainees' inclination to consistently perform EBP steps in practice in anticipation that they will direct this behavior to the unforeseeable (and thus unauditable) clinical problems they will encounter in the future.

Global Ratings

Since the American Board of Medicine revised its rating form to reflect the six new ACGME competencies, residency programs are gaining experience with faculty's global rating of residents' "practice-based learning and improvement," which includes EBP and quality improvement. In this evaluation, a faculty member rates each resident's overall competence (encompassing knowledge, skills, behaviors, and attitudes) on a 9-point scale. A recent factor analysis of rating forms,[131] including all six competencies, demonstrated that faculty raters actually discriminated only between two broad dimensions (medical knowledge and interpersonal skills)—the same "halo effect" seen on the original rating forms. Furthermore, the rating form, as currently configured, does not distinguish between the two dimensions of PBLI described in the introduction.

Recommendations

Rating scales of the ACGME competencies, as required by the ABIM, do not psychometrically isolate an individual trainee's competence in EBP from a global impression of performance.[131] Thus, educators should defer to additional instruments and strategies, dictated by the purpose of evaluation, learners' level and needs, EBP domain of interest, feasibility, format, and compatibility with programmatic and institutional contextual variables.

Evaluating EBP Knowledge and Skills

For evaluation of the competence of individual trainees, educators may utilize the instruments with established discriminative validity listed in Table 10-3. The robust psychometric properties support their use in both formative and summative evaluations. However, although these instruments can discriminate between different levels of expertise, testing has defined an accepted minimum threshold of EBP competence. Thus, I would not yet recommend them for top high-stakes summative evaluations.[25]

Educators can also take advantage of efficiencies of integrating EBP evaluation into the course of clinical care and teaching. Although I am unaware of any published experience, educators could assess EBP skills as part of a mini-clinical evaluation exercise (mini-CEX). These observations, described in Chapter 9, assess brief snapshots of real clinical encounters, show measurement characteristics similar to those of other performance assessments, permit evaluation based on a broader set of clinical settings and patient problems, and achieve sufficient reliability with multiple testing.[132] For example, a clinic preceptor supervising the patient encounter described in the introduction could prompt and then rate the resident's clinical question formulation, information gathering plan, or integration of the evidence for AAA screening into an informed decision-making discussion. Such items could be incorporated into customized mini-CEX forms. In addition, when the EBP "moment" cannot occur in real time, faculty can rate components of "filled" educational prescriptions (see Appendix 10-2), using them in this way to evaluate skills rather than behaviors. This approach should be restricted to formative evaluation until studies document its psychometric properties.

To determine the programmatic level impact of specific curricula, educators may turn to instruments with strong evidence of responsive validity, including four of the generally most robust instruments listed in Table 10-3[46–49] and the seven instruments listed in Table 10-4.[50–55] Educators should choose instruments with outcome measures aligned with their curricula's learning objectives.

EBP Attitudes

Assessing attitudes may uncover hidden but potentially remediable barriers to trainees' EBP skill development and performance. In addition to surveys (or sections of surveys)[40,75–77] educators may use focus groups or structured interviews to determine trainees' attitudes and experiences.[79–86]

EBP attitudes may also relate to trainees "inclination" or "readiness" for lifelong self-directed learning in medicine. Educators might use the SDLRS[88] or, if continued testing confirms its validity, the JSPLL[99,100] to inform program development, assist with individual trainee remediation, or serve as a barometer of the hidden curriculum related to EBP.

EBP Behaviors

Although EBP behaviors remain the most challenging domain, evaluators, nonetheless, must ensure that trainees implement their EBP skills in actual practice. The range of strategies to evaluate EBP behaviors appears in Table 10-5. A portfolio of educational prescriptions represents the most promising technology to document the performance of EBP steps in practice (see Appendix 10-2, for examples). With a simple system to dispense and collect the forms in place, the trainees can do most of the data entry. Internet-based systems may make tracking of information seeking and applying behavior more feasible. In addition, unlike many other approaches, the prescription serves as an education intervention as well, particularly if the trainee reflects upon the "EBP moment" and reviews it with a faculty member. Program directors (or regulatory bodies) might consider *requiring* documentation of a minimum number of "EBP episodes," much in the same way they currently do for technical procedures.

To document evidence-based practice performance, educators can borrow the quality data often already collected by health care organizations or team with institutional officials to leverage resources for nascent efforts. In addition, the American Board of Internal Medicine now offers practice improvement modules (PIMs) for residency programs and maintenance of certification credit for faculty who facilitate them.[133] Finally, as noted earlier in the chapter, we can put the residents to work collecting their own practice performance data (often with a fair measure of chagrin) in the context of a quality curriculum.[130]

ACKNOWLEDGMENTS
I wish to thank Drs. Sharon Straus and Scott Richardson for their thoughtful reviews of the manuscript.

BIBLIOGRAPHY

Articles

Fung MF, Walker M, Fung KF, et al: An internet-based learning portfolio in resident education: The KOALA multicentre programme. Med Educ 2000;34(6):474–479.

Green ML: Evaluating evidence-based practice performance. Evid Based Med 2006;11(4):99–101.

Green ML: Evidence-based medicine training in graduate medical education: Past, present and future. J Eval Clin Pract 2000;6(2):121–138.

Green ML, Ruff TR: Why do residents fail to answer their clinical questions? A qualitative study of barriers to practicing evidence-based medicine. Acad Med 2005;80(2):176–182.

Hatala R, Keitz SA, Wilson MC, Guyatt G: Beyond journal clubs: Moving toward an integrated evidence-based medicine curriculum. J Gen Intern Med 2006;21(5):538–541.

Richardson WS: Teaching evidence-based practice on foot. ACP J Club 2005;143(2):A10–A12.

Shaneyfelt T, Baum KD, Bell D, et al: Instruments for evaluating education in evidence-based practice: A systematic review. JAMA 2006;296(9):1116–1127.

Straus SE, Green ML, Bell DS, et al: Evaluating the teaching of evidence based medicine: conceptual framework. BMJ 2004;329(7473):1029–1032.

Textbooks

Fletcher RW, Fletcher SW: Clinical Epidemiology: The Essentials. Philadelphia, Lippincott Williams & Wilkins, 2005.

Guyatt G, Rennie D (eds): User's Guides To the Medical Literature: A Manual for Evidence-Based Clinical Practice. Chicago, AMA Press, 2002, (Internet version accessed July 16, 2007 at www.usersguides.org).

Haynes RB, Sacket DL, Guyatt GH, Tugwell P: Clinical Epidemiology: How to Do Clinical Practice Research, 3rd ed. Philadelphia, Lippincott Williams & Wilkins, 2005.

Heneghan C, Badenoch D: Evidence-based Medicine Toolkit. Oxford, Blackwell BMJ Books, 2006.

Straus SE, Richardson WS, Glasziou P, Haynes RB: Evidence-based Medicine: How to Practice and Teach EBM, 3rd ed. Edinburgh, Elsevier, 2005.

REFERENCES

1. Institute of Medicine: Crossing the Quality Chasm: A New Health System for the 21st Century. Washington, DC, National Academy Press, 2001.
2. Haynes RB, Devereaux PJ, Guyatt GH: Clinical expertise in the era of evidence-based medicine and patient choice. ACP J Club 2002;136(2):A11–A14.
3. Dawes M, Summerskill W, Glasziou P, et al: Sicily statement on evidence-based practice. BMC Med Educ 2005;5(1):1.
4. Covell DG, Uman GC, Manning PR: Information needs in office practice. Ann Intern Med 1985;103(4):596–599.
5. Gorman PN, Helfand M: Information seeking in primary care: How physicians choose which clinical questions to pursue and which to leave unanswered. Med Decision Making 1995;15(2):113–119.
6. Choudhry NK, Fletcher RH, Soumerai SB: Systematic review: The relationship between clinical experience and quality of health care. Ann Intern Med 2005;142(4):260–273.
7. McGlynn EA, Asch SM, Adams J, et al: The quality of health care delivered to adults in the United States. N Engl J Med 2003;348(26):2635–2645.
8. Hayward RA, Asch SM, Hogan MM, et al: Sins of omission. Getting too little medical care may be the greatest threat to patient safety. J Gen Intern Med 2005;20(8):686–691.
9. Davis DA, Thomson MA, Oxman AD, Haynes RB: Changing physician performance. A systematic review of the effect of continuing medical education strategies. JAMA 1995;274(9):700–705.
10. Davis D, O'Brien MA, Freemantle N, et al: Impact of formal continuing medical education: Do conferences, workshops, rounds, and

other traditional continuing education activities change physician behavior or health care outcomes? JAMA 1999;282(9):867–874.

11. Institute of Medicine: Health Professions Education: A Bridge to Quality. Washington, DC, National Academies Press, 2003.

12. American Association of Medical Colleges: Medical School Objectives Project: Medical Informatics and Population Health. Accessed July 16, 2007 at www.aamc.org/meded/msop/.

13. Accreditation Council for Graduate Medical Education: Outcomes Project: General Competencies. Accessed July 16, 2007 at www.acgme.org/outcome/comp/compFull.asp.

14. American Board of Medical Specialties: Maintenance of Certification. Accessed July 16, 2007 at www.abms.org/About_Board_Certification/MOC.aspx.

15. Smith CS, Morris M, Francovich C, et al: A qualitative study of resident learning in ambulatory clinic. Adv Health Sci Educ 2004;9:93–105.

16. Slotnick HB: How doctors learn: physicians' self-directed learning episodes. Acad Med 1999;74(10):1106–1117.

17. Schon DA: Educating the Reflective Practitioner. San Francisco, Jossey-Bass, 1987.

18. U.S. Preventive Services Task Force: Screening for abdominal aortic aneurysm: Recommendation statement. Ann Intern Med 2005;142(3):198–202.

19. Joint Committee on Standards for Educational and Psychological Testing of the American Educational Research Association; the American Psychological Association; and the National Council on Measurement in Education: Standards for Educational and Psychological Testing. Washington, DC, American Educational Research Association, 1999.

20. Downing SM: Validity: On the meaningful interpretation of assessment data. Med Educ 2003;37(9):830–837.

21. Downing SM, Haladyna TM: Validity threats: Overcoming interference with proposed interpretations of assessment data. Med Educ 2004;38(3):327–333.

22. Downing SM: Reliability: On the reproducibility of assessment data. Med Educ 2004;38(9):1006–1012.

23. Downing SM: Threats to the validity of clinical teaching assessments: What about rater error? Med Educ 2005;39(4):353–355.

24. Downing SM: Face validity of assessments: Faith-based interpretations or evidence-based science? Med Educ 2006;40(1):7–8.

25. Downing SM, Tekian A, Yudkowsky R: Procedures for establishing defensible absolute passing scores on performance examinations in health professions education. Teach Learn Med 2006;18(1):50–57.

26. Greenhalgh T, Macfarlane F: Towards a competency grid for evidence-based practice. J Eval Clin Pract 1997;3(2):161–165.

27. McGowan JJ, Berner ES: Proposed curricular objectives to teach physicians competence in using the World Wide Web. Acad Med 2004;79(3):236–240.

28. Straus SE, Green ML, Bell DS, et al: Evaluating the teaching of evidence based medicine: Conceptual framework. BMJ 2004; 329(7473):1029–1032.

29. Richardson WS, Wilson MC: On questions, background and foreground. Evidence-Based Healthcare Newsletter 1997;17:8–9.

30. Straus SE, Richardson WS, Glasziou P, Haynes RB: Evidence-based Medicine: How to Practice and Teach EBM, 3rd ed. Edinburgh, Elsevier, 2005.

31. Richardson WS, Wilson MC, Nishikawa J, Hayward RS: The well-built clinical question: A key to evidence-based decisions [editorial]. ACP J Club 1995;123(3):A12–A13.

32. Richardson WS: Ask, and ye shall retrieve. Evidence-Based Med 1998;3:100–101.

33. Rosenberg WM, Deeks J, Lusher A, et al: Improving searching skills and evidence retrieval. J R Coll Phys Lond 1998;32(6): 557–563.

34. Bergus GR, Randall CS, Sinift SD, Rosenthal DM: Does the structure of clinical questions affect the outcome of curbside consultations with specialty colleagues? Arch Fam Med 2000;9(6): 541–547.

35. McKibbon KA, Richardson WS, Walker-Dilks CM: Finding answers to well-built questions. Evidence-Based Med 1999; 4:164–167.

36. Cheng GY: A study of clinical questions posed by hospital clinicians. J Med Library Assoc 2004;92(4):445–458.

37. Centre for Evidence-based Medicine: Can clinicians actually practice EBM? Accessed July 16, 2007 at www.cebm.utoronto.ca/intro/canpract.htm.

38. Haynes RB: Of studies, syntheses, synopses, and systems: The "4S" evolution of services for finding current best evidence. ACP J Club 2001;134(2):A11–A13.

39. Guyatt GH, Meade MO, Jaeschke RZ: Practitioners of evidence based care: Not all clinicians need to appraise evidence from scratch but all need some skills. BMJ 2000;320(7240):954–955.

40. McColl A, Smith H, White P, Field J: General practitioner's perceptions of the route to evidence based medicine: A questionnaire survey. BMJ 1998;316(7128):361–365.

41. Green ML: Graduate medical education training in clinical epidemiology, critical appraisal, and evidence-based medicine: A critical review of curricula. Acad Med 1999;74(6):686–694.

42. Green ML: Evidence-based medicine training in internal medicine residency programs: A national survey. J Gen Intern Med 2000;15(2):129–133.

43. Hatala R, Guyatt G: Evaluating the teaching of evidence-based medicine. JAMA 2002;288(9):1110–1112.

44. Shaneyfelt T, Baum KD, Bell D, et al: Instruments for evaluating education in evidence-based practice: A systematic review. JAMA 2006;296(9):1116–1127.

45. Ramos KD, Schafer S, Tracz SM: Validation of the Fresno test of competence in evidence based medicine. BMJ 2003;326(7384): 319–321.

46. Fritsche L, Greenhalgh T, Falck-Ytter Y, et al: Do short courses in evidence based medicine improve knowledge and skills? Validation of Berlin questionnaire and before and after study of courses in evidence based medicine. BMJ 2002;325(7376):1338–1341.

47. Bennett KJ, Sackett DL, Haynes RB, et al: A controlled trial of teaching critical appraisal of the clinical literature to medical students. JAMA 1987;257(18):2451–2454.

48. Taylor R, Reeves B, Mears R, et al: Development and validation of a questionnaire to evaluate the effectiveness of evidence-based practice teaching. Med Educ 2001;35(6):544–547.

49. MacRae HM, Regehr G, Brenneman F, et al: Assessment of critical appraisal skills. Am J Surg 2004;187(1):120–123.

50. Smith CA, Ganschow PS, Reilly BM, et al: Teaching residents evidence-based medicine skills: A controlled trial of effectiveness and assessment of durability. J Gen Intern Med 2000; 15(10):710–715.

51. Green ML, Ellis PJ: Impact of an evidence-based medicine curriculum based on adult learning theory. J Gen Intern Med 1997;12(12):742–750.

52. Landry FJ, Pangaro L, Kroenke K, et al: A controlled trial of a seminar to improve medical student attitudes toward, knowledge about, and use of the medical literature. J Gen Intern Med 1994;9(8):436–439.

53. Linzer M, Brown JT, Frazier LM, et al: Impact of a medical journal club on house-staff reading habits, knowledge, and critical appraisal skills: A randomized control trial. JAMA 1988; 260(17):2537–2541.

54. Ross R, Verdieck A: Introducing an evidence-based medicine curriculum into a family practice residency—Is it effective? Acad Med 2003;78(4):412–417.

55. Villanueva EV, Burrows EA, Fennessy PA, et al: Improving question formulation for use in evidence appraisal in a tertiary care setting: A randomised controlled trial. BMC Med Inf Decision Making 2001;1(1):4.

56. Miller GE: The assessment of clinical skills/competence/performance. Acad Med 1990;65(9 Suppl):S63–S67.

57. Davidson RA, Duerson M, Romrell L, et al: Evaluating evidence-based medicine skills during a performance-based examination. Acad Med 2004;79(3):272–275.

58. Bradley P, Humphris G: Assessing the ability of medical students to apply evidence in practice: The potential of the OSCE. Med Educ 1999;33(11):815–817.

59. Berner ES, McGowan JJ, Hardin JM, et al: A model for assessing information retrieval and application skills of medical students. Acad Med 2002;77(6):547–551.

60. Fliegel JE, Frohna JG, Mangrulkar RS: A computer-based OSCE station to measure competence in evidence-based medicine skills in medical students. Acad Med 2002;77(11):1157–1158.

61. Schwartz A, Hupert J: Medical students' application of published evidence: Randomised trial. BMJ 2003;326(7388):536–538.

62. Schwartz A, Hupert J: A decision making approach to assessing critical appraisal skills. Med Teach 2005;27(1):76–80.

63. Cheng GY: Educational workshop improved information-seeking skills, knowledge, attitudes and the search outcome of hospital clinicians: A randomised controlled trial. Health Info Libraries J 2003;20(Suppl 1):22–33.

64. Bergus GR, Emerson M: Family medicine residents do not ask better-formulated clinical questions as they advance in their training. Fam Med 2005;37(7):486–490.

65. Burrows SC, Tylman V: Evaluating medical student searches of MEDLINE for evidence-based information: Process and application of results. Bull Med Libr Assoc 1999;87(4):471–476.

66. Gruppen LD, Rana GK, Arndt TS: A controlled comparison study of the efficacy of training medical students in evidence-based medicine literature searching skills. Acad Med 2005;80(10):940–944.

67. Vogel EW, Block KR, Wallingford KT: Finding the evidence: Teaching medical residents to search MEDLINE. J Med Library Assoc 2002;90(3):327–330.

68. Bradley DR, Rana GK, Martin PW, Schumacher RE: Real-time, evidence-based medicine instruction: A randomized controlled trial in a neonatal intensive care unit. J Med Libr Assoc 2002;90(2):194–201.

69. Toedter LJ, Thompson LL, Rohatgi C: Training surgeons to do evidence-based surgery: A collaborative approach. J Am Coll Surg 2004;199(2):293–299.

70. Haynes RB, McKibbon KA, Walker CJ, et al: Online access to MEDLINE in clinical settings: A study of use and usefulness. Ann Intern Med 1990;112(1):78–84.

71. McKibbon KA, Haynes RB, Dilks CJ, et al: How good are clinical MEDLINE searches? A comparative study of clinical end-user and librarian searches. Comput Biomed Res 1990;23(6):583–593.

72. Haynes RB, Johnston ME, McKibbon KA, et al: A program to enhance clinical use of MEDLINE. A randomized controlled trial. Online J Curr Clin Trials 1993;Doc(No 56):4005 words.

73. Forsetlund L, Bradley P, Forsen L, et al: Randomised controlled trial of a theoretically grounded tailored intervention to diffuse evidence-based public health practice. BMC Med Educ 2003;3(1):2.

74. Reiter HI, Neville AJ, Norman GR: Medline for medical students? Searching for the right answer. Adv Health Sci Educ 2000;5:221–232.

75. McAlister FA, Graham I, Karr GW, Laupacis A: Evidence-based medicine and the practicing clinician. J Gen Intern Med 1999;14(4):236–242.

76. Baum KD: The impact of an evidence-based medicine workshop on residents attitudes towards and self-reported ability in evidence-based practice. Med Educ Online 2003;8:4–10.

77. Young JM, Ward JE: Evidence-based medicine in general practice: Beliefs and barriers among Australian GPs. J Eval Clin Pract 2001;7(2):201–210.

78. Markey P, Schattner P: Promoting evidence-based medicine in general practice—The impact of academic detailing [see comment]. Fam Pract 2001;18(4):364–366.

79. Freeman AC, Sweeney K: Why general practitioners do not implement evidence: Qualitative study. BMJ 2001;323(7321):1100–1102.

80. Montori VM, Tabini CC, Ebbert JO: A qualitative assessment of 1st-year internal medicine residents' perceptions of evidence-based clinical decision-making. Teach Learn Med 2001;14(2):114–118.

81. Tracy CS, Dantas G, Upshur R: Evidence-based medicine in primary care: Qualitative study of family physicians. BMC Fam Pract 2003;4(1):6.

82. Putnam W, Twohig PL, Burge FI, et al: A qualitative study of evidence in primary care: What the practitioners are saying. CMAJ 2002;166(12):1525–1530.

83. Oswald N, Bateman H: Treating individuals according to evidence: Why do primary care practitioners do what they do? J Eval Clin Pract 2000;6(2):139–148.

84. Bhandari M, Montori V, Devereaux PJ, et al: Challenges to the practice of evidence-based medicine during residents' surgical training: A qualitative study using grounded theory. Acad Med 2003;78(11):1183–1190.

85. Green ML, Ruff TR: Why do residents fail to answer their clinical questions? A qualitative study of barriers to practicing evidence-based medicine. Acad Med 2005;80(2):176–182.

86. Lam WWT, Fielding R, Johnston JM, et al: Identifying barriers to the adoption of evidence-based medicine practice in clinical clerks: A longitudinal focus group study. Med Educ 2004;38(9):987–997.

87. Wiley K: Effects of a self-directed learning project and preference for structure on self-directed learning readiness. Nurs Res 1983;32(3):181–185.

88. Guglielmino LM: Development of the Self-Directed Learning Readiness Scale. Doctoral dissertation, University of Georgia. Dissertation Abs Int 1977;38:6467A. Accessed July 16, 2007 at www.guglielmino734.com/newpage3.htm.

89. Mourad SA, Torrance EP: Construct validity of the self-directed learning readiness scale. J Educ Gifted 1979;3(2):93–104.

90. Field LD: An investigation into the structure, validity, and reliability of Guglielmino's Self-Directed Learning Readiness Scale. Adult Educ Q 1989;39:125–139.

91. Bligh JG: Independent learning among general practice trainers: An initial survey. Med Educ 1992;26:497–502.

92. Hoban JD, Lawson SR, Mazmanian PE, et al: The Self-Directed Learning Readiness Scale: A factor analysis study. Med Educ 2005;39(4):370–379.

93. Delahaye BL, Smith HE: The validity of the learning preference assessment. Adult Educ Q 1995;45(3):159–173.

94. Russell JW: Learner preference for structure, self-directed learning readiness, and instructional methods. Doctoral dissertation, University of Missouri. Dissertation Abs Int 1988;49:1689.

95. Hall-Johnson K: The relationship between readiness for self-directed learning and participation in self-directed learning. Doctoral dissertation, Iowa State University. Dissertation Abs Int 1981;46(7A).

96. Harvey BJ, Rothman AI, Frecker RC: Effect of an undergraduate medical curriculum on students' self-directed learning. Acad Med 2003;78:1259–1265.

97. Shokar GS, Shokar NK, Romero CM, Bulik RJ: Self-directed learning: Looking at outcomes with medical students. Fam Med 2002;34(3):197–200.

98. Fung MF, Walker M, Fung KF, et al: An internet-based learning portfolio in resident education: The KOALA multicentre programme. Med Educ 2000;34(6):474–479.

99. Hojat M, Nasca TJ, Erdmann JB, et al: An operational measure of physician lifelong learning: Its development, components and preliminary psychometric data. Med Teach 2003;25(4):437.

100. Hojat M, Veloski J, Nasca TJ, et al: Assessing physicians' orientation toward lifelong learning. J Gen Intern Med 2006;21(9):931–936.

101. Whitcomb ME: Research in medical education: What do we know about the link between what doctors are taught and what they do? Acad Med 2002;77(11):1067–1068.

102. Osheroff JA, Forsythe DE, Buchanan BG, et al: Physicians' information needs: Analysis of questions posed during clinical teaching. Ann Intern Med 1991;114(7):576–581.

103. Green ML, Ciampi MA, Ellis PJ: Residents' medical information needs in clinic: Are they being met? Am J Med 2000;109(3):218–223.

104. Flynn C, Helwig A: Evaluating an evidence-based medicine curriculum. Acad Med 1997;72(5):454–455.

105. Stevermer JJ, Chambliss ML, Hoekzema GS: Distilling the literature: A randomized, controlled trial testing an intervention to improve selection of medical articles for reading. Acad Med 1999;74(1):70–72.

106. Cabell CH, Schardt C, Sanders L, et al: Resident utilization of information technology. J Gen Intern Med 2001;16(12):838–844.

107. Reckase MD: Portfolio assessment: A theoretical estimate of score reliability. Educ Meas Issues Pract 1995;14:12–31.

108. Khunti K: Teaching evidence-based medicine using educational prescriptions. Med Teach 1998;20:380–381.

109. Rucker L, Morrison E: The ''EBM Rx'': An initial experience with an evidence-based learning prescription. Acad Med 2000;75(5):527–528.

110. Green ML: Evaluating evidence-based practice performance (editorial). ACP J Club 2006;145:A8–A10.

111. Centre for Evidence-Based Medicine—University of Toronto: Educational Prescription. Accessed July 16, 2007 at www.cebm.utoronto.ca/practise/formulate/eduprescript.htm.

112. Centre for Evidence-Based Medicine—Oxford: Educational Prescription. Accessed November 2005 at www.cebm.net/downloads/educational_prescription.rtf.

113. Crowley SD, Owens TA, Schardt CM, et al: A web-based compendium of clinical questions and medical evidence to educate internal medicine residents. Acad Med 2003;78(3):270–274.

114. Campbell C, Gondocz T, Parboosingh J: Documenting and managing self-directed learning among specialists. Ann R Coll Phys Surg Can 1995;28:80–84.

115. Campbell C, Parboosingh J, Gondocz T, et al: A study of the factors that influence physicians' commitments to change their practices using learning diaries. Acad Med 1999;74 (10 Suppl):S34–S36.

116. Ellis J, Mulligan I, Rowe J, Sackett DL: Inpatient general medicine is evidence based. A-Team, Nuffield Department of Clinical Medicine. Lancet 1995;346(8972):407–410.

117. Michaud G, McGowan JL, van der Jagt R, et al: Are therapeutic decisions supported by evidence from health care research? Arch Intern Med 1998;158(15):1665–1668.

118. Gill P, Dowell AC, Neal RD, et al: Evidence based general practice: A retrospective study of interventions in one training practice. BMJ 1996;312(7034):819–821.

119. Lai TYY, Wong VWY, Leung GM: Is ophthalmology evidence based? A clinical audit of the emergency unit of a regional eye hospital. Br J Ophthalmol 2003;87(4):385–390.

120. Jemec GB, Thorsteinsdottir H, Wulf HC: Evidence-based dermatologic out-patient treatment. Int J Dermatol 1998;37(11):850–854.

121. Myles PS, Bain DL, Johnson F, McMahon R: Is anaesthesia evidence-based? A survey of anaesthetic practice. Br J Anaesth 1999;82(4):591–595.

122. Kingston R, Barry M, Tierney S, et al: Treatment of surgical patients is evidence-based. Eur J Surg 2001;167(5):324–330.

123. Kenny SE, Shankar KR, Rintala R, et al: Evidence-based surgery: interventions in a regional paediatric surgical unit. Arch Dis Child 1997;76(1):50–53.

124. Geddes J, Game D, Jenkins N, et al: What proportion of primary psychiatric interventions are based on evidence from randomised controlled trials? Qual Saf Health Care 1996;5(4):215–217.

125. Straus SE, Ball C, Balcombe N, et al: Teaching evidence-based medicine skills can change practice in a community hospital. J Gen Intern Med 2005;20(4):340–343.

126. Lucas BP, Evans AT, Reilly BM, et al: The impact of evidence on physicians' inpatient treatment decisions. J Gen Intern Med 2004;19(5 Pt 1):402–409.

127. Langham J, Tucker H, Sloan D, et al: Secondary prevention of cardiovascular disease: A randomised trial of training in information management, evidence-based medicine, both or neither: The PIER trial. Br J Gen Pract 2002;52(483):818–824.

128. Epling J, Smucny J, Patil A, Tudiver F: Teaching evidence-based medicine skills through a residency-developed guideline. Fam Med 2002;34(9):646–648.

129. Peabody JW, Luck J, Glassman P, et al: Measuring the Quality of Physician Practice by Using Clinical Vignettes: A Prospective Validation Study. Ann Intern Med 2004;141(10):771–780.

130. Holmboe ES, Prince L, Green ML: Teaching and improving quality of care in a primary care internal medicine residency clinic. Acad Med 2005;80(6):571–577.

131. Silber CG, Nasca TJ, Paskin DL, et al: Do global rating forms enable program directors to assess the ACGME competencies? Acad Med 2004;79(6):549–556.

132. Norcini JJ, Blank LL, Duffy FD, Fortna GS: The mini-CEX: A method for assessing clinical skills. Ann Intern Med 2003;138(6):476–481.

133. American Board of Internal Medicine: Practice Improvement Modules for Residency Training. Accessed July 16, 2007 at www.abim.org/cert/tet_pims.shtm.

134. Akl EA, Izuchukwu IS, El-Dika S, et al: Integrating an evidence-based medicine rotation into an internal medicine residency program. Acad Med 2004;79(9):897–904.

135. Bradley P, Herrin J: Development and validation of an instrument to measure knowledge of evidence-based practice and searching skills. Med Educ Online 2004;9:15–19.

136. Bradley P, Oterholt C, Herrin J, et al: Comparison of directed and self-directed learning in evidence-based medicine: A randomised controlled trial. Med Educ 2005;39(10):1027–1035.

137. Taylor R, Reeves B, Ewings P, Taylor R: Critical appraisal skills training for health care professionals: A randomized controlled trial. BMC Med Educ 2004;4(1):30.

138. McCluskey A, Lovarini M: Providing education on evidence-based practice improved knowledge but did not change behaviour: A before and after study. BMC Med Educ 2005;5(1):40.

139. MacRae HM, Regehr G, McKenzie M, et al: Teaching practicing surgeons critical appraisal skills with an Internet-based journal club: A randomized, controlled trial. Surgery 2004;136(3):641–646.

140. Weberschock TB, Ginn TC, Reinhold J, et al: Change in knowledge and skills of year 3 undergraduates in evidence-based medicine seminars. Med Educ 2005;39(7):665–671.

141. Emerson JD, Colditz GA: Use of statistical analysis in the New England Journal of Medicine. N Engl J Med 1983;309(12):709–713.

APPENDIX 10-1
Internet EBP Education Resources

Centre for EBM (Oxford): www.cebm.net/

Centre for EBM (Toronto): www.cebm.utoronto.ca/

Centre for Health Evidence (Alberta): www.cche.net/che/home.asp

Surgical Outcomes Research Center (McMaster University): www.fhs.mcmaster.ca/source/EBS/ebs-1.htm

Educational prescription (Oxford Centre for EBM): www.cebm.net/downloads/educational_prescription.rtf

EBM Tips electronic resources: www.ebmtips.net/risk001.asp

SGIM EBM Task Force: www.sgim.org/ebm-mission.cfm

The Fresno EBP Test[45]: bmj.bmjjournals.com/cgi/content/full/326/7384/319/DC1

The Berlin Test[46]: bmj.bmjjournals.com/cgi/content/full/325/7376/1338/DC1

The SDLRS[88]: www.guglielmino734.com/newpage3.htm

General practitioners' perceptions of the route to evidence-based medicine survey[40]: bmj.bmjjournals.com/cgi/content/full/316/7128/361/DC1

APPENDIX 10-2
Examples Of Educational Prescriptions

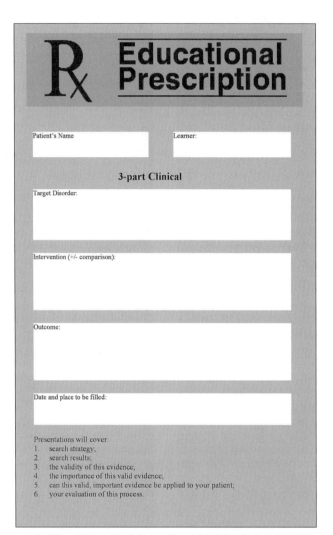

Figure 10-1 Educational prescription example. (From Centre for Evidence-Based Medicine: University of Toronto Educational Prescription. Accessed July 16, 2007 at www.cebm.utoronto.ca/practise/formulate/eduprescript.htm.)

| Resident(s): _____ | Faculty: _____ | "Rx" date _____ |
| | | "Fill" date _____ |

| 1. Rotation: | Wards | Elective | Geriatrics | Continuity clinic | Ambulatory office | Other: |
| | ICU | Emergency | Night float | | Ambulatory specialty | |

| 2. Context | Question conference | EBm curriculum | Resident report | General patient care | Other: |

3. Chnical scenario:

4. Question

| Patient | Intervention | Comparison | Outcome |

| 5. Clinical task: | Clinical findings | Diagnostic diagnosis | Prognosis | Prevention |
| | Etiology/harm | Diagnostic testing | Therapy | Manifestations of disease |

6. Information source that provided answer:	Clinical evidence	EBM on call	MEDLINE original study
	Cochrane Library/DARE	UpToDate	MEDLINE meta-analysis
	ACPJC on line	PIER	MEDLINE narrative review
	Rational clinical exam	Textbook	Consultant/colleague
	Info retriever (POEM or other source: _____)		Other:

7. The evidence (reference)

8. Your answer/results:

9. What did you learn from this experience? How will it change your clinical practice, If at all?

Faculty

Date returned: _____

Describe the main teaching point (EBM slice) you made for this exercise:

☐ None	
☐ Ask	
☐ Acquire	
☐ Appraise	
☐ Apply	

Figure 10-2 Educational prescription example. (From Green ML: Evaluating evidence-based practice performance [editorial]. ACP J Club 2006; 145:A8–A10; reprinted with permission.)

Competence in Improving Systems of Care Through Practice-Based Learning and Improvement

F. Daniel Duffy, MD, MACP, and Eric S. Holmboe, MD

The Institute of Medicine, in the Quality Chasm report, attributed much of the poor quality of U.S. health care to a flawed and broken system—not to failure of individuals within the system.[1] However, the health care system is not an abstract entity but the cooperative interaction between people and technology. Therefore, as the ACGME and ABMS have determined, it is critical that physicians,

critical people in the health care system, acquire competence in systems-based practice and practice-based learning and improvement.[2] Moreover, to implement changes in health care systems, physicians must become architects and engineers in helping to transform the systems to cross the quality chasm. The journey to acquire these competencies must begin early in training.

Commitment to quality and accountability is increasingly seen as a core professional value. The Physician Charter on Medical Professionalism, developed jointly by the ABIM Foundation (ABIMF), European Federation of Internal Medicine (EFIM), and the American College of Physicians (ACP) Foundation, explicitly listed active involvement in quality improvement as a core principle of professionalism.[3] Others have highlighted quality improvement as not only a professional obligation but also a civic responsibility.[4–7] These authors speak to a new set of beliefs and ethics physicians must embrace in order to bring about meaningful improvements in health care.

In response to the clear need to change residency education to meet this challenge, the Accreditation Council for Graduate Medical Education in the United States developed two new general competencies: practice-based learning and improvement (PBLI) and systems-based practice (SBP). These two competencies directly address the need to teach and evaluate students' and residents' ability to effectively incorporate quality improvement principles and methods into changing the systems in which they practice. In Chapter 10, we learned the principles and methods of evidence-based medicine as part of the PBLI competency. The ability to find reliable, evidence-based information at the "point of care" is an essential PBLI skill for all physicians. Knowledge, skills, and attitudes in applying evidence to change processes and systems that actually deliver the care, applying quality improvement methods, and working in interdisciplinary teams are also important elements of other competency frameworks, including medical school education.[8–10]

The Institute of Medicine (IOM) lists the ability to apply quality improvement methods and to employ evidenced-based medicine methods to deliver care through the coordinated effort of interdisciplinary teams as core competencies for all health care providers[11] (Box 11-1).

In order to teach and evaluate these new competencies, educators must have an understanding of key concepts and methods of quality improvement science and deep understanding that people working as a system deliver care, not just doctors. Such concepts are still new to many medical educators and practicing physicians. Therefore, we begin this chapter by providing an overview on quality science and systems thinking. We will specifically define what a "system" is; with a better understanding about quality and systems, we can next look at the knowledge, skills, and attitudes required for

competency. We will finish the chapter by discussing some of the emerging approaches to evaluating trainees. However, it is important to realize the tools and methods for the evaluation of these two competencies are in the very early stages of their development.

What Is a System?

When most physicians hear the word "system" they immediately think about large health care organizations such as health plans, hospital and physician networks, national health services, or the vague concept of all the people and operations that deliver the elusive service called health care. For physicians, the word "system" usually carries a pejorative connotation and is referenced as being in opposition to physician-level quality of care. This attitude arises from the professional value of autonomy and responsibility; unfortunately, it impedes progress in physicians gaining competence in practice-based learning and improvement and systems-based practice.

What we mean by system in this context is the organization of the people, their work processes, and the technical tools and methods they use to accomplish their common goals of good patient care. To get our minds around systems, it is helpful to use the Batalden model of concentric circles (Fig. 11-1) to represent levels of organization or relationship.[12]

At the inner circle is the dyadic patient-provider relationship. From the physician perspective, we think of this as the physician-patient relationship; however, from the patient's perspective it is actually a multitude of patient-other relationships that occur in the course of health care. The next concentric circle Batalden calls the clinical microsystem, which is the unit of organization in which patients receive their care. For primary or principal care this unit has recently been dubbed the

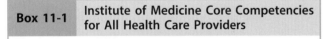

Box 11-1	Institute of Medicine Core Competencies for All Health Care Providers

Provide patient-centered care
Employ evidence-based medicine
Utilize informatics
Work in interdisciplinary teams
Apply quality improvement

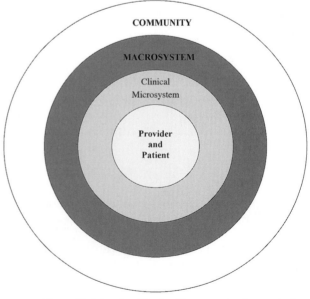

Figure 11-1 Levels of the health care system's organization.

MODEL FOR EFFECTIVE CHRONIC CARE: MACROSYSTEM

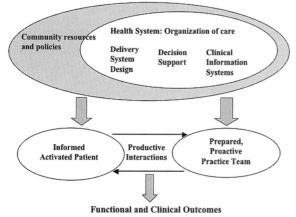

Figure 11-2 The macrosystem in the care of chronic disease. (Adapted from Wagner EH, Austin BT, Von Korff M: Organizing care for patients with chronic illness. Milbank Q 1996;74:511–542.)

"medical home."[13,14] This small organization of people and technology provides the care that patients receive. The third circle contains the network of the multiple microsystems that are tied together to provide the range of services needed for care. This circle is called the macrosystem. These third circle microsystems include laboratories, imaging services, consultation, diagnostic and therapeutic procedural services, patient education and counseling, pharmacy, and many more. The fourth circle contains the community. Wagner's chronic care model (Fig. 11-2) demonstrates how a macrosystem is needed to facilitate high-quality care for patients with chronic illness such as diabetes.[15,16]

For the purposes of discussing systems in the context of training, we will focus on the second level, the clinical microsystem, its functioning, and its relationship to the inner dyadic system and next level macrosystem that directly affects trainees' acquisition of knowledge, skills, and attitudes in practice-based learning and improvement and systems-based practice.

Components of a Clinical Microsystem

Nelson defined a microsystem as "a small group of people who work together on a regular basis to provide care to discrete subpopulations of patients and who share clinical and business aims, linked processes of care and information for the purpose of producing meaningful performance outcomes."[17] Examples of a clinical microsystem in the training environment would include ambulatory clinics, hospital wards, and surgical suites. Trainees must learn how these microsystems should function most efficiently and effectively, and how microsystems relate and interact with each other. Figure 11-3 shows how the steps doctors use to provide medical care, the clinical method, come together in a sequence of work processes and are

integrated with supporting processes, people, and technology to create a clinical microsystem. Let's break down these important components and steps further.

Patients with Needs

The circle on the far left of Figure 11-3 shows the population of *patients* with specific health care needs (acute care, prevention of future disease, and management of chronic care) who seek care from the particular microsystem. In primary care microsystems, some patients select a practice because it is convenient to home or work, and others choose a practice for financial reasons or because it has attractive cultural or social features. For many patients in poverty in the United States the training clinic is their only access to health care. Research has shown the population of patients in training clinics is more socioeconomically disadvantaged and experience higher levels of co-morbidity.[18]

The population of patients in other microsystems such as cardiology clinics or dialysis centers has been preselected by their medical conditions. The more specialized the microsystem, the more selection has occurred prior to the patient's access to the practice. The value to trainees of rotating among many different sources is to experience the differences in microsystems that provide care for specific populations of patients. It is important to understand the needs of the patient populations using the microsystem because the design of the work process must vary to efficiently and effectively meet their needs.

Clinical Processes

The sequential steps shown in the middle boxes of Figure 11-3 are the familiar components of the clinical method: (1) *access to the practice*—appointments, telephone or mail contact; (2) *workup and diagnosis*—the first medical task that requires strong clinical skills; (3) *treatment and monitoring*—the second important medical task; and (4) patient *self-care support*—the third medical task, which informs the patient about

Clinical Microsystem

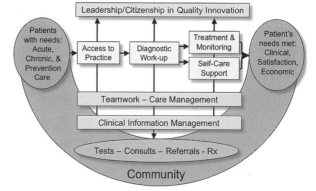

Figure 11-3 Clinical microsystem elements. See text for discussion.

their role in the care process and assists them in carrying it out.

Outcomes of Care

The circle on the right of Figure 11-3 shows the outcomes of the care that are of interest to everyone: meeting the patient population needs. The obvious goal is achieving desirable clinical outcomes (e.g., blood pressure control, acceptable A_{1c} levels for diabetes, and no bronchospasm for asthmatics) for an individual patient and for the population of patients seeking care from the practice.

In addition to clinical outcomes, other important measures of practice success include the patient rating of their satisfaction with their experience of care. Equally important is the physicians' and staff satisfaction with their work. The satisfaction of residents with the clinical experience, especially in outpatient microsystems, is an underappreciated factor in their ultimate career choice. A fourth important measure of the success of the practice is its economic viability and ability to provide care at an affordable price and achieve its business goals.[19] For training clinics, applying an insurance-based fee-for-service business model challenges clinics to provide care for the poor, uninsured, and disadvantaged populations.

Supporting Processes

The rectangles in Figure 11-3 represent important processes of the clinical microsystem that make the care directed by clinicians reliable, safe, and efficient. At the top of the diagram is leadership/citizenship in quality innovation. This category tops the list of supporting processes. In many training program microsystems, residents have a difficult time knowing who has leadership responsibility for its quality performance. Moreover, few microsystems explicitly tell residents that they have a role as a citizen, albeit a temporary one, for contributing to microsystem quality performance.

In addition to leadership and citizenship, healthy microsystems have a systematic process for making timely changes in microsystem processes in response to continuing advances in medical care and changes in the health care environment. Innovation processes include measurement of performance against goals for care and methods for envisioning improved processes, testing the most promising ones, and implementing those that work.

Recently, training programs have begun to look at performance measures of the quality of care delivered in primary care microsystems. In practice settings, the majority of the microsystems that have begun to measure performance are those linked to larger group practices that provide the measurement and improvement processes for the primary care microsystem, which participates passively in improvement activities.[20] However, at the heart of physician-level competence in practice-based learning and improvement is the attitude of wanting performance measurement and the personal capacity to use performance measurement to apply quality improvement (QI) practices such as root-cause analysis or failure mode effects analysis to developing ideas for redesigning a process of care, testing its impact on the practice to determine if the change improved performance on the measures.[21]

The rectangle below the clinical method in Figure 11-3 is labeled teamwork and care management. This process, performed by nonphysician staff, assures proactive care of patients to treat chronic conditions and to assure preventive care is delivered. The microsystem designs the most efficient sequence of tasks to be performed and assigns staff to roles and responsibilities to execute them. This standardization produces reliable, safe, efficient, effective proactive care for patients who will benefit. Each team member has a role and responsibility for the seamless hand-off of the patients or information along the train of steps in managing their care.

Proactive care management is guided by the microsystem's definition of quality and an understanding of how it is measured. All the physicians and staff members involved in the steps leading to care management use an individualized and integrated patient care plan to remind them of the next steps and to document execution of their tasks. Care management processes are well defined in hospitals, some procedure laboratories, surgical suites, and emergency rooms, but are only recently being defined for primary care office practices.

When rotating through a microsystem, residents must be instructed in their roles and responsibilities for tasks in the care management process. By experiencing different microsystems, residents will learn how teamwork occurs to achieve goals for different patient problems.

The lower rectangle in Figure 11-3 shows the clinical information management process that ties the entire microsystem together and connects it to the external consultants, laboratories, and pharmacies (shown in the oval at the bottom of the diagram) that are necessary for providing integrated care for the patient. An effective information management system is essential for the reliable execution and coordination of care. Complete interoperability of electronic clinical information systems is a dream rather than a reality. However, a microsystem's success depends in large part on the effectiveness of its information management system, whether that system is purely paper-telephone-fax-mail or a combination of paper with electronic systems for practice management, medical records, patient data tracking (registry), electronic prescribing, ordering, and test and consultation tracking. Regardless of the level of computerization of the microsystem's information, its flow can be managed by using a system of templates, flowsheets, order forms, request forms, medical record pages, prescriptions, telephone notes, and others that are passed along, collated, and filed by members of the microsystem.

Supplier Microsystems

The oval at the bottom of Figure 11-3 indicates the external microsystems that supply vital services to patients in the practice. These microsystems include laboratory services, imaging service, pharmacy, a variety of consulting services for hospitalization, and diagnostic and therapeutic services. The practice's clinical information management system must connect clinical data collected within the practice microsystem with these external services; there must be processes for tracking and recording the information returned from these external services. Important interpersonal tasks of any microsystem are managing these external service relationships to assure quality patient care through reliable coordination and follow-through on care provided by multiple microsystems.

Systems and Adaptations

As we have learned, a system is a set of interdependent parts sharing a common purpose. Interdependence means that the parts of the system work in a coordinated manner and understand their dependency on each other. It is a system and not the individual that ultimately produces results. When the parts lack a common purpose and interdependence, or act with autonomy, as so often happens in medicine, the system weakens and ultimately may collapse.

Common purpose is not a platitude to provide high-quality care, it is a clear statement of goals that are tied to specific quality measures that guide those who work together in intentionally seeking to improve them through changes in the way they work together. Clinical environments continually change; therefore, for a care system of people and methods to thrive, it must have the capacity to adapt. Change and adaptation are essential properties of healthy systems and arise from the capacity of the individuals whose work maintains the system to evolve.[22] This does not mean we should praise students and residents to continually devise "work-arounds" to get their work done in the dysfunctional systems they too often encounter in the clinical setting. Rather, adaptation here refers to the ability of all individuals to identify when a change in the environment has occurred, to determine the impact of the change in reaching health care team and patient quality goals, and to develop a plan for an improved way of working together. Thus, quality improvement is not a "science fair project" which is intermittently applied to the system or which takes time-out from regular work to make a change. Quality improvement means that changes occur every day in a managed and systematic way, and our students and residents must be explicitly trained in how to participate in making these changes for improvement.

Innovation in Medical Care

Innovation in medical care depends on physician competence in SBP and PBLI. One of the most important goals of medical education is to show trainees how competence in PBLI and SBP "fit" together to advance medical science to provide high-quality, effective care that responds to changes in the health care environment. With an

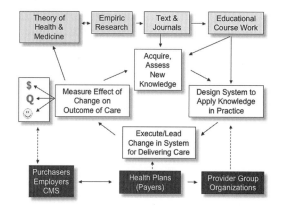

Figure 11-4 An integrated model of system-based practice and practice-based learning and improvement. See text for discussion.

understanding of how the clinical microsystem delivers care, let's turn our attention to how practice-based learning and improvement change the systems of practice to innovate processes of care.

A Model of Understanding SBP and PBLI

Figure 11-4 shows an integrated model for understanding how competence in system-based practice and practice-based learning and improvement create the innovations in practice that improve the quality outcomes of care. In this model we've incorporated three basic processes: (1) discovery and dissemination of new knowledge; (2) translating new knowledge into practice to make measurable improvements delivered by the microsystem (where physicians do their work to deliver care); and (3) integrating the delivery of care with the needs of patients and the health care marketplace as part of the macrosystem.

The steps in tier 1 of the process involve developing new knowledge about health, disease, and medicine that is grounded in sound theory supported by scientific empiric research. The results of this research are published in the medical literature as scientific papers and as distilled guidelines for care. These guidelines are based on the prevailing theories supported by scientific evidence or, at times, expert opinion. These skills were explored in detail by Dr. Green in Chapter 10.

An important stimulus for developing new theories that drive research for new knowledge are the observations made by astute clinicians dealing with real patients in practice. This essential step is a by-product of the practice system. Development of new hypotheses has been traditionally the role of the clinical investigator—the clinician scientist who sees patients in the context of delivering care, develops a question, and then returns to the laboratory to test the theoretical answer to that question in a research experiment. Training programs have a professional obligation to teach this competence to future generations of physicians.

Tier 3 of this diagram shows the important role of the macroenvironment in financing and managing the health care in the United States. Obviously, the financiers in other countries will be organized differently, but the concept remains the same. Purchasers of health care (mostly employers and the government in the United States) are increasingly interested in having credible measures of the outcomes of care. They want to know the quality and cost of the services they are buying for their employees or citizens. In the United States, purchasers directly influence health plans to manage payment contracts with physicians and hospitals to provide the services that purchasers want for their charges. Trainees must develop, at a minimum, a basic understanding of this macroenvironment and how it will affect them in practice, regardless of the macrosystem in which they practice.

The circle of steps in the middle of the model shows the tasks of physician competence in systems-based practice and practice-based learning and improvement. Although this is a perpetual cycle, let's begin at the top of the cycle in the center of the diagram. This step is the physician acquiring and assessing new information and knowledge. This is a traditional part of medical professionalism: "keeping up." It involves reading the scientific publications and participating in continuing medical education activities for learning the "how-to" aspects of medical care. This is where the physician applies or seeks knowledge at the point of care.

Following the cycle clockwise, the next box depicts a completely new task: design of systems to apply the new knowledge. This has not been a part of traditional medical education; it has come into recent focus in health care through the work of industrial engineers such as Demming and Juran and translated into medicine by Berwick.[23–25] Translation of new knowledge and methods into the work flow of medical practice is the purpose of system design. It is a specific subcompetence within the overall competence of systems-based practice.

The third task in the practice system change cycle is to execute/lead change in systems for delivering care. This task has been an aspiration of medical professionalism, but there has been little education in the management and interpersonal skills that are needed to actually accomplish the task.

The fourth task in the cycle is measurement of the outcome of care. This task is also new for physicians as well. Although physicians have learned statistical analysis to understand scientific reports, they have not applied measurement principles and practice to understand the processes and outcomes of care within their own practices. This critical step is important for quality outcomes (Q in the figure), patient satisfaction (☺), and improved efficiency ($). With this model as our backdrop, we can now turn our attention to further defining these two competencies and how to begin to evaluate a trainee's competence.

Understanding that medical care is delivered by systems of people and technology, and that improving the systems involves learning from experience in practice, the ACGME defined two new competencies for

---

Box 11-2   Definitions for Practice-Based Learning and Improvement and Systems-Based Practice

Practice-Based Learning and Improvement
Residents must demonstrate the ability to investigate and evaluate their care of patients, to appraise and assimilate scientific evidence, and to continuously improve patient care based on constant self-evaluation and lifelong learning. Residents are expected to develop skills and habits to be able to meet the following goals:
- Identify strengths, deficiencies, and limits in one's knowledge and expertise;
- Set learning and improvement goals;
- Identify and perform appropriate learning activities;
- Systematically analyze practice using quality improvement methods and implement changes with the goal of practice improvement;
- Incorporate formative evaluation feedback into daily practice;
- Locate, appraise, and assimilate evidence from scientific studies related to their patients' health problems;
- Use information technology to optimize learning;
- Participate in the education of patients, families, students, residents, and other health professionals.

Systems-Based Practice
Residents must demonstrate an awareness of and responsiveness to the larger context and system of health care as well as the ability to call effectively on other resources in the system to provide optimal health care. Residents are expected to
- Work effectively in various health care delivery settings and systems relevant to their clinical specialty;
- Coordinate patient care within the health care system relevant to their clinical specialty;
- Incorporate considerations of cost awareness and risk-benefit analysis in patient and/or population-based care as appropriate;
- Advocate for quality patient care and optimal patient care systems;
- Work in interprofessional teams to enhance patient safety and improve patient care quality;
- Participate in identifying system errors and implementing potential system solution.

From Accreditation Council for Graduate Medical Education (ACGME) Outcomes Project, Competencies. Accessed at www.acgme.org/outcome/comp/compFull.asp, July 16, 2007.

---

graduating residents. These expectations are shown in Box 11-2. PBLI depends on the use of performance measurement, determining the meaning of the measures, and changing personal practice and the processes performed by the system of care. Competence in PBLI is not possible in the absence of performance data. Chapter 5 covered the issues and methods of medical records audit, a skill needed for PBLI. SBP acknowledges that medical care is delivered not only through the efforts of individual physicians but by a coordinated group of professionals working in teams and using standardized clinical care methods and technology.

These competencies describe essential capabilities of individual physicians that are necessary to work in, learn from, and continually improve the systems of people and technology that deliver care to patients. Like other core competencies these require specific knowledge, attitudes, and skills that must be learned, practiced, and ultimately mastered to become a competent physician. To help educators determine if a trainee has attained competence, we present two frameworks. The first framework, developed by Ogrinc and colleagues, is based on managed care principles, closely related to PBLI and SBP, and provides useful developmental benchmarks from medical school through residency based on the Dreyfus model of professional development.[26,27] Their framework is presented in Tables 11-1 and 11-2 and provides a useful guide for what to evaluate and when it falls in the educational continuum. In this framework, medical students focus the majority of their efforts in acquiring knowledge about quality improvement science and skills before moving into application of that knowledge and skills. However, one study did find medical students could successfully perform medical record audits in a practicing physician's office and assist in quality improvement in that office.[28]

Regardless of the experiences obtained in medical school, residents by graduation must be able to "do" basic quality improvement, demonstrating the capacity to use outcome and process measurement and systematic redesign processes to improve microsystems of care. We present an expanded framework for the minimum level of knowledge, skills, and attitudes that should be obtained by the end of residency and continue to advance during fellowship training.

Knowledge

Residents should understand a specific taxonomy of terms and set of concepts about SBP and PBLI. These can be assessed through faculty questions, self-directed exercises, and as part of examinations of knowledge. Some of the basic concepts include the following:

- The concept of microsystems and macrosystems (defined earlier in the chapter) should be clear.
- Reliable and safe care requires deliberate design to standardize processes of care, prevent variability within and between microsystems, and to eliminate waste and errors.
- Safety and reliability are built into the design of work processes and are not solely qualities of physicians. The lone ranger "work harder" approach to quality and safety may actually reduce the safety and reliability of system of care.
- Knowledge about statistics, measurement of clinical care, use of clinical workflow processes diagrams, design of rapid-cycle tests of change, and implementing effective changes into clinical care processes are needed for PBLI.

Attitude

SBP and PBLI demand a fundamental change in traditional attitudes about physician autonomy and responsibility for the processes and outcomes of medical care. These competences require physicians to adopt the attitude that they have an essential, but insufficient, role in providing highly reliable, quality care. Physicians must adopt the belief that coordinated, systematized teams of people with their own roles, responsibilities, and specific training are essential for quality medical care. Physicians must develop the attitudes needed for responsible teamwork and leadership for system change and improvement. The traditional skills and attitudes of respect for data, application of statistical methods to understand the meaning of data, and careful attention to details in conducting experiments (rapid-cycle tests of change) expand the traditional internal medicine attitudes about the scientific method and apply them to PBLI.

Skills

The skills of PBLI include critical questioning, literature searching, and analysis of findings; use of electronic informational resources to answer clinical questions at the point of care for the benefit of patients; use of statistics applied to process and outcome measurement; applying root-cause analysis to a quality problem; using failure mode effects analysis to evaluate and test a change idea; designing and executing rapid-cycle tests of change; implementing successful change ideas; and training others for specific roles and tasks in processes.

Skills for SBP include the following:

- Skill in teamwork, communication, and interpersonal interaction needed to maintain effective relationships
- Using health information technology
- Developing and agreeing on the use of evidence-based protocols to standardize workflow in the processes of care
- Organizing and transferring clinical information throughout the system both within a microsystem (e.g., consultations) and between microsystems (e.g., discharge from hospital to home)
- Developing and maintaining networks of consultants and clinical services
- Managing backup processes when things don't go as planned
- Organizing, giving, and receiving feedback
- Standardizing hand-off processes, including sign-outs, transfer between wards, etc.
- Designing systems with redundancy and failsafe methods and technology
- Diagramming the processes of clinical workflow; and applying new technological tools and methods

It is important to realize this list represents minimum, not optimal, competencies. For graduating residents and fellows to successfully enter independent practice today, regardless of geographic location, they must obtain these competencies. In order to achieve them, the curriculum must provide them with the appropriate experiences and opportunities.

Table 11-1 Origin Developmental Competencies in Practice-Based Learning and Improvement

Level of Training (Dreyfus Model)	Customer Knowledge	Practice-Based Learning and Improvement		
		Measurement	Making a Change	Developing New, Locally Useful Knowledge
Beginning medical student (novice)	Demonstrate how quality improvement principles are useful, to both patients and medical students	Understand the variation inherent in health care systems Introductory assessment of health summary statistics for populations of patients	Understand basic change concepts In an educational or personal improvement process, identify where change can be applied	Understand how the introductory concepts of improvement science are used to improve outcomes in own life or medical education Understand improvement science as synergistic with other scientific methods of building knowledge
Advanced medical student (advanced beginner)	Be able to map the process of care from a patient's point of view for a clinical encounter	Identify outcome and process measures appropriate for a clinical problem	Be able to recommend changes in clinical processes for a group of patients	Apply the introductory concepts of improvement science to patient-focused outcomes
Beginning resident (advanced beginner)	Demonstrate an appreciation of the patients' needs and explore how these needs can be met	Begin to measure and describe the processes and outcomes of care for the resident's own patients	Identify places in the resident's own practice that can be changed to affect the processes and outcomes of care	Apply continuous improvement to one's own patient panel
Advanced resident (competent)	Identify needs within the resident's patient population (i.e, medical or surgical panel) and initiate changes to meet those needs	Be able to use balanced quality measures to show that changes have improved the care for the resident's patients	Demonstrate how to use several cycles of change to improve the care delivery system	Apply continuous improvement to a discrete population or have several efforts directed at different subpopulations

Adapted from Ogrinc G, Headrick LA, Mutha S, et al: A framework for teaching medical students and residents about practice-based learning and improvement, synthesized from a literature review. Acad Med 2003;78:748–756.

Table 11-2 **Ogrinc Developmental Competencies in Systems-Based Practice**

Level of Training (Dreyfus Model)	Health Care as a System	Collaboration	Social Context and Accountability
Beginning medical student (novice)	Understand the basic components of a health care system Demonstrate how outcomes are dependent on systems	Describe why an interdisciplinary approach is necessary for continuous improvement in health care	Describe the links between quality and costs in health care systems Describe approaches to assessing community health needs
Advanced medical student (advanced beginner)	Describe the system and process of care for a group of patients in a defined setting	Display skill in communication and collaborative work with health professionals from other disciplines	Identify and understand the implications of health care resource allocation
Beginning resident (advanced beginner)	Describe a system of care for a population of patients with which the resident interacts	Describe how an effective interdisciplinary team functions	Describe the business case for quality in health care Identify methods to improve care for populations in their practice
Advanced resident (competent)	Understand and describe the reactions of a system when perturbed by change that is initiated by the resident	Contribute to an interdisciplinary team effort to improve care	Describe the business case for quality in health care for specific quality improvement goals in their own practice Identify community resources to improve care for individuals within their practice

Basics of the Core Curriculum for SBP and PBLI

Training residents to become competent in SBP and PBLI involves two educational methods: (1) interactive education to learn the terms, concepts, and principles involved in the competencies, and (2) clinical experience in applying this knowledge on every clinical rotation so that attitudes may emerge and skills may be honed.

Interactive Education

Ideally national educational programs in these topics will be developed and delivered over the Internet so that students and residents, as well as practicing physicians, may rapidly develop common knowledge about these new competencies. Programmed educational experiences might be accompanied by self-assessment questions to assure that learning of the facts and concepts has occurred.

Education in PBLI and SBP is evolving rapidly, but Web-based educational experiences are limited. However, the recently constituted Academy of Post Graduate Health Care Education currently supports a Web-based teaching site called the Healthcare Improvement Skills Center (www.improvementskills.org). This site contains a self-directed, clinically based, teaching program consisting of six modules covering the important basic concepts of quality improvement

such as team building, how to identify a problem, what is a PDSA cycle, and core quality improvement statistical concepts. The site is also free. Useful educational resources can also be found at the Institute for Healthcare Improvement (www.ihi.org) and other Web sites listed in Appendix 11-1. We strongly encourage educators to take advantage of these sites and not try to reinvent a quality training program from scratch.

Clinical Experience

SBP

One goal for an internal medicine resident rotating on each service would be to understand how the particular service fits into the overall system of care for patients with internal medicine problems. The same holds true for residents in other specialties. Regardless of residents' ultimate careers, this broad knowledge about systems of care will be needed. Components of SBP can be learned during the orientation to every clinical rotation when faculty makes clear how the microsystem(s) of the rotation interconnect with other microsystems to form a network or system of care.[12,17,29–31] The orientation should include an explicit description of the characteristics of the patients served, specific methods and technology used, and the specific roles of the people who work together in the microsystem. A process diagram of the patient flow through the microsystem can be explicitly displayed and the specific role, responsibilities, and tasks that the resident can be expected to perform while working in the microsystem should be taught. In this way, SBP becomes explicit. One very simple but useful exercise is to have all students and residents create a flowchart of how a patient moves through one of multiple microsystems. For example, what are all the steps necessary for a newly diagnosed diabetic to be seen in the clinic and obtain laboratory tests, preventive screenings, immunizations, medications, glucose monitoring, and referrals? In our experience, few residents can accurately complete such a flowchart.

Another useful exercise is creating a work process diagram on what is required to deliver a single component of care. For example, what are the required work steps to get the results of an urgent computed tomographic scan for a patient with acute abdominal pain in the emergency department or to administer a beta-blocker to a patient with acute chest pain and electro-cardiographic changes? These simple exercises can be profoundly helpful.

Finally, we provide in Appendix 11-1 a systems survey developed by one of the authors (in collaboration with the National Committee for Quality Assurance) specifically designed for the primary care outpatient clinic setting. This survey asks for extensive detail about how the clinic microsystem is organized and how it operates to deliver care. In a study conducted by the American Board of Internal Medicine using a practice improvement module (see following discussion), participating residency programs that had the residents complete the survey independently found substantial discordance between what the residents believed existed (or not) and the actual state of the clinic microsystem. If applicable to your setting and specialty, you may also find this to be a useful learning exercise for your trainees.

PBLI

While rotating on each service, residents should apply point-of-care learning methods and the application of EBM (evidence-based medicine) principles at the bedside. Residents should participate as active members of interdisciplinary teams that are working on improving the quality of care provided by the microsystem. This is not to be misconstrued as doing a "QI project," but should be meaningful participation in the team meetings, rapid-cycle tests of change, performance measurement and analysis, root-cause analysis, and implementation strategies for successful change ideas applied to a particular microsystem. After rotating among many different clinical services and experiencing their microsystems, residents should have a portfolio of PBLI experiences and activities that should add up to an aggregate, in-depth, first-hand experience in PBLI.

Teamwork in PBLI and SBP

You've probably noticed that working effectively in interdisciplinary teams has been a consistent theme in PBLI and SBP.[32,33] Working in teams is a new paradigm for physicians. We are only now beginning to understand the core competencies involved in working effectively in teams. Several definitions are in order. Many physicians incorrectly equate the concepts of multidisciplinary and interdisciplinary teams. When working in a multidisciplinary team or environment, each discipline contributes its particular expertise independently to an individual patient's care, and it is the physician who is most responsible for determining the contribution of other disciplines and coordination of services. However, in an interdisciplinary team approach, members work closely together and communicate frequently to optimize patient care, the team is organized around solving a common set of problems for the benefit of patients, and frequent consultation among the team members is the norm, not the exception. Interdisciplinary work embraces two important principles:

1. Idea dominance
   - A clear and recognizable idea must serve as the focus for teamwork.
   - The patient is at the center of that focus.
   - The team must also be able to recognize success and achievements as a team.
2. Professional role and role blurring
   - Most of us learn our roles through the process of professional socialization within our discipline, helping to further define our profession-specific "cognitive maps," or in other words, how we view and interpret our world. These preconceived "maps" of roles are based on learned culture, beliefs, and cognitive approaches learned in training for our specific discipline.
   - In order to function in an interdisciplinary world, we must learn to give up, when necessary, our preconceived cognitive maps. We must also be willing to "blur" our preconceived professional role if someone else on the team is better equipped to lead or perform a specific task.

Baker and colleagues at the Agency for Healthcare Research and Quality (AHRQ) performed a systematic review of what's known about effective teamwork across professions.[34] From this review, they have created a list of core competencies in teamwork educators can use to teach and assess trainees. These competencies are shown in Table 11-3.

Evaluation of Competence in SBP and PBLI

We spent a substantial proportion of this chapter describing what trainees should know, do, and feel, and how some of that learning might occur. Obviously the next task is to determine if a trainee acquired the necessary knowledge, skills, and attitudes in PBLI and SBP.[27,35,36] Unfortunately, the state of the art in the evaluation of these two competencies is limited. Yet, some early work does help to point the way. Given the current state of evaluation in PBLI and SBP,

Table 11-3 **Team-Based Competencies**

Competencies	Definition	Behavioral Examples	KSA
Team leadership	Ability to direct and coordinate the activities of other team members, assess team performance, assign tasks, develop team KSAs, motivate team members, plan and organize, and establish a positive atmosphere	Facilitate team problem solving Provide performance expectations and acceptable interaction patterns Synchronize and combine individual team member contributions Seek and evaluate information that impacts team functioning Clarify team member roles Engage in preparatory meetings and feedback sessions with the team	Knowledge, skill
Mutual performance monitoring	Ability to develop common understandings of the team environment and apply appropriate task strategies in order to accurately monitor teammate performance	Identifying mistakes and lapses in other team member actions Providing feedback regarding team member actions in order to facilitate self-correction	Skill
Back-up behavior	Ability to anticipate other team member's needs through accurate knowledge about their responsibilities Ability to shift workload among members to achieve balance during high periods of workload	Recognition by potential backup providers that there is a workload distribution problem in their team Shifting of work responsibilities to underutilized team members Completion of the whole task or parts of tasks by other team members	Knowledge, skill
Adaptability	Ability to adjust strategies based on information gathered from the environment through the use of compensatory behavior and reallocation of intra-team resources Altering a course of action or team repertoire in response to changing conditions (internal or external)	Identify cues that a change has occurred, assign meaning to that change, and develop a new plan to deal with the changes Identify opportunities for improvement and innovation for habitual or routine practices Remain vigilant to changes in the internal and external environment of the team	Skill
Team/collective orientation	Propensity to take other's behavior into account during group interaction and the belief in the importance of team goals over individual member's goals	Taking into account alternative solutions provided by teammates and appraising that input to determine what is most correct Increased task involvement, information sharing, strategizing, and participatory goal setting	Attitude
Shared mental models	An organizing knowledge structure of the relationships between the task the team is engaged in and how the team members will interact	Anticipating and predicting each other's needs Identify changes in the team, task, or teammates and implicitly adjusting strategies as needed	Knowledge
Mutual trust	The shared belief that the team members will perform their roles and protect the interests of their teammates	Information sharing Willingness to admit mistakes and accept feedback	Attitude
Closed-loop communication	The exchange of information between a sender and a receiver irrespective of the medium	Following up with the team members to ensure message was received Acknowledging that a message was received Clarifying with the sender of the message that the message received is the same as the intended message sent	Skill

From Baker DP, Salas E, King H, et al: The role of teamwork in the professional education of physicians: Current status and assessment recommendations. Jt Comm J Qual Patient Saf 2005;31:185–202.

few, if any, summative assessment methods currently exist. Most educators have designed experiences that combine learning with formative assessment activities. We will break them down into different "learning by doing" approaches.

Most hospitals, and some larger clinics, have existing quality improvement committees and ongoing programs.

Thus, it may be possible to add, or "embed," the students and trainees into existing initiatives. To date, little has been written about this approach. Weingart and colleagues created a multifaceted 3-week elective for their residents consisting of four separate activities.[37] Two activities had the residents participate in an existing hospital quality committee and an investigation of a medical error or complaint. However, the residents' skills were not specifically evaluated in these two activities.

There are several potential disadvantages to the "embedding" approach. First, the trainee will often not be able to join the hospital (or clinic) quality initiative/project at the beginning, or sustain a continued presence on the project given the rotational nature of most current training programs. However, this approach might work for more senior trainees once they have acquired the core knowledge, skills, and attitudes around QI. This approach may be particularly well suited for subspecialty fellows, provided they successfully attained competence, as defined earlier, during residency. Other work has shown that residents can also be excellent sources of information and recommendations for change when looking to reduce errors and improve safety practices.[38] More research is needed to determine how best to embed trainees into existing quality improvement activities.

Quality Improvement Projects/ Programs

Individual Quality Improvement Projects

Multiple studies demonstrate the value of trainees developing a quality improvement project using the rapid cycle test of change approach.[39–41] This is usually executed as an elective rotation where the resident identifies a problem, then develops a plan to improve the quality problem identified. The resident is also asked to describe how he would implement and study the intervention chosen (do and study steps of the PDSA cycle).[42] In the process of developing the rapid cycle for change, they acquire knowledge about important QI concepts and principles. Djuricich, Ogrinc, and others have found that some of the projects developed by the residents can actually be implemented and lead to real change.[21,43] Ogrinc and colleagues developed an instrument called QIKAT (Quality Improvement Knowledge Assessment Test) that is a reliable method to evaluate the quality of the project described by the resident. Research has shown residents clearly enjoy the experience, and their knowledge in quality improvement does increase.[21]

The strengths of the individual project approach are its strong focus on learning and applying, hypothetically, the steps and tools of quality improvement. The QIKAT tool allows faculty to assess the degree of understanding of the steps and concepts of PBLI and SBP. Another strength of the QIKAT tool is the capacity to use written text for assessment of the trainee. The weakness of this approach is the potential lack of real-time experience in implementing and working on an actual quality improvement initiative. As you might have already surmised, it simply would not be feasible to implement *all* resident quality improvement projects at the group level using this approach, and in fact such

an approach runs counter to the concept of interdisciplinary quality improvement. We think this approach is best suited as a first exposure activity in residency, followed by participation in a real-time quality improvement initiative.

Long and colleagues took this individual approach one step further by having the residents conduct a chart audit of their own practice and compare the results with evidence-based standards; then they had the residents identify and implement a quality improvement intervention in their own practice. Thus, this approach adds some real-time experience. Residents are assigned a faculty facilitator to help them with their improvement intervention. Each resident also presents projects to faculty and peers in a conference setting. The resident's project is subsequently assessed using a simple "yes/no" checklist for the presence of 11 different items in the resident's project.[44]

Longitudinal Resident-Based Quality Improvement

In this approach, residents come in and out of an ongoing quality improvement initiative. One example comes from the Yale Primary Care Internal Medicine residency program. During an ambulatory rotation, the second-year residents spend a half day over 4 weeks performing a medical record audit of their own patients from an ambulatory clinic in conjunction with a 4-week structured reading syllabus about quality improvement.[45] Prior to each abstraction session, each resident meets with a faculty member for 30 minutes to discuss the readings and, more important, to perform self-reflection and assessment about what the residents learned about themselves and the microsystem as a result of their medical record audit. At the end of the 4 weeks, the residents must each write a one-page summary of the experience describing what they learned about themselves, their clinic, and what they would recommend for improvements. They finish the rotation by listing up to five "commitment to change(s)" (CtC) they wish to make in their clinical practice.[46–49] Six months later the residents receive a copy of their original CtCs and are asked to reflect by writing how successful they were in making the change(s).

As new residents come on, they contribute to the "pool" of data that is periodically shared with the other residents at a designated quarterly conference throughout the academic year. A summary quality report card is posted publicly. A small study of this approach did find high satisfaction among the residents and modest improvements in patient care. Residents particularly liked the self-audit activity. The weaknesses of this approach are the limited nature of the activity to a single rotation, and lack of ongoing feedback data at the individual level. From an evaluation perspective, faculty can assess whether the resident completed the required activities, the quality of the summary report and commitment to change statements, and the results of their audits. However, more research is needed before such information could be used for summative purposes.

Programs with robust information technology systems have used the classic audit with feedback approach, and as noted in Chapter 5, medical record audit alone does lead to modest changes in behavior.[50,51] However, we do not consider the provision of data alone to constitute a meaningful quality improvement activity. Receiving and reviewing data is simply part of the needs assessment activity that should be performed as the initial steps in the process for system improvement.

Group Quality Improvement Projects

It is possible to build quality improvement initiatives around the training program as a group process. One example is the internal medicine residency program at Southern Illinois University in Springfield, Illinois. This program develops interdisciplinary projects that include residents from the outset. These residents, despite moving from rotation to rotation, stay with their quality improvement team until the initiative ends. Because each team contains multiple residents, the team is always assured some residents can contribute to the initiative during the life cycle of the project. This program has experienced significant changes in quality measures at the patient level, but work is ongoing to determine the effects on resident competence. Other residency programs have also reported positive impacts by involving residents in group initiatives.[40]

Other tools now available to training programs in internal medicine, family medicine, and many subspecialties are Web-based practice improvement modules. The development of these Web-based tools was catalyzed by a recent requirement from the American Board of Medical Specialties to evaluate performance in practice as part of maintenance of certification programs in the United States. The American Board of Internal Medicine was one of the first boards to develop Web-based practice improvement modules (PIMs). PIMs take physicians step by step through some combination of a medical record audit, patient survey, and practice system assessment. All medical record data are entered in a Web-based abstraction instrument, and patients use a telephone (interactive voice response technology) or the Web to complete the patient survey. The ABIM requires each resident to abstract at least five of their own charts as part of the group initiative. The PIM is based on the quality improvement framework popularized by the Institute of Healthcare Improvement[52] and the practice system analysis is based on the Wagner Chronic Care Model.[15,16] The practice system survey includes questions about the specific information management processes, patient access and reminder systems, and patient activation for self-care (see Appendix 11-1). All this information is collected and then submitted to the ABIM via the Internet.[53]

The patient survey asks about practice access, communication and interpersonal skills of the physician, education, and self-activation in the care of their condition. Using a prespecified scoring algorithm, ABIM then analyzes the data from the three sources and returns to the residency group a summary report of their performance via the Web. The residents interact with this summary report to select opportunities for improvement which are then automatically aggregated to develop a quality improvement plan. After a period of 2 to 6 months, the training program is reminded to submit an impact statement via the Web describing the effects of their quality improvement interventions. The PIM program automatically sends e-mail reminders to the program to keep on schedule with data submission, planning, and reporting.

The ABIM piloted its preventive cardiology PIM among 15 different residency programs in 2004 as part of a feasibility study. Programs found the medical record audit was relatively easy for the residents to do, and as noted already, lessons learned from the systems survey were often eye-opening. The biggest challenge the programs faced was completing the patient surveys, mostly because so many of their patients were socioeconomically disadvantaged and needed help completing the surveys. All programs found the comprehensive report they received from the PIM to be valuable and catalyzed a number of quality improvement interventions in the program. The types of interventions used in these programs can be seen in Appendix 11-2.

Other Approaches to Evaluate Individual Residents

A number of other tools covered in this textbook can be used to evaluate competency in PBLI and SBP. We will briefly review them here in the context of these two competencies. The reader is referred to the specific chapters on these tools for more detailed information.

Multisource Feedback

Multisource feedback (MSF) can be very useful in evaluating the critical communication and teamwork skills needed for PBLI and SBP. Patient surveys can target important behaviors around transitions of care (such as referral or discharge) and patient activation needed to produce improved outcomes of care, especially for chronic conditions. Nursing and peer surveys can target many of the team-based competencies highlighted in Table 11-3.

Standardized Patients

A number of studies have used unannounced standardized patients (SPs) to assess clinical behaviors, including recommendation of evidence-based care with a high degree of reliability. Thus, SPs can be a good way to assess the quality of care at the patient-provider level. The major limitations of this approach are cost and the lack of ability to assess actual quality improvement knowledge, skills, and attitudes. Thus, SPs are best suited to assess the quality of care.

Portfolios

Portfolios provide a "holistic" approach to competency assessment. Any activity involving PBLI and SBP can be incorporated into a portfolio with trainee reflection. Self-assessment and self-reflection are a major strength of the portfolio process. Successful engagement in quality improvement and change must include these two skills. As Linda Headrick has pointed out, the PDSA cycle of improvement is in fact a model for effective continuous professional development.[54] Medical school and residency, with or without a fellowship, is only the beginning of a life course of improvement and change. Portfolios by their very design facilitate these behaviors.

Clinical Vignettes

Clinical vignettes are in essence a form of written assessment. Trainees are given a series of clinical scenarios (vignettes) and asked what the next steps in care should be. Peabody and colleagues found vignettes to be as accurate as standardized patients and more complete than a medical record audit.[55,56] Results on a set of clinical vignettes correlated highly with the trainees' performance with unannounced SPs. However, like SPs, clinical vignettes can mostly demonstrate capability at the quality level and again provides less information to assess QI skills.

Evaluating PBLI and SBP: An Example

We'd like to close this chapter by providing an example of how a program can use multiple tools to evaluate PBLI and SBP. We will start with a clinical scenario involving a surgical and family medicine resident.

> A 74-year-old woman with diabetes and hypertension presents to her family medicine clinic for follow-up after hospital discharge. Two weeks ago the patient underwent a left-sided colectomy for localized colon cancer. Her postoperative course was complicated by persistently high blood sugar levels treated with sliding scale insulin, and a prolonged ileus. She lives at home with her 73-year-old husband who suffers from Parkinson's disease and angina.
>
> As the resident walks into the clinic room, she notices a large ecchymosis on the patient's left shoulder and upper arm. When the patient is asked what happened, she responds she fell in her tub. She says she didn't lose consciousness, but just felt terribly weak. She is also unsure what medication she is taking, and the resident, who was on another rotation at a different hospital, doesn't have any information from the current hospitalization or surgery. The patient cannot remember any of the names of her doctors.

Unfortunately, this scenario is all too common, but presents examples of how faculty and others could evaluate competence in PBLI and SBP. For example, did the surgery resident know who the key individuals are in safely and effectively helping this patient with the transition at discharge from hospital to home, and how to communicate key information about the patient to the receiving caregivers? Were understandable discharge instructions given to the patient and other caregivers, such as a visiting nurse? Did the surgical team assess the patient for fall risk at discharge? These are just a few measurable skills.

Educators can use vignettes like these to teach specific knowledge, skills, and attitudes in these two competencies. The surgery and family medicine residents could complete a flowchart of all the important steps required for a safe hospital discharge of a postoperative patient. The communication skills of the surgery resident can be assessed through multisource instruments. Finally, is this a common problem at this hospital? Either resident could conduct a root cause analysis about what led to this patient's fall, and then develop a quality improvement rapid cycle test of change to improve discharge practices working with the quality committee of the hospital. The project developed by the resident could then be evaluated using QIKAT.[21] So you can see how the suboptimal experiences of a single patient can lead to multiple opportunities to both teach and evaluate the competencies of practice-based learning and improvement and systems-based practice.

Conclusion

A competency-based curriculum and evaluation method provide a guideline (even a checklist) for assessing the knowledge, attitude, and skills that can be acquired over 36 months of internal medicine residency training. Before entering any of the focused practice settings of initial or subspecialty training, a competent physician should demonstrate a portfolio of learning experiences and evaluative evidence of competence in SBP and PBLI.

It may not be necessary to conduct formal lectures or workshops in these topics; they ought to be learned through independent study, Web-based learning, and self-assessment programs. By working in many real microsystems, residents should gain the knowledge, attitudes, and skills needed for competence in SBP and PBLI. What must be added to the current curriculum is explicit discussion on each rotation about the interdependence of the network of microsystems that make up a local and regional health care system.

Likewise, our long-term goal should be to move away from doing "QI projects" just to satisfy the residency curriculum. In fact, such activity would not only be wasteful of the resident's time but not helpful to the institution. Instead, residents should learn PBLI through active, real-time participation in the ongoing quality improvement activities in every microsystem they rotate through. A portfolio that contains a catalog of experiences and evidence of competence that is kept by the resident can serve as a self-directed guide to acquiring these competencies and may be the best approach, but much work lies ahead.

ANNOTATED BIBLIOGRAPHY

1. Institute of Medicine: Educating Health Professionals: A Bridge to Quality. Washington, DC, National Academy Press, 2003.

   This 2003 report from the Institute of Medicine followed the Crossing the Quality Chasm report, and covers competencies vital to working effectively in systems. Examples of effective systems and competencies are provided throughout.

2. Ogrinc G, Headrick LA, Mutha S, et al: A framework for teaching medical students and residents about practice-based learning and improvement, synthesized from a literature review. Acad Med 2003;78:748–756.

   This paper provides a useful developmental framework and is highlighted in Tables 2a and 2b. The paper describes how the framework was created and how educators can use it to improve medical student and resident education in quality and systems.

3. Langley GJ, Nolan KM, Nolan TW, et al: The Improvement Guide. A Practical Approach to Enhancing Organizational Performance. San Francisco, Jossey-Bass, 1996, pp 3–11.

   This book is a must read for anyone involved in teaching about practice-based learning and improvement and systems-based practice. This book lays out in understandable detail how to implement rapid cycles of change using the plan-do-study-act approach. The topics discussed in this book are core skills for physicians of the future.

4. Baker DP, Salas E, King H, et al: The role of teamwork in the professional education of physicians: Current status and assessment recommendations. Jt Comm J Qual Patient Safety 2005;31:185–202.

   This paper describes the core competencies trainees will need in order to work effectively in teams (see Table 11-3). The paper provides a nice review of research about teamwork in other fields, notably aviation. A more comprehensive review of teamwork can be found by Baker and colleagues at the Agency for Healthcare Research and Quality (AHRQ) Web site (www.ahrq.gov).

5. Kilo CM, Leavitt M:Medical Practice Transformation with Information Technology. Chicago, Health Information Management Systems Society, 2005.

   Although the title suggests this paperback is mostly about using technology, the book actually describes how an effective systems-based medical practice should function. This is important for educators to understand; trainees cannot learn effectively about systems-based practice if they do not gain experience working in an effective medical practice. The book specifically covers principles for transforming practices and changing the clinical environment. This book can be purchased at www.himss.org.

REFERENCES

1. Institute of Medicine. Crossing the Quality1 Chasm. Washington, DC, National Academy Press, 2001.
2. Accreditation Council for Graduate Medical Education. The Outcomes Project. Accessed July 16, 2007 at www.acgme.org/Outcome.
3. Blank L, Kimball H, McDonald W, Merino J:Medical professionalism in the new millennium: A physician charter 15 months later. Ann Intern Med 2003;138:839–841.
4. Becher EC, Chassin MR:Taking health care back: The physician's role in quality improvement. Acad Med 2002;77:953–962.
5. Brennan TA:Physicians' Professional Responsibility to Improve the Quality of Care. Acad Med 2002;77:973–980.
6. Goode LD, Clancy CM, Kimball HR, et al: When is "good enough"? The role and responsibility of physicians to improve patient safety. Acad Med 2002;77:947–952.
7. Gruen RL, Pearson SD, Brennan TA:Physician-citizens-public roles and professional obligations. JAMA 2004;291:94–98.
8. United Kingdom Medical Council: Good Medical Practice. Accessed July 16, 2007 at www.gmc-uk.org/guidance/good_medical_practice/index.asp.
9. Royal College of Physicians and Surgeons of Canada: The CanMEDS 2005 Physician Competency Framework. Accessed July 16, 2007 at http://rcpsc.medical.org/canmeds/CanMEDS2005/index.php.
10. Association of American Medical Colleges: Medical School Outcomes Project. Accessed July 16, 2007 at www.aamc.org/meded/msop/.
11. Institute of Medicine: Educating Health Professionals: A Bridge to Quality. Washington, DC, National Academy Press, 2003.
12. Batalden PB, Nelson EC, Edwards WH, et al: Microsystems in healthcare. Part 9: Developing small clinical units to attain peak performance. Jt Comm J Qual Safety 2003;29:575–585.
13. American College of Physicians: The advanced medical home: A patient-centered, physician guided model of care. Accessed July 16, 2007 at www.acponline.org/hpp/adv_med.pdf.
14. Grumbach K, Bodenheimer T:A primary care home for Americans: Putting the house in order. JAMA 2002;288:889–893.
15. Wagner EH, Austin BT, Von Korff M:Organizing care for patients with chronic illness. Milbank Q 1996;74:511–542.
16. Von Korff M, Gruman J, Schaefer J, et al: Collaborative management of chronic illness. Ann Intern Med 1997;127:1097–1102.
17. Nelson EC, Batalden PB, Huber TP, et al: Microsystems in Healthcare. Part 1: Learning from high performing front-line clinical units. Jt Comm J Qual Safety 2002;28:472–493.
18. Bowen JL, Salerno SM, Chamberlain JK, et al: Changing habits of practice. Transforming internal medicine residency education in ambulatory settings. J Gen Intern Med 2005;20:1181–1187.
19. Demming WE: The New Economics for Industry, Government, Education, 2nd ed. Cambridge, Mass., The MIT Press, 1994, pp 92–115.
20. Audet AM, Doty MM, Shamasdin J, Schoenbaum SC:Measure, learn, and improve: Physicians' involvement in quality improvement. Health Affairs 2005;24:843–853.
21. Ogrinc G, Headrick LA, Morrison LJ, Foster T:Teaching and assessing resident competence in practice-based learning and improvement. J Gen Intern Med 2004;19:496–500.
22. Bowen JL:Adapting residency training. Training adaptable residents. West J Med 1998;168:371–377.
23. Berwick DM:Broadening the view of evidence-based medicine. Qual Safety Health Care 2005;14(5):315–316.
24. Barach P, Berwick DM:Patient safety and the reliability of health care systems. Ann Intern Med, 2003;138(12):997–998.
25. Leape LL, Berwick DM, Bates DW:What practices will most improve safety? Evidence-based medicine meets patient safety. JAMA, 2002;288(4):501–507.
26. Ogrinc G, Headrick LA, Mutha S, et al: A framework for teaching medical students and residents about practice-based learning and improvement, synthesized from a literature review. Acad Med 2003;78:748–756.
27. Batalden P, Leach D, Swing S, et al: General competencies and accreditation in graduate medical education. Health Affairs 2002;21(5):103–111.
28. Gould BE, Grey MR, Huntington CG, et al: Improving patient care outcomes by teaching quality improvement to medical students in community-based practices. Acad Med 2002;77:1011–1018.
29. Nelson EC, Batalden PB, Homa K, et al: Microsystems in healthcare. Part 2: Creating a rich information environment. Jt Comm J Qual Safety 2003;29:5–15.
30. Wasson JH, Godfrey MM, Nelson EC, et al: Microsystems in healthcare. Part 4: Planning patient-centered care. Jt Comm J Qual Safety 2003;29:227–237.
31. Batalden PB, Nelson EC, Mohr JJ, et al: Microsystems in health care: Part 5. How leaders are leading. Jt Comm J Qual Safety 2003;29:297–308.
32. Cooper H, Carlisle C, Gibbs T, Watkins C:Developing an evidence-based for interdisciplinary learning: a systematic review. J Adv Nurs 2001;35:228–237.
33. Moore SM, Alemi F, Headrick LA:Interdisciplinary learning in continuous improvement of healthcare: Four perspectives. Jt Comm J Qual Safety 1996;22:165–187.
34. Baker DP, Salas E, King H, et al: The role of teamwork in the professional education of physicians: Current status and assessment recommendations. Jt Comm J Qual Patient Safety 2005; 31:185–202.
35. Lynch DC, Swing SR, Horowitz SD, et al: Assessing practice-based learning and improvement. Teach Learn Med 2004;16:85–92.

36. Hayden SR, Dufel S, Shih R:Definitions and competencies for practice-based learning and improvement. Acad Emerg Med 2002;9:1242–1248.
37. Weingart SN, Tess A, Driver J, et al: Creating a quality improvement elective for medical house officers. J Gen Intern Med 2004;19:861–867.
38. Volpp KG, Grande D:Residents' suggestions for reducing errors in teaching hospitals. N Engl J Med, 2003;348(9):851–855.
39. Ziegelstein RC, Fiebach NH:"The mirror" and "the village": A new method for teaching practice-based learning and improvement and systems-based practice. Acad Med 2004;79:83–88.
40. Sutherland JE, Hoehns JD, O'Donnell B, Wiblin RT:Diabetes management quality improvement in a family practice residency program. J Am Board Fam Pract 2001;14:243–251.
41. Coleman MT, Nasraty S, Ostapchuk M, et al: Introducing practice-based learning and improvement ACGME core competencies into a family medicine residency curriculum. Jt Comm J Qual Safety 2003;29:238–247.
42. Langley GJ, Nolan KM, Nolan TW, et al: The Improvement Guide. A Practical Approach to Enhancing Organizational Performance. San Francisco, Jossey-Bass, 1996, pp 3–11.
43. Djuricich AM, Ciccarelli M, Swigonski NL:A continuous quality improvement curriculum for residents: addressing core competency, improving systems. Acad Med, 2004;79(10 Suppl):S65–S67.
44. Lough JRM, Murray TS:Audit and summative assessment: A completed audit cycle. Med Educ 2001;35:357–363.
45. Holmboe ES, Prince L, Green M:Teaching and improving quality of care in a primary care internal medicine residency clinic. Acad Med, 2005;80(6):571–577.
46. Mazmanian PE, Mazmanian PM:Commitment to change: Theoretical foundations, methods, and outcomes. J Cont Educ Health Prof 1999;19:200–207.
47. Jones DL:Viability of the commitment-for-change evaluation strategy in continuing medical education. Acad Med 1990; 65:S37–S38.
48. Pereles L, Gondocz T, Lockyer JM, et al: Effectiveness of commitment contracts in facilitating change in continuing medical education intervention. J Cont Educ Health Prof 1997;17:27–31.
49. Mazmanian PE, Johnson RE, Zhang A, et al: Effects of a signature on rates of change: A randomized controlled trial involving continuing education and the commitment-to-change model. Acad Med 2001;76:642–646.
50. O'Brien T, Oxman AD, Davis DA, et al: Audit and feedback versus alternative strategies: Effects on professional practice and health care outcomes. Cochrane Database Syst Rev 2000;2:1–15.
51. Veloski J, Boex JR, Grasberger MJ, et al: Systematic review of the literature on assessment, feedback and physicians' clinical performance: BEME Guide No. 7. Med Teach, 2006;28(2):117–128.
52. Institute for Healthcare Improvement. Accessed July 16, 2006 at www.ihi.org.
53. Holmboe ES, Meehan TP, Lynn L, et al: The ABIM diabetes practice improvement module: A new method for self assessment. J Cont Educ Health Prof 2006;26:109–119.
54. Aron DC, Headrick LA:Educating physicians prepared to improve care and safety is no accident: It requires a systematic approach. Qual Safety Health Care 2002;11(2):168–173.
55. Peabody JW, Luck J, Glassman P, et al: Measuring the quality of physician practice by using clinical vignettes: A prospective validation study. Ann Intern Med 2004;141(10):771–780.
56. Dresselhaus TR, Peabody JW, Lee M, et al: Measuring compliance with preventive care guidelines: Standardized patients, clinical vignettes, and the medical record. J Gen Intern Med, 2000; 15(11):782–788.
57. Headrick LA:Improving complex systems of care. Collaborative Education to Improve Patient Safety. Washington, DC, HRSA/ Bureau of Health Professions, 2000, pp 75–88.

USEFUL WEB SITES

Provided here is a list of three useful Web sites where educators can find valuable experiences or tools for practice-based learning and improvement and systems-based practice.

Academy of Post Graduate Health Care Education.

As mentioned in the chapter, the Academy of Post Graduate Health Care Education has developed six Web-based educational modules about quality improvement. Each module is case-based and covers important principles and concepts of quality improvement science. Each module concludes with a series of self-assessment multiple-choice questions with feedback. The modules can be accessed at www.qualityimprovementskills.org. The site is free.

Institute for Healthcare Improvement (IHI).

The IHI is a valuable resource for tools and guidance, including templates for rapid cycle of change, root cause analysis, and failure modes effects analysis. The IHI has also has a specific site for health professions education (www.ihi.org/IHI/Topics/HealthProfessionsEducation/) with a paper by Linda Headrick on learning to improve complex systems of care.[57] The IHI also has a sister site about clinical microsystems: www.clinicalmicrosystems.org. On this site is an in-depth toolkit called "The Green Book" with a wealth of tools for improving systems of care.

Achieving Competence Today (ACT).

ACT is a national initiative of The Robert Wood Johnson Foundation through the Partnerships for Quality Education initiative. The ACT model is designed to prepare health care trainees across disciplines and has three main components (from the ACT Web site):

1. An intensive, action-based learning curriculum that teaches learners about systems and practice improvement

2. Interdisciplinary learning through collaboration on a quality improvement project

3. Connecting the learners with the institution's senior quality leadership
More information about the ACT curriculum can be found at www.actcurriculum.org.

Appendix 11-1
Systems Survey for Residency Outpatient Practice

Many physicians have not been trained how to understand or influence the design of their practice systems. Yet recent information about health care quality makes it clear that the structure of the practice system is as important as physician knowledge, attitudes, and skills in determining outcomes of care. Therefore, clinicians need to learn how to influence the systems in which they deliver care. Influencing systems involves acquiring new competencies in system-based practice and practice-based learning and improvement discussed in this chapter.

What do we mean by "practice systems"? We use the concept of the clinical microsystem developed by Paul Batalden and his colleagues[12] at Dartmouth Medical School:

Clinical microsystems are the front-line units that provide most health care to most people. They are the places where patients, families and care teams meet. Microsystems also include support staff, processes, technology and recurring patterns of information, behavior and results. Central to every clinical microsystem is the patient.

In other words, a clinical microsystem is the organization of people (doctors, staff, and patients) and the ways they collaborate and communicate to achieve common aims for quality care. We encourage you to visit their Web site at www.clinicalmicrosystem.org to learn more and review their comprehensive guide on tools you can use in your training programs.

The survey provided in this appendix was developed in collaboration between Dr. F. Daniel Duffy at the American Board of Internal Medicine, and Sarah Scholle, Phyllis Torda, and other staff members at the National Committee on Quality Assurance (NCQA). Information about the NCQA Provider Practice Connections, a recognition program that uses a version of this survey, can be found at www.ncqa.org to see how an organization uses this type of instrument for practicing physicians.

This survey is provided as a self-assessment tool. Simply circle (or write in where indicated) the appropriate response for each question. Be sure to carry what you choose or write in for each condition throughout the survey where indicated.

You can calculate a simple system score by adding up the numbers circled for each section. A lower score is a better score; higher scores identify areas for improvement. However, when choosing an intervention to improve your system, look for the more feasible opportunities first.

Identifying Important Conditions Seen in the Practice

1. What are the most important conditions in the practice's patient population?

Condition 1
1. Diabetes
2. Cardiovascular disease
3. Depression
4. Asthma
5. Hypertension
6. Heart failure
7. Arthritis
8. Other: _____

If you selected "Other," please type the condition

Condition 2
1. Diabetes
2. Cardiovascular disease
3. Depression
4. Asthma
5. Hypertension
6. Heart failure
7. Arthritis
8. Other: _____

If you selected "Other," please type the condition

Condition 3
1. Diabetes
2. Cardiovascular disease
3. Depression
4. Asthma
5. Hypertension
6. Heart failure
7. Arthritis
8. Other: _____

If you selected "Other," please type the condition

2. Does your practice use practice data or other information to identify the most important conditions seen in your practice's patient population?
   1. Yes
   2. No
   3. Don't know
   4. Not applicable

3. What are the most important risk factors that occur in the practice's patient population?
   Risk Factor 1:_____
   Risk Factor 2:_____
   Risk Factor 3:_____

4. Does your practice use practice data or other information to identify the most important risk factors seen in your practice's patient population?
   1. Yes
   2. No
   3. Don't know
   4. Not applicable

Patient Tracking and Registry Function

1. Does your practice use an electronic data system that includes searchable patient information? This can be a practice management system, registry, or other electronic system.
   1. Yes
   2. No

2. For patients seen in the last 3 months, please indicate whether each type of information is available and for what proportion of your patients.

Name
1. Yes, system has data for ≥75% of patients
2. Yes, system has data but for <75% of patients
3. No, data is not available electronically
4. Don't know

Date of birth
1. Yes, system has data for ≥75% of patients
2. Yes, system has data but for <75% of patients
3. No, data is not available electronically
4. Don't know

Gender
1. Yes, system has data for ≥75% of patients
2. Yes, system has data but for <75% of patients
3. No, data is not available electronically
4. Don't know

Marital status
1. Yes, system has data for ≥75% of patients
2. Yes, system has data but for <75% of patients
3. No, data is not available electronically
4. Don't know

Language preference
1. Yes, system has data for ≥75% of patients
2. Yes, system has data but for <75% of patients
3. No, data is not available electronically
4. Don't know

Voluntarily self-identified race/ethnicity
1. Yes, system has data for ≥75% of patients
2. Yes, system has data but for <75% of patients
3. No, data is not available electronically
4. Don't know

Address
1. Yes, system has data for ≥75% of patients
2. Yes, system has data but for <75% of patients
3. No, data is not available electronically
4. Don't know

Telephone number(s)
1. Yes, system has data for ≥75% of patients
2. Yes, system has data but for <75% of patients
3. No, data is not available electronically
4. Don't know

E-mail address (when available)
1. Yes, system has data for ≥75% of patients
2. Yes, system has data but for <75% of patients
3. No, data is not available electronically
4. Don't know

External ID, such as insurance ID or Social Security number
1. Yes, system has data for ≥75% of patients
2. Yes, system has data but for <75% of patients
3. No, data is not available electronically
4. Don't know

Insurance payer ID
1. Yes, system has data for ≥75% of patients
2. Yes, system has data but for <75% of patients
3. No, data is not available electronically
4. Don't know

Emergency contact information
1. Yes, system has data for ≥ 75% of patients
2. Yes, system has data but for < 75% of patients
3. No, data is not available electronically
4. Don't know

Past and current diagnoses
1. Yes, system has data for ≥75% of patients
2. Yes, system has data but for <75% of patients
3. No, data is not available electronically
4. Don't know

Dates of previous clinical visits
1. Yes, system has data for ≥75% of patients
2. Yes, system has data but for <75% of patients
3. No, data is not available electronically
4. Don't know

Billing codes for services
1. Yes, system has data for ≥ 75% of patients
2. Yes, system has data but for < 75% of patients
3. No, data is not available electronically
4. Don't know

3. Does your practice use an electronic data system that includes clinical patient information in searchable, coded data fields? This can be a registry, electronic medical record or other electronic system.
   1. Yes
   2. No

4. For patients seen in the last 3 months, please indicate whether each type of information is available and for what proportion of your patients.

Status of appropriate preventive services (immunizations, screenings, counseling)
1. Yes, system has data for ≥75% of patients
2. Yes, system has data but for <75% of patients
3. No, data is not available electronically
4. Don't know

Allergies and adverse reactions
1. Yes, system has data for ≥75% of patients
2. Yes, system has data but for <75% of patients
3. No, data is not available electronically
4. Don't know

Blood pressure
1. Yes, system has data for ≥75% of patients
2. Yes, system has data but for <75% of patients
3. No, data is not available electronically
4. Don't know

Height
1. Yes, system has data for ≥75% of patients
2. Yes, system has data but for <75% of patients
3. No, data is not available electronically
4. Don't know

Weight
1. Yes, system has data for ≥75% of patients
2. Yes, system has data but for <75% of patients
3. No, data is not available electronically
4. Don't know

Body mass index (BMI)
1. Yes, system has data for ≥75% of patients
2. Yes, system has data but for <75% of patients
3. No, data is not available electronically
4. Don't know

Laboratory test results
1. Yes, system has data for ≥75% of patients
2. Yes, system has data but for <75% of patients
3. No, data is not available electronically
4. Don't know

Report of imaging results
1. Yes, system has data for ≥75% of patients
2. Yes, system has data but for <75% of patients
3. No, data is not available electronically
4. Don't know

Report of pathology results
1. Yes, system has data for ≥75% of patients
2. Yes, system has data but for <75% of patients
3. No, data is not available electronically
4. Don't know

Presence or absence of advance directives
1. Yes, system has data for ≥75% of patients
2. Yes, system has data but for <75% of patients
3. No, data is not available electronically
4. Don't know

5. Does your practice use an electronic system to generate lists to identify patients who need follow-up care?
   1. Yes
   2. No

6. Does your practice's electronic system generate the following lists?

   ### Patients who need pre-visit planning, such as obtaining tests prior to the visit
   1. Yes
   2. No
   3. Don't know

   ### Patients who need their records reviewed by a clinician; reasons may include abnormal test results or missed visits
   1. Yes
   2. No
   3. Don't know

   ### Patients on a particular medication
   1. Yes
   2. No
   3. Don't know

   ### Patients who are due for preventive care services
   1. Yes
   2. No
   3. Don't know

   ### Patients who are due for specific tests
   1. Yes
   2. No
   3. Don't know

   ### Patients who are due for follow-up visits, such as for a chronic condition
   1. Yes
   2. No
   3. Don't know

7. Does your practice send reminders to patients by mail, telephone, or electronic mail about the following kinds of services?

   ### Preventive services, such as immunizations and screening tests
   1. Yes, and the process works well
   2. Yes, but the process could use improvement
   3. No
   4. Don't know

Diagnostic or follow-up testing, such as periodic lipid testing or dilated eye examinations for diabetics
1. Yes, and the process works well
2. Yes, but the process could use improvement
3. No
4. Don't know

Follow-up visits
1. Yes, and the process works well
2. Yes, but the process could use improvement
3. No
4. Don't know

8. Does your practice use a patient registry for the following?

   ### Condition 1
   1. Yes
   2. No
   3. Don't know

   ### Condition 2
   1. Yes
   2. No
   3. Don't know

   ### Condition 3
   1. Yes
   2. No
   3. Don't know

   ### Tracking preventive service needs (e.g., screening, immunizations, counseling for behavior change)
   1. Yes
   2. No
   3. Don't know

   ### Tracking patients whose conditions require visits to multiple clinicians, frequent hospitalizations or emergencies
   1. Yes
   2. No
   3. Don't know

Care Management and Patient Self-Care Education

1. Have all the clinicians in your practice who see patients with the following conditions agreed to practice in a consistent style, based on written, evidence-based guidelines (when applicable)?

   ### Condition 1
   1. Yes
   2. No
   3. Don't know

   ### Condition 2
   1. Yes
   2. No
   3. Don't know

   ### Condition 3
   1. Yes
   2. No
   3. Don't know

Ordering appropriate screening tests

1. Yes
2. No
3. Don't know

Giving appropriate immunizations

1. Yes
2. No
3. Don't know

Relevant risk assessments

1. Yes
2. No
3. Don't know

Counseling for behavior change

1. Yes
2. No
3. Don't know

2. Does your practice use guideline-based reminders, flowsheets, checklists, or other templates to remind physicians about needed services at the point of care for the following conditions? These can range from pop-ups within an electronic medical record or paper notes attached to the front of the chart. Please indicate whether electronic or paper tools are used.

Condition 1

1. Yes, electronic
2. Yes, paper-based
3. No
4. Don't know

Condition 2

1. Yes, electronic
2. Yes, paper-based
3. No
4. Don't know

Condition 3

1. Yes, electronic
2. Yes, paper-based
3. No
4. Don't know

Ordering appropriate screening tests

1. Yes, electronic
2. Yes, paper-based
3. No
4. Don't know

Giving appropriate immunizations

1. Yes, electronic
2. Yes, paper-based
3. No
4. Don't know

Performing relevant risk assessments

1. Yes, electronic
2. Yes, paper-based
3. No
4. Don't know

Counseling for behavior change

1. Yes, electronic
2. Yes, paper-based
3. No
4. Don't know

3. Does your practice use the following charting tools to organize and document clinical information in the medical record? Tools may be electronic or paper-based. For patients seen in the last 3 months, please indicate whether each type of information is available and for what proportion of your patients.

Template for integrated treatment plan

1. Yes, the tool is filled out for $\geq$75% of patients
2. Yes, the tool is used but for <75% of patients
3. No, the tool is not used
4. Don't know

Algorithm to recommend adjustments in treatment to achieve goal

1. Yes, the tool is filled out for $\geq$75% of patients
2. Yes, the tool is used but for <75% of patients
3. No, the tool is not used
4. Don't know

Problem list

1. Yes, the tool is filled out for $\geq$75% of patients
2. Yes, the tool is used but for <75% of patients
3. No, the tool is not used
4. Don't know

List of prescribed medications, including both chronic and short-term

1. Yes, the tool is filled out for $\geq$75% of patients
2. Yes, the tool is used but for < 75% of patients
3. No, the tool is not used
4. Don't know

List of over-the-counter medications, supplements, and alternative therapies

1. Yes, the tool is filled out for $\geq$ 75% of patients
2. Yes, the tool is used but for <75% of patients
3. No, the tool is not used
4. Don't know

Structured template for narrative progress notes

1. Yes, the tool is filled out for $\geq$75% of patients
2. Yes, the tool is used but for <75% of patients
3. No, the tool is not used
4. Don't know

Flow sheet for monitoring tests

1. Yes, the tool is filled out for $\geq$75% of patients
2. Yes, the tool is used but for <75% of patients
3. No, the tool is not used
4. Don't know

Questionnaire for patient symptoms or functional level

1. Yes, the tool is filled out for $\geq$75% of patients
2. Yes, the tool is used but for <75% of patients
3. No, the tool is not used
4. Don't know

Patient self-monitoring log
1. Yes, the tool is filled out for ≥75% of patients
2. Yes, the tool is used but for <75% of patients
3. No, the tool is not used
4. Don't know

Structured template for recording risk factors
1. Yes, the tool is filled out for ≥75% of patients
2. Yes, the tool is used but for <75% of patients
3. No, the tool is not used
4. Don't know

Structured template for recording screening test results
1. Yes, the tool is filled out for ≥75% of patients
2. Yes, the tool is used but for <75% of patients
3. No, the tool is not used
4. Don't know

Structured history and physical examination form to document stage of disease
1. Yes, the tool is filled out for ≥75% of patients
2. Yes, the tool is used but for <75% of patients
3. No, the tool is not used
4. Don't know

4. In addition to the care that you provide, are the following types of care management routinely provided by others to your patients with Condition 1? "Others" can include your practice staff, your medical group, or a health plan or other external disease management organization.

Perform pre-visit planning to assure that all needed information is available at the time of the visit
1. Yes
2. No
3. Don't know

Review and individualize the care management plan for patients with Condition 1
1. Yes
2. No
3. Don't know

Help patients with Condition 1 set individualized treatment goals
1. Yes
2. No
3. Don't know

Assess and document the progress of patients with Condition 1 toward treatment goals
1. Yes
2. No
3. Don't know

Review all prescribed medications, supplements, and alternative therapies for patients with Condition 1 at each visit
1. Yes
2. No
3. Don't know

Review self-monitoring results for patients with Condition 1 and incorporate the results into the record
1. Yes
2. No
3. Don't know

Assess barriers when patients with Condition 1 have not met treatment goals
1. Yes
2. No
3. Don't know

Assess barriers when patients with Condition 1 have not filled, refilled, or taken prescribed medications
1. Yes
2. No
3. Don't know

Follow up when patients with Condition 1 have not kept important appointments
1. Yes
2. No
3. Don't know

Review longitudinal data in tabular or graphical form of targeted clinical measurements for patients with Condition 1 (e.g., blood pressure, BMI, LDL levels)
1. Yes
2. No
3. Don't know

Complete after-visit follow-up (e.g., by a nurse or care manager) for patients with Condition 1
1. Yes
2. No
3. Don't know

5. Does your practice routinely use the following activities to encourage patient self-management for patients with Condition 1?

Uses tool to assess self-management capabilities, including readiness to change and patient preferences (when relevant) for patients with Condition 1
1. Yes
2. No
3. Don't know

Provides educational resources for patients with Condition 1 in the language or medium that the patient understands
1. Yes
2. No
3. Don't know

Instructs patients with Condition 1 in self-management techniques and periodically observes their technique
1. Yes
2. No
3. Don't know
4. Not relevant

Provides a convenient method for patients with Condition 1 to record and report self-monitoring results

1. Yes
2. No
3. Don't know
4. Not relevant

Provides or connects patients with Condition 1 to self-management support programs

1. Yes
2. No
3. Don't know

Provides or connects patients with Contition 1 to classes taught by qualified instructors

1. Yes
2. No
3. Don't know
4. Not relevant

Provides or connects patients with Condition 1 to other self-management resources where needed, such as Internet sites

1. Yes
2. No
3. Don't know

6. Does your practice have systematic processes to assess patients' communication needs?

Identify and prominently display in the medical record the language preferred by the patient, if other than English

1. Yes, and the process works well
2. Yes, but the process could use improvement
3. No
4. Don't know

Assess other communication barriers (e.g., hearing, vision, literacy)

1. Yes, and the process works well
2. Yes, but the process could use improvement
3. No
4. Don't know

7. Do the members of your staff function as a team by sharing responsibility for managing patient care in the following ways?

Nonphysician staff reminds patients of appointments and collects information prior to appointments

1. Yes, and the process works well
2. Yes, but the process could use improvement
3. No
4. Don't know

Nonphysician staff executes standing orders for medication refills, ordering tests, and providing routine preventive services

1. Yes, and the process works well
2. Yes, but the process could use improvement
3. No
4. Don't know

Nonphysician staff educates patients about self-care

1. Yes, and the process works well
2. Yes, but the process could use improvement
3. No
4. Don't know

Nonphysician staff coordinates care with external disease management or case management organizations

1. Yes, and the process works well
2. Yes, but the process could use improvement
3. No
4. Don't know

8. Does the practice provide the following care management services for patients who see multiple physicians or who have frequent admission to other facilities, including hospitals, skilled nursing facilities, or emergency rooms? These services can be performed by the practice on its own, or in conjunction with an external care management organization.

Identifies patients who have been discharged from or received care from other facilities, including hospitals, skilled nursing facilities, and emergency rooms

1. Yes, and the process works well
2. Yes, but the process could use improvement
3. No
4. Don't know

Determines which patients require pro-active contact (other than patient-initiated visits) or who are at risk for adverse outcomes by reviewing information from other facilities, such as discharge summaries or ongoing updates

1. Yes, and the process works well
2. Yes, but the process could use improvement
3. No
4. Don't know

Contacts patients after discharge from other facilities

1. Yes, and the process works well
2. Yes, but the process could use improvement
3. No
4. Don't know

Provides or coordinates follow-up care to patients who have been discharged

1. Yes, and the process works well
2. Yes, but the process could use improvement
3. No
4. Don't know

Coordinates care with external disease management or case management organizations, as appropriate

1. Yes, and the process works well
2. Yes, but the process could use improvement
3. No
4. Don't know

Communicates with patients receiving ongoing disease management or high-risk case management
1. Yes, and the process works well
2. Yes, but the process could use improvement
3. No
4. Don't know

Communicates with case managers for patients receiving ongoing disease management or high-risk case management
1. Yes, and the process works well
2. Yes, but the process could use improvement
3. No
4. Don't know

Systematically sends clinical information to other facilities at the time of a planned admission
1. Yes, and the process works well
2. Yes, but the process could use improvement
3. No
4. Don't know

Access and Coordination

1. Does your practice have written policies for the following processes to support patient access and communication with the practice?

Assigning patients to a personal clinician
1. Yes, and the process works well
2. Yes, but the process could use improvement
3. No
4. Don't know

Coordinating visits to multiple clinicians or for diagnostic tests during one trip
1. Yes, and the process works well
2. Yes, but the process could use improvement
3. No
4. Don't know

Determining through triage how soon a patient needs to be seen
1. Yes, and the process works well
2. Yes, but the process could use improvement
3. No
4. Don't know

Maintaining the capacity to schedule patients the same day they call
1. Yes, and the process works well
2. Yes, but the process could use improvement
3. No
4. Don't know

Scheduling same-day appointments based on the practice's triage of the patient's condition
1. Yes, and the process works well
2. Yes, but the process could use improvement
3. No
4. Don't know

Scheduling same-day appointments based on patient request
1. Yes, and the process works well

2. Yes, but the process could use improvement
3. No
4. Don't know

Providing telephone advice on clinical issues during office hours by physician, nurse or other clinician within a specified time
1. Yes, and the process works well
2. Yes, but the process could use improvement
3. No
4. Don't know

Returning urgent phone calls within a specified time, with clinician support available 24/7
1. Yes, and the process works well
2. Yes, but the process could use improvement
3. No
4. Don't know

Providing secure e-mail consultation with physicians or other clinicians, responding to clinical issues within a specified time
1. Yes, and the process works well
2. Yes, but the process could use improvement
3. No
4. Don't know

Providing an interactive practice Web site that allows patients to address nonurgent needs, such as scheduling appointments, obtaining test results, or renewing prescriptions
1. Yes, and the process works well
2. Yes, but the process could use improvement
3. No
4. Don't know

Making language services available for patients with limited English proficiency
1. Yes, and the process works well
2. Yes, but the process could use improvement
3. No
4. Don't know

2. Does your practice measure its performance in the following areas against written standards for patient access?

Scheduling visits with the personal clinician
1. Yes
2. No

Appointment scheduling
1. Yes
2. No

Providing telephone advice during office hours
1. Yes
2. No

Returning urgent phone calls within a specified time; clinician support available 24/7
1. Yes
2. No

Responding to e-mail and/or interactive Web requests
1. Yes
2. No

Making language services available for patients with limited English proficiency
1. Yes
2. No

Electronic Prescribing

1. Does your practice use an electronic prescription writer?
   1. Yes
   2. No

2. Can the electronic prescription writer used by your practice do the following?

Print prescriptions at the office/clinic or send a fax or electronic message to a pharmacy
1. ≥75%
2. <75%
3. No
4. Don't know

Link to patient-specific demographic and clinical information
1. ≥75%
2. <75%
3. No
4. Don't know

Connect to a pharmacy
1. ≥75%
2. <75%
3. No
4. Don't know

Connect to the patient's pharmacy benefit manager
1. ≥75%
2. <75%
3. No
4. Don't know

Receive requests for prescription renewals electronically
1. ≥75%
2. <75%
3. No
4. Don't know

Automatically provide information on medications that could be substituted, including generic medications
1. ≥75%
2. <75%
3. No
4. Don't know

Automatically provide information on alternative drugs on the patient's specific formulary, including generic medications
1. ≥75%
2. <75%

3. No
4. Don't know

3. Does your practice have an electronic prescription reference program that provides information to clinicians at the time the clinician is writing the prescription? Please indicate whether the program provides general information or patient-specific information.

Alert to clinically important drug-drug interactions
1. Yes, program provides general information
2. Yes, program provides patient-specific information
3. No, practice does not have an electronic prescription reference program
4. Don't know

Recommend appropriate dosing
1. Yes, program provides general information
2. Yes, program provides patient-specific information
3. No, practice does not have an electronic prescription reference program
4. Don't know

Recommend therapeutic monitoring for specific drugs
1. Yes, program provides general information
2. Yes, program provides patient-specific information
3. No, practice does not have an electronic prescription reference program
4. Don't know

Alert to drug-disease interactions
1. Yes, program provides general information
2. Yes, program provides patient-specific information
3. No, practice does not have an electronic prescription reference program
4. Don't know

Alert to drug-allergy possibility
1. Yes, program provides general information
2. Yes, program provides patient-specific information
3. No, practice does not have an electronic prescription reference program
4. Don't know

Provide drug-patient history alerts
1. Yes, program provides general information
2. Yes, program provides patient-specific information
3. No, practice does not have an electronic prescription reference program
4. Don't know

Alert to duplication of drugs in a therapeutic class
1. Yes, program provides general information
2. Yes, program provides patient-specific information
3. No, practice does not have an electronic prescription reference program
4. Don't know

Alert to drugs to avoid in the elderly
1. Yes, program provides general information
2. Yes, program provides patient-specific information

3. No, practice does not have an electronic prescription reference program
4. Don't know

Provision of patient-appropriate medication information

1. Yes, program provides general information
2. Yes, program provides patient-specific information
3. No, practice does not have an electronic prescription reference program
4. Don't know

Test Tracking

1. Does your practice have a system other than the paper medical chart for:

Tracking all laboratory tests ordered or done within the practice, until results are available to the clinician, flagging overdue results

1. Yes, through an electronic system
2. Yes, through a paper-based system
3. No
4. Don't know

Tracking all imaging tests ordered or done within the practice, until results are available to the clinician, flagging overdue results

1. Yes, through an electronic system
2. Yes, through a paper-based system
3. No
4. Don't know

Flagging abnormal test results, bringing them to a clinician's attention

1. Yes, through an electronic system
2. Yes, through a paper-based system
3. No
4. Don't know

Following up with patients for all abnormal test results

1. Yes, through an electronic system
2. Yes, through a paper-based system
3. No
4. Don't know

2. Does your practice use an electronic system for the following services?

Ordering laboratory tests

1. Yes
2. No
3. Don't know

Ordering imaging tests

1. Yes
2. No
3. Don't know

Retrieving laboratory results directly from laboratory facility

1. Yes
2. No
3. Don't know

Retrieving imaging text reports directly from the imaging facility

1. Yes
2. No
3. Don't know

Retrieving images directly from the imaging facility

1. Yes
2. No
3. Don't know

Ensuring that appropriate clinical personnel receive and respond to current and historical test results (for review and comparison)

1. Yes
2. No
3. Don't know

Flagging orders for duplicate tests

1. Yes
2. No
3. Don't know

Generating alerts when potentially inappropriate tests are ordered

1. Yes
2. No
3. Don't know

Referral Tracking

1. Does your practice have a system other than the paper chart to track critical referrals until the consultation report returns to the practice? Please indicate if the system is paper, electronic, or both.
   1. Yes, electronic only
   2. Yes, paper only
   3. Yes, combination of paper and electronic
   4. No
   5. Don't know

2. Does the system track the following information?

Referring clinician

1. Yes
2. No
3. Don't know

Reason for referral and relevant clinical findings

1. Yes
2. No
3. Don't know

Whether referral report has been received

1. Yes
2. No
3. Don't know

Administrative information such as whether the referral requires health plan approval

1. Yes
2. No
3. Don't know

3. Does the practice have a paper-based or electronic system that provides information about the following at the time of referral?

Duplicate requests for referrals

1. Yes
2. No
3. Don't know

Available quality performance reports on consultants or facilities

1. Yes
2. No
3. Don't know

4. Does the electronic report which accompanies a referral request include the following information?

Reason for consultation

1. Yes
2. No
3. Don't know

Pertinent physical findings

1. Yes
2. No
3. Don't know

Pertinent clinical data

1. Yes
2. No
3. Don't know

Support person

1. Yes
2. No
3. Don't know

Functional status

1. Yes
2. No
3. Don't know

Family history

1. Yes
2. No
3. Don't know

Social history

1. Yes
2. No
3. Don't know

Plan of care

1. Yes
2. No
3. Don't know

Health care providers

1. Yes
2. No
3. Don't know

Interoperability

1. Does your practice use an electronic medical record?
   1. Yes
   2. No

2. Do your practice's electronic systems store and manipulate patient data in a structured computable manner using nationally accepted standard code sets based on the following criteria?

There is a unique identifier for patients in all systems

1. Yes
2. No
3. Don't know

All providers in the practice use unique identifiers (e.g., a National Provider Identifier)

1. Yes
2. No
3. Don't know

The electronic system uses and maintains clinical information using standardized codes (e.g., ICD, CPT, DRG, SNOMED(r))

1. Yes
2. No
3. Don't know

The electronic system uses and maintains codes (e.g., LOINC(r) codes) to identify clinical observation and diagnostic results and allergies

1. Yes
2. No
3. Don't know

The electronic system maintains medication and allergy data (e.g., RxNorm or NDC codes)

1. Yes
2. No
3. Don't know

3. Do your practice's electronic systems have the capability to receive the following types of data and to integrate them into the system by both patient and ordering provider?

Prescription data

1. Yes
2. No
3. Don't know

Laboratory tests and results

1. Yes
2. No
3. Don't know

Imaging tests and results

1. Yes
2. No
3. Don't know

Medical histories from other practitioners

1. Yes
2. No
3. Don't know

Inpatient data (e.g., DRG, discharge status)
1. Yes
2. No
3. Don't know

Physical findings from other practitioners
1. Yes
2. No
3. Don't know

Self-monitored information from patients who have their own electronic health or personal health record (PHR)
1. Yes
2. No
3. Don't know

4. Do your practice's electronic systems have the capability to automatically transmit the following types of data to external organizations in a secure manner?

Clinical information to other providers including health plans
1. Yes
2. No
3. Don't know

Clinical information to patients who have their own personal health records (PHRs)
1. Yes
2. No
3. Don't know

Prescription information (ordered, current use, dispensed) to patients and other providers
1. Yes
2. No
3. Don't know

Diagnostic information, including tests ordered and results, to patients and other providers
1. Yes
2. No
3. Don't know

Orders to service providers, such as home health providers or physical therapists
1. Yes
2. No
3. Don't know

Appointments requested with other providers and sites
1. Yes
2. No
3. Don't know

Performance Monitoring and Quality Improvement

1. Does your practice measure or receive results on the following types of performance for individual physicians?

Clinical processes of care
1. Yes
2. No
3. Don't know

Clinical outcomes
1. Yes
2. No
3. Don't know

Service data
1. Yes
2. No
3. Don't know

Patient experience of care
1. Yes
2. No
3. Don't know

Patient safety
1. Yes
2. No
3. Don't know

2. Does your practice measure or receive results on the following types of performance for the practice as a whole?

Clinical processes of care
1. Yes
2. No
3. Don't know

Clinical outcomes
1. Yes
2. No
3. Don't know

Service data
1. Yes
2. No
3. Don't know

Patient experience of care
1. Yes
2. No
3. Don't know

Patient safety
1. Yes
2. No
3. Don't know

3. Does your practice or medical group conduct or participate in formal quality improvement activities?
1. Yes
2. No
3. Don't know

4. Do your quality improvement activities include:

Holding team meetings
1. Yes
2. No
3. Don't know

Setting goals based on performance data from the practice
1. Yes
2. No
3. Don't know

Taking action where identified to improve performance of individual physicians
1. Yes
2. No
3. Don't know

Taking action where identified to improve performance of the practice as a whole
1. Yes
2. No
3. Don't know

Performing rapid change cycles
1. Yes
2. No
3. Don't know

5. Does your practice have the ability to link clinical and management data electronically for the following purposes?

To create internal reports based on nationally accepted performance measures?
1. Yes
2. No
3. Don't know

To transmit data electronically for nationally recognized quality of care measures to health plans, local quality collaboratives, government agencies, or other entities?
1. Yes
2. No
3. Don't know

Quality Culture of the Practice

1. To what extent does the practice have the technical expertise needed to guide the practice in quality improvement strategies?
   1. Not at all
   2. Somewhat
   3. Mostly
   4. To a great extent

2. To what extent does the practice management look for system errors rather than assign blame to individuals when something goes wrong?
   1. Not at all
   2. Somewhat
   3. Mostly
   4. To a great extent

3. To what extent does the practice staff look for system errors rather than assign blame to individuals when something goes wrong?
   1. Not at all
   2. Somewhat
   3. Mostly
   4. To a great extent

4. To what extent do physicians in the practice look for system errors rather than assign blame to individuals when something goes wrong?
   1. Not at all
   2. Somewhat
   3. Mostly
   4. To a great extent

5. To what extent does the practice culture encourage questioning decisions or actions when someone sees a problem, regardless of their role or training on the team?
   1. Not at all
   2. Somewhat
   3. Mostly
   4. To a great extent

6. To what extent does the practice have an effective process for staff education and training when implementing changes in policies or procedures?
   1. Not at all
   2. Somewhat
   3. Mostly
   4. To a great extent

7. To what extent does everyone on the staff know how the practice is doing in terms of practice performance and clinical outcomes?
   1. Not at all
   2. Somewhat
   3. Mostly
   4. To a great extent

8. Does the practice have clear clinical leadership that supports quality improvement by setting well-defined quality goals and allocating resources needed to achieve the goals?
   1. Not at all
   2. Somewhat
   3. Mostly
   4. To a great extent

Practice/Personal Characteristics

1. About the Practice

   Which of the following best describes your medical practice structure?
   1. Solo physician medical practice
   2. Single specialty medical group or partnership
   3. Multispecialty group or partnership (including staff or group model HMOs)
   4. Institutional practice (e.g., VAMC, public health organization)
   5. Community health center
   6. Residency teaching clinic
   7. Hospital department group practice
   8. Academic faculty practice
   9. Other

How many years has your medical practice, more or less as it is at present, been in existence?
1. <1 year
2. 2–5 years
3. 6–10 years
4. 11–15 years
5. 16–20 years
6. 20 or more years
7. Don't know

At the present time, what is the total number of physicians (both fulltime and part time) practicing in your medical practice across all its locations?
1. 1
2. 2
3. 3
4. 4
5. 5
6. 6–10
7. 11–20
8. 21–25
9. 26–50

10. 51 or more
11. Don't know

At the present time, what is the total number of nurse practitioners or physicians assistants (both full time and part time) practicing in your medical practice across all its locations?
1. 1
2. 2
3. 3
4. 4
5. 5
6. 6–10
7. 11–20
8. 21–25
9. 26–50
10. 51 or more
11. Don't know
12. None

APPENDIX 11-2
Agency for Healthcare Research and Quality Taxonomy of Quality Improvement Strategies

Nine types of QI strategies are outlined here along with key substrategies. These categories are broad and, in some cases, combine multiple interventions. The authors explored this heterogeneity in their analyses to assess the possibility of making inferences and judgments about the success of the strategy as a whole, or whether further subdivision would be needed.

Where relevant, the analyses also take into consideration the fact that many interventions are multifaceted and employ more than one type of QI strategy.

1. Provider reminder systems—the investigators defined a reminder system as any patient- or clinical encounter–specific information, provided orally, in writing, or by computer, to prompt a clinician to recall information, or intended to prompt consideration of a specific process of care (e.g., "This patient last underwent screening mammography 3 years ago"). The reminder also may include information prompting the clinician to follow evidence-based care recommendations (e.g., to make medication adjustments, or to order appropriate screening tests). The phrase "clinical encounter–specific" in the definition serves to distinguish reminder systems from audit and feedback, in which clinicians typically receive performance summaries relative to a process or outcome of care spanning multiple encounters (e.g., all type 2 diabetic patients seen by the clinician during the past 6 months).

2. Facilitated relay of clinical data to providers—this term is used to describe the transfer of clinical information collected directly from patients and relayed to the provider, in instances in which the data are not generally collected during a patient visit, or using some format other than the existing local medical record system (i.e., the telephone transmission of a patient's blood pressure measurements from a specialist's office). The EPOC group uses the term "patient mediated" to describe such interventions, but the authors regard the above label as more descriptive. Some overlap with provider reminder systems was expected, but the strategies were kept separate at the abstraction stage. This decision allowed for the possibility that the data could be subsequently analyzed with and without collapsing the two strategies.

3. Audit and feedback—the researchers defined audit and feedback as any summary of clinical performance for health care providers or institutions, performed for a specific period of time and reported either publicly or confidentially to the clinician or institution (e.g., the percentage of a provider's patients who achieved or did not achieve some clinical target, such as blood pressure or HbA_{1c} control over a certain period).

Benchmarking is a term referring to the provision of performance data from institutions or providers regarded as leaders in the field. These data serve as performance targets for other providers and institutions. The authors included benchmarking as a type of audit and feedback, so long as local data were provided for comparison with the benchmark data.

4. Provider education—this term is used to describe a variety of interventions including educational workshops, meetings (e.g., traditional continuing medical education [CME]), lectures (in person or computer-based), educational outreach visits (by a trained representative who meets with providers in their practice settings to disseminate information with the intent of changing the providers' practice). The same term also is used to describe the distribution of educational materials (electronically published or printed clinical practice guidelines and audiovisual materials). The investigators further captured information about the intensity (i.e., duration and number of educational sessions) and format (i.e., lectures delivered live, via teleconference, or prerecorded) in a free-text mode, for each of these substrategies. Early plans to capture these and other predictors in a structured form were abandoned after the authors and their technical advisors agreed the judgments were too subjective. This was due in large part to a relative lack of detail surrounding the interventions in the vast majority of studies.

5. Patient education—this strategy is centered on in-person patient education, either individually or as part of a group or community, and through the introduction of print or audiovisual educational materials. Patient education may be the sole component of a particular quality improvement strategy, or it can be one part of a multifaceted QI strategy. It should be noted that the authors evaluated only those strategies in which patient education was regarded as one component of a multifaceted strategy. A future volume in this series may address the topic of patient education as a singular intervention, along with its relative effects on a variety of chronic diseases.

6. Promotion of self-management—this strategy includes the distribution of materials (i.e., devices for blood pressure or glucose self-monitoring) or access to a resource that enhances the patients' ability to manage their conditions, the communication of useful clinical data to the patient (e.g., most recent HbA_{1c} or lipid panel levels), or follow-up phone calls from the provider to the patient, with recommended adjustments to care. The authors expected some overlap with regard to patient education (strategy 5) and patient reminders (strategy 7). They elected to keep the strategies separate at the abstraction stage, to allow for the possibility that the data could be analyzed after the fact, with and without collapsing the two strategies.

7. Patient reminders—such reminders are defined as any effort directed by providers toward patients that encourages them to keep appointments or adhere to other aspects of the self-management of their condition.

8. Organizational change—this strategy includes any intervention having features consistent with at least one of the following descriptions, each of which represents a substrategy of organizational change that was abstracted for incorporation in the analysis:
   a. Disease management or case management—the coordination of assessment, treatment, and referrals by a person or multidisciplinary team in collaboration with, or supplementary to, the primary care provider.
   b. Team or personnel changes—adding new members to a treatment team (e.g., the addition of a diabetes nurse, a clinical pharmacist, or a nutritionist to a clinical practice), creating multidisciplinary teams within a practice, or revising the roles of existing team members (e.g., a clinic nurse is given a more active role in patient management), or the simple addition of more nurses, pharmacists, or physicians to a clinical setting.
   c. Communications, case discussions, and the exchange of treatment information between distant health professionals (i.e., telemedicine).
   d. Total quality management (TQM) or continuous quality improvement (CQI) techniques for measuring quality problems, designing interventions and their implementation, along with process re-measurements.
   e. Changes in medical records systems—adopting improved office technology (e.g., computer-based records, patient tracking systems).

   Although the definition used for this strategy is consistent with prior reviews[52] the authors recognized the potential heterogeneity of included interventions and accordingly planned to analyze this strategy with respect to the aforementioned substrategies.

9. Financial, regulatory or legislative incentives—this strategy encompassed any intervention having features consistent with at least one of the following descriptions:
   a. Positive or negative financial incentives directed at providers (e.g., regarding adherence to some process of care or achievement of target patient outcome).
   b. Positive or negative financial incentives directed at patients.
   c. System-wide changes in reimbursement (e.g., capitation, prospective payment, shift from fee-for-service to salary).
   d. Changes to provider licensure requirements.
   e. Changes to institutional accreditation requirements.

Simulation-Based Assessment

Ross J. Scalese, MD, and S. Barry Issenberg, MD

Although the seminal article about simulation in medical education appeared nearly 40 years ago,[1] it is only in the last decade that we have witnessed a significant increase in the use of simulation technology for teaching and assessment in the health professions. This represents a bold departure from the traditional approach, a system that for hundreds of years has centered on real patients for training as well as testing. Multiple factors have contributed to this evolution. Changes in health care delivery have resulted in shorter hospital stays and clinic visits, greater numbers of patients, and higher acuity of illnesses; at academic medical centers this has resulted in reduced patient availability as learning and assessment opportunities, as well as decreased time for clinical faculty to teach and evaluate trainees.[2,3] Simulators, by contrast, can be readily available at any time and can reproduce a wide variety of clinical conditions and situations on demand. Unlike real patients, simulators are never "off the ward" to undergo diagnostic tests or treatment at the time trainees or examinees arrive to perform their evaluations; simulators do not become tired or embarrassed or behave unpredictably, and therefore they provide a standardized experience for all.[4]

In addition, technological advances in diagnosis and treatment, such as newer imaging modalities and endoscopic or laparoscopic procedures, require development of psychomotor and perceptual skills that are different from traditional approaches and which, therefore, require new techniques for teaching, learning, and assessment.[5] Concurrent progress in simulation technology, such as high-tech virtual reality catheterization or endoscopy simulators that are increasingly realistic, offers advantages for such instruction, skills acquisition, and evaluation.

At the same time, recent international reports[6-9] have focused increased attention on the problem of medical errors and the need to improve patient safety, not only through prevention of mistakes by individuals, but also through correction of faults in the systems of care.[10] Other fields with high-risk performance environments have long and successfully incorporated simulation technology into their training and assessment programs—for example, flight simulators for pilots and astronauts, war games and training exercises for military personnel, management games for business executives, and technical operations scenarios for nuclear power plant personnel—not only to develop and test individual skills and effective collaboration in teams, but also to build a culture of safety.[11-13] Adopting these models in medical education, specialties such as anesthesiology, critical care, and emergency medicine have led the way in using simulation modalities, especially for teaching and testing the skills needed to manage rare or critical incidents. Trainees can make mistakes and learn to recognize and correct them in the simulated environment without fear of punishment or harm to real patients.

Closely related to these safety issues are important ethical questions about the appropriateness of "using" real (even standardized) patients as training or assessment resources. Such debate often centers on instructional or evaluation settings that involve sensitive tasks (e.g., pelvic examination) or risk of harm to patients (e.g., endotracheal intubation or other invasive procedures). Use of patient substitutes, such as cadavers or animals, has attendant ethical concerns of its own; additional challenges, including cost, availability, and maintenance of an adequately realistic clinical context, have also limited the use of cadaveric and animal tissue models for clinical skills training and assessment. Simulators, on the other hand, circumvent most of these obstacles and, thus, recently have come into widespread use for teaching and evaluation at all levels of health care professional education.

Finally, all of these influences driving the increased use of simulation are operating within a broader new context: "While student learning is clearly the goal of education, there is a pressing need to provide evidence that learning or mastery actually occurs."[14] As noted in Chapter 1, this statement reflects a recent worldwide shift in focus toward outcomes-based education throughout the health care professions. This paradigm change derives in part from attempts by academic institutions and professional organizations to self-regulate and set standards for quality assurance, but chiefly it represents a response to public demand for assurance that doctors are competent.[15] Accordingly, medical schools, postgraduate training programs, hospital and health care system credentialing committees, and licensing and specialty boards (including their high-stakes certification examinations) are all placing greater emphasis on using simulation modalities for the assessment of competence across multiple domains.[16–23]

Medical simulations, in general, aim to imitate real patients, anatomic regions, or clinical tasks, and to mirror the real-life situations in which medical services are rendered. These simulations range from static anatomic models and single task trainers (such as venipuncture arms and intubation mannequin heads) to dynamic computer-based systems that can respond to user actions (such as full-body anesthesia patient simulators); from individual trainers for evaluating the performance of a single user to interactive role-playing scenarios involving groups of people; and from relatively low technology standardized patient (SP) encounters to very high-tech virtual reality surgical simulators.

In setting a framework for the discussion to follow, our use of the term "assessment" will generally refer to simulation-based *summative* assessment, rather than *formative* assessment. The intention, however, is not to downplay the latter's importance. On the contrary,

provision of individualized feedback plays a role crucial to achieving effective educational outcomes from simulation-based interventions[24]: trainees receive guidance toward future improvement based on evaluation of their past performance and, thus, teaching and learning are intimately related to this type of assessment. Common examples of summative assessments, on the other hand, include examinations at the end of a clinical clerkship, or after a year of residency training, or prior to specialty certification. These evaluations usually involve higher stakes than tests undertaken for formative purposes; they can determine pass/fail decisions or whether clinical performance meets accepted standards of care for professional licensure.

The subsequent discussion also employs two other terms that we will use almost interchangeably: *simulation* refers broadly to any device or set of conditions—including SP-based examinations—that attempts to present evaluation problems authentically, whereas a *simulator*, more narrowly defined, is a simulation *device*. Most of our considerations will apply to simulations in general, but the section on available technologies will focus specifically on simulators.

Psychometric Properties and Related Considerations

Previous chapters have discussed essential concepts of psychometrics relevant to various assessment methods, including reliability and validity. Although we often speak of these as properties intrinsic to an evaluation tool itself, it is important to remember that they actually characterize the inferences drawn from test scores obtained using an assessment method under a specific set of circumstances or for a particular purpose.[25] Moreover, when considering these properties as they pertain to simulation technology, evaluators must distinguish between the measurement characteristics of the simulator per se and those of the assessment overall. This is because simulators themselves usually do not comprise an entire assessment, but rather serve as tools to complement existing evaluation methods, present clinical findings, and facilitate standardization. For example, simulators often serve effectively as one of several tools used in the brief examining stations of an objective structured clinical examination (OSCE). These examinations often utilize checklists or global rating scales in conjunction with simulations, and they have their own measurement characteristics. Thus, we can discuss separately the reliability and validity of a simulation itself versus those of a rating scale versus those of an OSCE in its entirety; at the same time it is worthwhile to consider the interrelated way in which, say, the reliability of the simulation influences that of the OSCE.

Reliability

Viewed in a simplified way, for assessments in general, *reliability* refers to the reproducibility and consistency of an evaluation method and, more specifically applied to medical simulations, involves the ability of the simulator to present the same clinical findings, task, or scenario repeatedly and accurately over multiple occasions and to any number of examinees. If we consider that the clinical assessment equation contains three variables—the patient, the examiner, and the examinee—then to devise an evaluation in which the examinee's performance represents a true measure of his or her clinical competence, we must control for (or maximize the reliability of) the first two variables.[4] Examiner training and the use of other reliable evaluation tools (checklists, rating scales, etc.) allow for standardization of the "examiner" component. Simulators, on the other hand, by virtue of their programmability, can standardize many aspects of the "patient" variable, offering a uniform, reproducible experience to multiple examinees. This generally high degree of reliability is one of the inherent strengths of simulators for assessment and is especially important for high-stakes examinations. Reliability coefficients for the use of a simulator in a particular examination setting are relatively straightforward to calculate.[26–29]

Validity

By contrast, we cannot directly measure *validity* or calculate a "validity coefficient"; rather, we accumulate evidence in support of validity from various empirical studies.[30] We can define the term "validity" as the degree to which a test measures what it was intended to measure, but this simplified notion belies the many types of validity discussed in the educational literature. For instance, we can speak of "construct validity" as it relates to a simulator used for assessment: if it is a valid test of, say, endoscopic skills, experts with the most experience in real endoscopy should perform best on the simulated task, novices with no real-life endoscopy experience should perform least well on the simulator, and the group with some experience in actual endoscopy should perform at a level somewhere between that of the other two groups. Alternatively, we might infer "predictive validity" of a particular catheterization simulator, if the same radiology residents who perform better on simulator-based skills testing later perform better, as rated by trained expert examiners, during actual interventional radiology procedures. Consensus opinion of a panel of experts can provide evidence of "content validity": experienced cardiologists agree that the findings on a cardiology patient simulator are representative of those in patients with actual cardiac diseases, or surgeons with expertise in a particular procedure determine that skills assessed on a surgical simulator represent the key steps in performing the real task.

Fidelity

Any discussion of simulation entails use of another important term, *fidelity*, which describes some aspect of the reality of the experience, or the likeness of the simulation to the real-life circumstances it was designed to duplicate. (The assessment literature refers to the closely related concept of "face validity.") Of course, the fidelity of a simulator is never completely identical to "the real thing." Some reasons are obvious: engineering limitations, other psychometric requirements, ethical and safety considerations, and time and cost constraints.[31] Again, fidelity describes the extent to which the appearance and behavior of the simulation imitate the appearance and behavior of the real system, but several authors have offered clarification of past inconsistency and imprecision in use of the term, highlighting an important distinction between physical (or engineering) fidelity and functional (or psychological) fidelity.[32] The latter refers to the degree to which the simulated task duplicates the skills in the real task (i.e., behavior); simulations can achieve high-level psychological fidelity with relatively low-technology methods (e.g., SP scenarios). Engineering fidelity refers to the degree to which the simulation device or training environment reproduces the physical characteristics of the real task (i.e., appearance); simulators with high-level engineering fidelity often employ high-tech components (e.g., full-body patient simulators or virtual reality simulations), making them expensive to purchase, operate, and maintain. Thus, as with choosing simulators for educational purposes, evaluators must match the fidelity of a simulation with its intended use as an assessment tool. "The highest possible fidelity may be unnecessary or even introduce undesired complexity for teaching [or evaluating] a particular skill and may result in unacceptably expensive simulations, making the methodology an unfeasible teaching [or assessment] tool."[3]

Feasibility

Therefore, another important consideration when discussing the use of simulators for assessment is *feasibility*, which generally relates to the cost-effectiveness of using a particular device as an evaluation tool. A later section of this chapter addresses the various costs (for the device, training, personnel, maintenance, etc.) to be tallied; in addition, the reckoning of a simulation's feasibility for assessment must include not only whether we *can* afford a simulator in terms of resources required, but also whether we *should* acquire and implement it for a particular evaluation (is any demonstrable improvement in testing with the simulator compared with a traditional method *worth* the expenditure of money, time, etc.?).[3]

Scoring

Finally, there are important considerations relevant to developing scoring rubrics for simulation-based assessments. Several common criteria are available for generating scores for performance during trainee evaluations, and the optimal choice depends on whether the competency tested relates more to a *process* (such as completing an orderly and thorough "code

Table 12-1 **Scoring Criteria and Examples**

Criteria Type	Example
Explicit process (measure)	A case-specific checklist to record action steps during suturing on a skin wound simulator (see Table 12-2)
Implicit process (judge)	A global rating scale (with well-defined anchor points) that allows an evaluator to observe and judge the quality of suturing performed on a skin wound simulator (see Table 12-3)
Explicit outcome (measure)	Observing and recording specific indicators of patient [simulator] status (alive, cardiac rhythm, blood pressure) after an ACLS "code"
Implicit outcome (judge)	A global rating scale (with well-defined anchor points) that allows an evaluator to observe and judge the quality of the overall patient status after an ACLS "code"
Combined (explicit process and outcome)	Task-specific checklist for performing bedside cardiac exam and observation/recording of correct identification and interpretation of physical findings

blue" resuscitation) or an *outcome* (such as the status of the [simulated] patient after said cardiopulmonary resuscitation). In some cases, such as summative assessments to determine if examinee performance meets a minimum acceptable level or standard of care, process criteria form a more appropriate basis for the evaluation, with measurement against a checklist of explicit process criteria being the most commonly employed technique. In other instances, we might deem the final result or "bottom line" (Did the examinee make the right diagnosis? Is the patient alive?) more important than the method of achieving that result, in which case outcome criteria may be more relevant. Tables 12-1 to 12-3 illustrate how we can assess processes and outcomes with simulators.[25]

As mentioned briefly earlier in this section and detailed in previous chapters, the checklists and global rating scales based on these criteria and used along with simulators in performance-based clinical examinations have their own reliability and validity characteristics, which depend (among other factors) on rater training, the specific skill under evaluation, and the purpose of the particular assessment.

Strengths and Best Applications

Earlier we highlighted the reliability of simulations as one of the principal advantages in their use for assessment: because of their programming, simulators are

highly standardized, thereby minimizing the variability inherent in actual clinical encounters. This reproducibility and consistency in presenting evaluation problems in the same manner for every examinee is extremely important, especially when high-stakes decisions hinge on these assessments.

Another strength of simulators as evaluation tools is the ability of some devices to simulate a wide range of patients or clinical problems for testing, and to do so on demand. This transforms the planning for assessments from an *ad hoc* process (dependent on finding patients with specific conditions of interest) to a proactive scheme with great flexibility for evaluators.

In considering the best applications of simulation technology for assessment purposes, we can use the new outcomes-based educational paradigm for our discussion. The Accreditation Council for Graduate Medical Education (ACGME) describes six domains of clinical competence: (1) patient care, (2) medical knowledge, (3) practice-based learning and improvement, (4) interpersonal and communication skills, (5) professionalism, and (6) systems-based practice.[34] (Other international organizations and accreditation bodies have outlined analogous core competencies.[35–37]) Evaluators may use simulations to assess various knowledge, skills, and attitudes within these domains. During a ward rotation for internal medicine residents, for example, faculty may test aspects of trainees' *patient care* (using a cardiology patient simulator, demonstrate the ability to perform a focused cardiac examination and identify the presence of a third heart sound in a "patient" presenting with dyspnea); *medical knowledge* (using a full-body simulator during a simulated case of ventricular fibrillation, verbalize the correct steps in the algorithm for treatment of ventricular fibrillation); or *interpersonal and communication skills* and *professionalism* (during a simulation integrating an SP with a plastic mannequin arm, demonstrate how to draw blood cultures while explaining to the patient the indications for the procedure). This last example highlights the fact that real clinical encounters often require practitioners to bring to bear their abilities in multiple domains simultaneously. Formal assessments have traditionally focused on isolated clinical skills (e.g., perform a procedure on a simulator at one station in an

Table 12-2 **Explicit Process Criteria—Suturing**

Process	Not Done or Incorrect	Done Correctly
Held instruments correctly		X
Spaced sutures 3–5 mm	X	
Tied square knots		X
Cut suture to correct length		X
Apposed skin without excessive tension on sutures	X	

Table 12-3 **Implicit Process Criteria—Suturing**[33]

Time and Motion				
1	2	3	4	5
Many unnecessary or repetitive movements		Efficient time/motion, but unnecessary and repetitive movements	Clear economy of movements and maximum efficiency	
Instrument Handling				
1	2	3	4	5
Repeatedly makes tentative or awkward moves with instruments through inappropriate use		Consistent use of instruments, but occasionally appears stiff or awkward	Fluid movement with instruments	

From Kalu PU, Atkins J, Baker D, et al: How do we assess microsurgical skill? Microsurgery 2005;25(1):25–29.

OSCE, obtain a history or deliver bad news with an SP at another station). More recently, very innovative work features evaluations more reflective of actual clinical practice by combining simulation modalities—for instance, a trainee must interact (gather some history, obtain consent, explain the procedure) with a male SP who is draped below the waist *while* inserting a urinary bladder catheter into a simulator placed beneath the drape—for simultaneous assessment of technical and communication skills.[38]

Additionally, within any of the domains of competence, one can assess learners at four different levels, according to the pyramid model conceptualized by Miller[39] (see Chapter 1):

1. *Knows* (knowledge)—recall of basic facts, principles, and theories
2. *Knows how* (applied knowledge)—ability to solve problems, make decisions, and describe procedures
3. *Shows how* (performance)—demonstration of skills in a controlled setting
4. *Does* (action)—behavior in real practice

Various assessment methods are more or less well suited to evaluation at different levels of competence; for example, written instruments, such as examinations consisting of multiple-choice questions, are efficient tools for assessing what a student "knows." On the other hand, the ACGME Toolbox of Assessment Methods[40] suggests that simulations are instruments most appropriate for evaluation of those outcomes that require trainees to demonstrate or "show how" they are competent to perform various skills. For example, in the *patient care* domain, the toolbox ranks simulations among "the most desirable" methods for evaluating ability to perform medical procedures and "the next best method" for demonstrating how to develop and carry out patient management plans; within the *medical knowledge* competency, evaluators can devise simulations to assess trainees' investigatory/analytic thinking or knowledge/application of basic sciences; simulations are "a potentially applicable method" to evaluate how practitioners analyze their own practice for needed improvements (*practice-based learning and improvement*); and in the realm of *professionalism*, simulations are among the methods listed for assessing ethically sound practice.[40]

Weaknesses and Challenges

As mentioned previously, costs are often among the most significant challenges to implementing a simulation program, whether for teaching or assessment. Simulators—especially those utilizing sophisticated technologies, such as computer-enhanced mannequins or virtual reality systems—can be expensive: beyond the initial purchase price, we must also factor in the ongoing costs to operate, store, maintain, and update the devices. For example, high-fidelity patient simulators can range in price anywhere from around $30,000 up to $250,000, and service agreements for the most full-featured models can cost an additional $7,000 to $11,000 per year.

In addition to these obvious direct financial expenditures, assessment planners should not underestimate the human resources (and associated indirect costs) required in any evaluation program, including those employing simulation-based methods. Even for relatively low-tech simulations (e.g., those utilizing SPs for assessment of communication skills), there are costs associated with recruiting and training personnel for role-playing, supervision, and evaluation (Chapter 8). The ability to save faculty time is an often-touted advantage of simulation technology as an instructional tool (i.e., when trainees can use the method for independent learning). When simulation modalities are used for testing, however, often the same does not hold true. Although some simulators have built-in measurement/recording functions that can provide assessment data, we noted earlier that most tests use simulators in conjunction with other evaluation instruments, such as checklists or rating scales, and these require scoring. Thus, we may not save faculty or staff time; in fact, for such assessments to be reliable, examiners must receive adequate training, and even raters with expertise in the domain under evaluation—who presumably need less training than, say, nonmedical personnel employed for the purposes of a given examination—require time for familiarization with a particular measurement tool and standardization of scoring. Their time is a valuable commodity.

Development of scenarios for use in simulator-based examinations can also be time- and resource-intensive.

Ideally, pilot testing of these evaluation schemes should occur, and this has associated costs that accrue even before implementation of the final assessment project. All of these factors pose even greater challenges in large-scale (e.g., national) testing programs and high-stakes (e.g., professional licensure) examinations.

Another drawback of some simulators for assessment is lack of portability: they may be bulky, and their computer or other hardware components may be delicate, limiting testing to dedicated centers and controlled environments. This imposes significant disadvantages if we are trying to assess, say, the skills of paramedics or military personnel in a realistic field setting. Along similar lines, many devices simulate only specific conditions or procedures; although such models may have very high fidelity within their limited domains, the lack of flexibility with some simulators to design testing for a wide range of clinical contexts or skills is a limitation of these evaluation tools.

These considerations lead again to questions raised earlier about feasibility: can we design valid and reliable tests of a desired outcome using a particular device? Can (or *should*) we justify the expense of a simulator for a given assessment? High-tech devices have a certain allure—we all want to have "the latest and greatest" gadget—but program planners must consider the cost-effectiveness of any method, including, ultimately, whether the decisions based on such evaluations will better identify those health care providers who are competent for safe practice with real patients. Rational allocation of resources for assessment programs—whether at the level of medical schools, residency training programs, credentialing bodies, or certification boards—demands *evidence* that the investment will yield valuable results.

In this respect, systematic review of the extant research on medical simulations has demonstrated some shortcomings: many of the published articles are descriptive reports, rather than comparative studies of simulation-based techniques versus traditional methods,[24] and most lack the scientific rigor to support meaningful analysis.[41] In addition, much of the research on simulation-based assessment, including the good earlier work on evaluations utilizing SPs,[42,43] focuses on psychometric properties and scoring. Although issues such as a test's validity are certainly important, most of these studies offer evidence of face, construct, or content validity, while not addressing the perhaps more important question of predictive validity (i.e., will performance on a given assessment predict future performance in actual practice?). Only recently have reports of newer simulation devices for testing (e.g., virtual reality systems for minimally invasive surgery) spoken to such important considerations.[44,45] These types of studies, however, pose dilemmas of their own: in trying to gather evidence of predictive validity, is it ethical to let sub-par performers identified in a simulation exercise later carry out tasks, especially invasive procedures, on live patients?

Available Technologies

There are numerous medical simulators commercially available today and, keeping pace with remarkable technological and engineering advances that allow creation of higher fidelity devices, that number is increasing rapidly. Therefore, this chapter cannot provide a comprehensive listing of all the technologies available to educators and evaluators, and any such compendium would quickly become outdated; rather, we will attempt to provide an overview of the range and types of simulators currently available, as well as some references for those seeking to obtain more detailed information about particular systems (see Appendix 12-1 and disclosure at the end of this chapter). To organize our approach to the large number of available simulators, we will discuss current technologies for various medical disciplines broadly grouped into three categories (each briefly introduced here and then detailed in the sections that follow): part task trainers, computer-enhanced mannequin (CEM) simulations, and virtual reality (VR) simulators.[46]

Part task trainers consist of representations of body parts/regions with functional anatomy for teaching and evaluating particular skills, such as plastic arms for venipuncture or suturing, or head/neck/torso mannequins for central line placement or endotracheal intubation. In most cases, the interface with the user is passive (i.e., the user performs some procedure with no response from the model). These generally have lower engineering fidelity and do not require sophisticated technological components, making them less expensive, yet they can reproduce the tasks to be assessed with moderate to high degrees of psychological fidelity.

Computer-enhanced mannequins consist of life-sized (often full-body) mannequins connected to computers, which reproduce not only the anatomy but also normal and pathophysiologic function. The interface with the user can be active or even interactive. In the former case, the simulator responds in a preprogrammed way to user actions (e.g., if in ventricular fibrillation, the heart rhythm will change to sinus rhythm whenever the user shocks the mannequin); with interactive programming, the simulator response will vary according to user actions (for the previous example, the heart rhythm will return to sinus rhythm only when a certain energy level is used for defibrillation; for another example, heart rate and blood pressure will change appropriately, depending on the specific dose of a particular drug administered intravenously). Such high-fidelity simulators often contain high-tech components, making them more costly. Assessment using CEMs can focus on individual skills (e.g., ability of a paramedic to intubate) or the effectiveness of teams (e.g., an emergency department resuscitation scenario). Championed initially by anesthesiologists, the advent of these CEMs led the recent expansion in use of simulation technology in medical education.

Virtual reality simulations are even newer innovations in which a computer display simulates the physical world, and user interactions are with the computer (or some extension thereof) within that simulated (virtual) world. Existing technologies now allow for very high-fidelity simulations, ranging from desktop computer-generated environments (much like those in three-dimensional [3D] computer games) to highly immersive VR (e.g., CAVE simulations where the user wears goggles and sensor-containing gloves or sits within a specially designed display). Sound and visual feedback are often highly realistic in these simulations, with recent progress in haptic (touch feedback) technology improving the tactile experience as well; the (usually high) cost is commensurate with the level of technological sophistication in these VR systems. Like assessments with CEMs, we can use VR simulations to evaluate both individual and collaborative skills. Moreover, one potential advantage of assessment in the virtual environment is that examinees need not be collocated with team members or even with the examiner; just as with educational programs delivered via the Internet or teleconferencing, "distance testing" in realistic clinical contexts is now possible.

Part Task Trainers

Simulators that reproduce nearly every anatomic region or clinical task are available today for assessment across various medical specialties and different health care professions.[47] The simplest of these consist of foam pads that simulate soft tissue and overlying skin for learning and evaluating venipuncture or injection technique. Slightly more sophisticated models include vessels filled with mock blood for practice and assessment of cannulation technique; simulations of various anatomic regions allow testing of skills ranging from peripheral to central intravenous line placement, as well as arterial catheter placement.

There are numerous simulators for evaluation of general examination skills. For example, ocular examination simulators consist of a mannequin head whose eyes have variable pupil sizes for testing funduscopic technique, allowing examinees to use a real ophthalmoscope for diagnosis of normal eyegrounds, as well as many pathologic retinal findings of common diseases (demonstrated via changeable funduscopic slides). In similar fashion, ear examination simulators test trainees with actual otoscopes and realistic changeable plastic auricles, requiring identification of normal and pathologic middle ear findings, in addition to allowing procedures such as foreign body removal. Breast trainers simulate realistic anatomy for assessing examination technique and ability to diagnose pathologic findings (cyst, lipoma, fibroadenoma, carcinoma); some even allow evaluation of procedural skills, such as cyst aspiration.

For assessment of surgical skills: there are multilayered pads for suturing techniques, some even with filled veins for cutdown procedures. Various trainers exist for performance of minor skin and other procedures, including local anesthetic injection, shave biopsy, linear and elliptical incision/closure, cyst and

lipoma removal, subcuticular suturing and knot tying, and ingrown toenail removal. Still other models allow testing of more advanced surgical skills, such as incision/closure of the abdominal wall, and bowel or vascular anastomosis. Another simulator provides the anatomy of the lower abdomen and perineum for performing diagnostic peritoneal lavage.

For anesthesia, emergency medicine, critical care, or other specialties: there are numerous airway trainers, usually consisting of representations of the head and neck (with or without torso/lungs attached) for assessing airway management skills; many of these task trainers can simulate variations in tongue, dentition, and other upper airway anatomy and vary conditions under which examinees can perform bag-valve-mask ventilation, placement of oral-pharyngeal or laryngeal mask airways, nasal or oral endotracheal intubation, and needle cricothyroidotomy.

For related skills, Laerdal Medical created Resusci Anne,[48] one of the earliest mannequin simulators, for teaching and practicing cardiopulmonary resuscitation, and this is still widely used for assessment of these critical lifesaving techniques. Although it mimics a full-sized adult, rather than just one body part or region, it is still essentially a task trainer, with functional anatomy for performing ventilation and chest compressions but no (patho)physiologic functions or interactive features. Child- and infant-sized mannequins are available for analogous pediatric skills assessment.

For assessment of general examination skills as well as more specialized orthopedics, sports medicine, or rheumatologic examinations and procedures: part trainers that mimic accurate anatomy and landmarks for nearly every joint area (e.g., shoulder, elbow, wrist and hand, knee) allow evaluation of examination technique, as well as joint and soft tissue injections; specially wired needles for these procedures provide indicators of proper placement.

For internal medicine, pediatrics, neurology, and anesthesia skills evaluation: there are part task trainers scaled to both adult and infant sizes for evaluation of lumbar puncture and various spinal injection techniques.

In the realm of obstetric skills evaluation assessment there are several birthing trainers for assessment of vaginal delivery technique. These provide partial (pelvis/perineum/thighs) maternal anatomy as well as neonate models that present a variety of scenarios, including normal delivery in various maternal positions, shoulder dystocia, breech presentation, and forceps delivery. Related task trainers allow assessment of technique for episiotomy suturing or umbilical vein cannulation/cord blood sampling.

For evaluation of urologic and gynecologic skills there are trainers that simulate the pelvis/perineum of both male and female patients. One can assess technique for digital rectal examination and insertion of a proctoscope, as well as ability to identify abnormal findings, such as rectal polyp or carcinoma and various prostate pathologies. Some trainers mimic anatomy for procedures such as bladder catheterization, while others focus on assessment of female pelvic examination technique, allowing both bimanual and speculum examinations, and requiring identification of normal and abnormal uterine and ovarian findings.

To one such simulator, the Pelvic ExamSIM[49] adds sensors that record timing, location, and pressure used in palpation during a female pelvic examination. Newer task trainers like this have begun to incorporate computerized features that may aid in assessment. For other examples, some airway trainers provide feedback on performance via indicators of depth of ventilation or amount of cricoid pressure. Resusci Anne and similar Laerdal trainers have optional built-in systems to assess frequency/volume of ventilation, depth of chest compressions, and hand placement. Although these technological enhancements have the potential to allow more detailed analysis of examinee performance, they do not alter the simulator interface with the user, which remains essentially passive.

Harvey, the Cardiopulmonary Patient Simulator,[50] is perhaps the most sophisticated example of such computerized task trainers: among the very earliest computer-enhanced mannequin simulators[51] and still in production after several "generations" of further development and refinement, this is the longest continuous high-fidelity simulation project in medical education. Unlike some of the other life-sized mannequin simulators described in the following section, however, Harvey is not interactive and does not permit performing physical interventions (defibrillation, intubation, etc.). Rather, it was designed to teach and evaluate bedside physical diagnosis skills: as such, Harvey features blood pressure; arterial, venous, and precordial pulses; as well as heart and lung sounds—all synchronized realistically to simulate 30 different cardiac conditions. The mannequin is portable and can speak via a wireless microphone from an operator; otherwise, no outside personnel or programming are required, as the computer is self-contained within the unit and digitally coordinates all the findings once a specific disease code is entered on the control pad. As the bedside examination of heart and lungs represents a fundamental skill set irrespective of medical specialty, Harvey has been employed for evaluation across many disciplines and at multiple levels of training, from medical students at the end of rotations[52] to physicians-in-training on high-stakes certification examinations.[23] Numerous studies have validated the use of Harvey as an assessment tool.[2]

Computer-Enhanced Mannequin Simulators

The previously described static models reproduce specific anatomy or a particular clinical task and, therefore, are most applicable to focused domains, whereas other devices use computer technology with programming that enables the simulator to present a wide range of (patho)physiology and to respond dynamically to user actions. These computer-enhanced mannequins are adaptable to a host of simulation scenarios and, thus,

are more generally applicable to multiple disciplines. As mentioned previously, those specialties with high-risk performance environments (particularly, anesthesiology) led the recent expansion in medical simulation by incorporating these technologies into their training and evaluation programs; following the example of flight simulators in commercial aviation, the focus has been on emergency or crisis management skills—both of individuals and teams—and most of the simulators described in this section can facilitate assessments in this realm. Thanks to the flexibility of CEMs in simulating numerous and varied conditions on demand, other medical specialties, plus many nursing and allied health professions education programs, have also adopted these methods for training and testing. Among the various types of simulators, CEMs have been perhaps the best validated as assessment instruments.[53]

Sim One was the earliest such CEM: introduced in 1967 (only 1 year before Harvey), it was a full-sized mannequin with computer controls that interfaced with an anesthesia machine and simulated hemodynamic, cardiac, and airway problems.[1] This prototypical simulator no longer exists, but—despite computer and other technological advancements that have allowed significant improvements in later systems—the general concept and design of Sim One still serve as a template for current human patient simulators.

A present-day "descendant" of the high-fidelity anesthesia simulators, and perhaps the most sophisticated among CEMs, is the Human Patient Simulator (HPS) from Medical Education Technologies, Inc. (METI).[54] This adult-sized mannequin simulates not only blood pressure, multiple peripheral arterial pulses, and breath and heart sounds, but also muscle twitch from nerve stimulation, pupillary reflexes, salivation, lacrimation, and bleeding from several anatomic sites. A system included with the simulator (or conventional external monitors) can display vital signs, electrocardiogram, oxygen saturation, and other physiologic parameters in real time; these recordings are particularly useful when the HPS is used for assessment. In addition, the simulator responds appropriately to the administration of multiple medications and to a host of procedures, including intubation and ventilation, chest compressions and defibrillation/cardioversion, needle or tube thoracostomy, and arterial and venous cannulation. The HPS contains multiple preprogrammed patient profiles and can simulate numerous scenarios involving these patients; educators and evaluators have developed many more customized programs for use in particular settings, and these are often freely available online or from simulation users groups.[55]

The comprehensive and realistic simulations possible with the HPS make the system relatively expensive. In addition, the accompanying hardware limits portability or use of the simulator outside controlled environments (e.g., simulating military or emergency medical services in the field). For this reason, METI also produces the Emergency Care Simulator (ECS)[56]: less complex hardware and software allow fewer preprogrammed patients and scenarios and fewer automatic responses by the simulator to interventions. Consequently, an operator must enter more information and commands during the simulation, but the ECS is portable and considerably less expensive than the HPS. Pediatric versions, PediaSIM and PediaSIM-ECS,[57] scaled to the size and physiology of a 20-kg child, offer capabilities for high-fidelity simulations analogous to their adult-sized counterparts.

Building on their earlier task trainers, Laerdal Medical has also developed a number of mannequin simulators with varying degrees of fidelity for teaching and assessing airway and resuscitation skills. Although not as comprehensive as the METI HPS system, SimMan[58] is a full-sized adult mannequin with a realistic airway that can reproduce various conditions for assessing intubation techniques. It also has peripheral pulses with oxygen saturation, and electrocardiographic and other monitoring capabilities for evaluation of advanced cardiac and (especially with optional moulage accessories) trauma life support skills. In addition to intubation and chest compressions/defibrillation, SimMan also permits invasive procedures testing, ranging from peripheral venipuncture to needle or tube thoracostomy and cricothyroidotomy. SimBaby[59] is an infant-sized mannequin with analogous functionality for assessing pediatric emergency skills. Allowing not as full a range of procedures or scenarios, AirMan[60] is a simpler system, consisting of a head and torso mannequin only, that nonetheless focuses in similar fashion on airway and advanced cardiac resuscitation skills; as with other simulators, this less complex technology makes AirMan even less expensive than SimMan. Perhaps because of familiarity with the simpler Laerdal mannequins (such as Resusci Anne), and because it seems to strike the best balance between versatile functionality and affordability, SimMan is often the initial high-fidelity CEM system acquired by new simulation or clinical skills centers and is consequently in widespread use at many institutions worldwide.

Similar in functional capabilities to SimMan, HAL[61] is another CEM that can be used to assess emergency medical skills; its monitoring and programming components come in the form of a wireless tablet computer. The same company also manufactures Noelle,[62] which consists of life-sized female adult and neonate mannequins for assessment of obstetric skills, including delivery and postpartum/natal care; although they can function alone as (relatively inexpensive) task trainers, with additional computer interactive components, they can simulate a wide range of scenarios involving emergency care and management of complications in pregnancy and childbirth. Users can assess maternal and fetal/neonatal vital signs, oxygenation status, and ultrasound via two separate monitors; implement emergency procedures such as intubation, CPR, or defibrillation/cardioversion of mother and child; administer medications via peripheral/umbilical intravenous or intraosseous routes; and perform various delivery procedures as well as episiotomy repair.

Virtual Reality Simulators

Rather than demonstrating skills on simple task trainers or patient simulator mannequins, examinees can now also perform required techniques on "virtual" patients. VR systems are already commercially available (and more are under development) that simulate a wide variety of procedures, ranging from relatively simple nonoperative techniques (e.g., intravenous cannulation[63]) to more complex surgeries (e.g., laparoscopic cholecystectomy[64]), and from percutaneous catheter-based approaches (e.g., carotid artery stenting[65]) to endoscopic methods (e.g., flexible sigmoidoscopy[66]). Beyond these applications for assessment of procedural skills, however, VR simulators can facilitate evaluation of other patient management and communication skills, for both individuals and teams: in a "virtual emergency department" for trauma resuscitation scenarios[67] or a "virtual delivery room" for neonatal examinations,[68] we can remotely and simultaneously assess multiple participants, as they take part in the treatment of virtual patients in a computer-generated environment.

Nevertheless, the most common uses of VR simulators for testing purposes are for evaluation of competence in performing procedures, including medical examinations, nonoperative invasive techniques, and surgeries. Among the latter two categories, percutaneous catheter-based and endoscopic interventions, as well as minimally invasive or limited access surgical procedures, share common characteristics that not only make them difficult to learn, but also render them particularly adaptable to VR simulation. These techniques require psychomotor and perceptual skills that are quite different from traditional open approaches, because practitioners must (1) perform complex invasive procedures based on indirect and limited viewing of two-dimensional images representing the 3D task; (2) overcome reduced depth perception and sometimes poor quality of such imaging, especially the gray-scale fluoroscopic displays used in some procedures; (3) manipulate delicate instruments at a distance from the operative site, with consequent limitations in tactile feedback and degree of movement; and (4) compensate for the "fulcrum effect" of handling instruments in this way, whereby proprioceptive and visual feedback often conflict.[69] The same limitations that pose challenges for learners of these real procedures, however, actually simplify modeling of the simulated task: for example, the circumscribed field of view and restricted degree of movement when performing endoscopy require less comprehensive visual and tactile simulation in the corresponding virtual procedure.

This is not to say that incredibly lifelike simulations are not already possible with current VR technology; indeed, recent advances—many led by the video gaming industry—in computer processing speed, 3D rendering, and other technologies have significantly improved the authenticity of these simulations. In addition to their increasingly realistic audiovisual content, the most sophisticated VR systems for assessing procedural skills also feature haptic (touch and pressure feedback) technology to convey "the feel" of the procedure, instruments, or anatomic structure under examination. As examples of such technology, PHANTOM[70] haptic devices allow users to palpate and manipulate virtual objects via mechanical jointed arms that provide force feedback: a thimble, stylus, or actual surgical instruments affixed to the end of the apparatus allow simulation of the tactile sensation (pressure, resistance, etc.) involved, for instance, in palpating internal organs or making incisions and suturing. The haptic mechanism interfaces with a computer that generates the visual components of the experience. Although many are not yet commercially available, PHANTOM haptic devices already have applications in multiple medical disciplines,[71–75] as well as in other health professions such as dentistry[76] and veterinary medicine.[77,78]

In addition to haptic technologies, VR simulation developers have created tracking devices, such as head-mounted sensors or the CyberGlove,[79] to detect position and follow movement of the participant's head or hands; these innovations not only enhance the realism of the user's interaction with the virtual world, but (along with built-in recording functions of some simulators themselves) also allow measurement of certain parameters, such as economy of movement and instrument handling, which are important in technical assessments of surgical skill.[80,81]

As first predicted a little more than a decade ago,[82] nearly all branches of surgery now utilize various forms of VR technology for teaching, learning, and assessing various competencies. In neurosurgery, for instance, applications of VR methods to simulate ventricular shunt placement encompass simple Web-based visual models[83] as well as more complex devices incorporating haptic feedback.[84,85] VR simulations for other neurosurgical skills already exist,[86–88] and ongoing development of more systems is likely.[89] Examples include virtual temporal bone dissection simulations,[90] which not only neurosurgeons but also otolaryngologists could use to assess their trainees' technique. VR devices are available that simulate a spectrum of additional ENT procedures, ranging from noninvasive examinations, such as palpation of head and neck malignancies,[74] to endoscopic approaches for sinus surgery.[91,92]

Plastic and reconstructive surgeons have utilized virtual patients for some time now,[93,94] but mostly to plan the surgical approach and model the intended cosmetic result, rather than to assess the skills of, say, a novice prior to performing a procedure for the first time on real patients. Some VR applications for testing, however, do exist in this domain: one system generates scores for user technique during simulated cleft lip repair.[95] Other VR tools can be useful for assessing performance of various osteotomy and fusion procedures employed in multiple specialties, including not only plastics, but also oral-maxillofacial surgery and orthopedics.[96,97]

The minimally invasive analogue among orthopedic surgery procedures is arthroscopy. Accordingly, there are VR platforms that simulate diagnostic and therapeutic arthroscopy techniques: the Procedicus Virtual Arthroscopy (VA) simulator[98] is already commercially available, with modules for both knee[99] and shoulder[100] procedures. This system tracks data for performance assessment, including time to locate specific structures, efficiency of scope movement, number of collisions with any tissue, and number of injuries (collisions beyond a threshold force).[100] Several other groups are developing alternative virtual arthroscopy simulators, particularly for the knee joint.[75,101,102] Still other VR systems simulate various open orthopedic procedures, including arthroplasty, reduction of fractures, and amputation.[103]

More than a decade ago, ophthalmologists developed a VR device with haptic feedback mechanisms as well as stereo views of the operation—a key component in eye surgery—to simulate a cataract extraction procedure; the system design included capability for playback of the surgery and analysis of operative technique from multiple viewpoints (including from inside the eye).[104] Since then, further work with VR technology has created ophthalmic simulators that can facilitate assessment of a number of skills, ranging from simple ocular examination[105] to more complex procedures such as retinal photocoagulation,[106] vitreoretinal surgery,[107,108] phacoemulsification,[109] and capsulorhexis.[110,111] Currently, the only commercially available ophthalmologic VR simulator is EYESI[112]: the system consists of a stylized mannequin head with cut-outs where the "virtual eyes" would be located, realistic foot pedals for equipment control, a position-tracking stylus to simulate the appearance and feel of various instruments, and a surgical microscope to which the computer transmits appropriate stereo images of the operative field.[113] Documentation options for objective assessment are available with this simulator, and several different procedure modules permit evaluation of a range of intraocular surgical skills.

For general surgery, VR systems can simulate performance of procedures ranging in difficulty from simple suturing[114] to diagnostic peritoneal lavage,[115] and from other trauma evaluations/treatments[116,117] to laparoscopic surgeries such as cholecystectomy.[45] Several virtual reality simulators for assessment of laparoscopic skills are commercially available,[118–120] but perhaps the most extensively studied is the Procedicus Minimally Invasive Surgical Trainer (MIST).[121] This simulator consists of a structural frame supporting two mechanical arms that hold standard laparoscopic instruments and link to a computer whose monitor displays the movement of these instruments in real time. Although the graphics are 3D, some of the modules utilize simple geometric shapes rather than more realistic representations of the anatomy or tissues involved. Nonetheless, the user can perform tasks of progressive complexity that represent key skills employed in laparoscopic surgery, including withdrawal and insertion of the instruments, stretching and clipping of soft tissues, use of diathermy, intracorporeal knot tying, manipulating needles, and continuous or interrupted suturing. The system records data that enable evaluation of performance, comprising scores for time to complete the task, number of errors, efficiency of instrument movements, and economy in the use of diathermy; the computer can also separately analyze right- and left-hand performance to assess ambidextrous skills. Scores for task completion on the MIST correlate with expert ratings during laparoscopic cholecystectomy carried out on live animals.[81] Moreover, studies demonstrate transfer of skills from the simulated task to the actual operation performed on real patients (so-called "VR to OR"),[44,45] offering important evidence of this virtual reality simulator's validity.

Surgeons utilize many of these same skills to perform laparoscopic procedures other than cholecystectomy; not surprisingly then, the MIST has found applications beyond general surgery, for assessment of competence in various disciplines such as gynecology[122] and urology.[123] Moreover, other VR systems allow evaluation of different procedural skills in these surgical specialties: in gynecology, for instance, realistic simulations exist to assess performance of laparoscopic salpingectomy for ectopic pregnancy[124] or hysteroscopy.[125,126] For the latter procedure, commercially available devices such as the Hysteroscopy AccuTouch System[127] provide modules to assess not only general skills (such as navigation through the cervical canal, fluid management, and uterine visualization), but also performance of specific procedures such as myomectomy using a loop electrode; the system tracks time and precision in completing psychomotor tasks and generates metrics that can aid in performance evaluations.

Other VR devices can accurately model genitourinary procedures, ranging from prostate examination[73] to cystoscopy and ureteroscopy.[128–130] One such simulator, the URO Mentor,[131] is very versatile in the range of diagnostic and therapeutic endourologic procedures it is capable of reproducing, including cystoscopic biopsy and tumor resection, as well as ureteroscopic treatment of strictures/obstructions via balloon dilation, catheter or stent placement, stone extraction, or intracorporeal lithotripsy.[132] Developers are creating additional modules for procedures such as transurethral resection of the prostate (TURP). The simulator supports use of both flexible and rigid endoscopes with working channels for tool insertion; the user can control instruments (e.g., catheters, guidewires, baskets, forceps, lithotripters, electrodes, stents, balloons) with actual tool handles that function realistically, while the computer displays a virtual representation of the operating end of these devices. Haptic technology provides a lifelike feel during scope insertion and instrument manipulation. Examinees can demonstrate endoscopy skills with direct visualization of pathologic lesions, or show their ability to perform real-time fluoroscopy with correct C-arm positioning and injection of contrast agents. The system tracks multiple parameters to aid in performance assessment, including time to complete key steps in the procedure, x-ray exposure time, and number of errors (such as perforations or laser misfires).

The PERC Mentor[133]—as a stand-alone system or as an add-on to the URO Mentor (in which one unit comprises both devices)—simulates related techniques for performing percutaneous renal access procedures. The platform consists of a stylized mannequin representing the patient's back and bilateral flanks: cartridges with layers to simulate the feel of skin, subcutaneous tissues, and ribs—interchangeable for practice on normal or obese patients—enable the user to carry out actual percutaneous punctures using various real needles, while simultaneously manipulating a virtual C-arm and following fluoroscopic images to pass guidewires and access the proper renal calyx. Again, the simulator has a built-in capability to record data for use in assessment exercises, such as time to perform important steps in the procedure, total x-ray exposure time, number of attempts to puncture the collecting system, and number of improper hits to other structures (e.g., ribs, blood vessels, other internal organs). Researchers are developing additional modules to simulate procedures such as percutaneous transhepatic cholangiography. Obviously, evaluation of skills required to perform such fluoroscopically guided percutaneous techniques is germane not only to urologists, but also to other specialists, such as vascular surgeons and interventional radiologists and cardiologists.

Along these lines, VR simulators exist that can aid the assessment of competence in performing angiography and endovascular procedures. Similar in design and capabilities to other devices by the same manufacturer (described above), the ANGIO Mentor[134] simulates a range of carotid, renal, and lower extremity artery diagnostic and therapeutic interventions, including cine and digital subtraction angiography, angioplasty, and stenting. High-end haptic mechanisms realistically mimic use of guidewires, balloons, stents, and other devices. The system includes dynamic indicators of patient status (e.g., vital signs, ECG, oxygen saturation, intra-arterial pressure gradients, and even virtual neurologic examination) that change appropriately with drug administration and procedural maneuvers, thereby allowing assessment of trainees' medical decision making and ability to manage complications. The simulator tracks a set of parameters and generates statistical reports on individual or group performance to aid in evaluation.

The Procedicus Vascular Intervention System Trainer (VIST)[135] is another system for assessing endovascular procedure skills. In addition to renal, iliac, and carotid artery techniques, this platform also simulates a range of interventional cardiology procedures, including cardiac catheterization with coronary angiography, angioplasty, and stenting, as well as biventricular pacemaker lead placement. The user manipulates real tools and devices passed through an introducer in the stylized mannequin; haptic mechanisms reproduce the tactile feedback, while simulated fluoroscopic images display the anatomy and results of interventions in real time. Studies have demonstrated the reliability[69] and validity[136–138] of this system as a test of ability to perform various endovascular techniques, leading to the landmark decision by the U.S. Food and Drug Administration (FDA), when it approved a carotid stenting system, to require would-be practitioners of this procedure to document adequate proficiency through participation in a training/evaluation program involving VR simulation.[65] The professional societies representing physicians who perform these endovascular procedures subsequently issued a consensus statement supporting the use of VR simulation for training and assessment of clinical competence in these domains.[139]

Other nonoperative invasive procedures amenable to VR simulation include various endoscopic techniques. Employed chiefly by surgeons and interventional medicine subspecialists, such as pulmonologists and gastroenterologists, these procedures include bronchoscopy, esophagogastroduodenoscopy (EGD), sigmoidoscopy, and colonoscopy. The Endoscopy AccuTouch System[140] is a haptic VR device that allows simulation of all these endoscopic procedures on a single platform. The bronchoscopy modules allow assessment of basic endoscopic and inspection skills, as well as various techniques for specimen collection (endobronchial sampling, transbronchial needle aspiration, and bronchoalveolar lavage); the system also simulates the more difficult navigation through pediatric airways. Similarly, the upper and lower gastrointestinal modules permit evaluation of basic endoscopic skills (instrument handling, navigation, and inspection of mucosa for lesions), as well as performance of more complex techniques, ranging from biopsies and polypectomy to cholangiopancreatography.

As mentioned at the beginning of this section, we have provided only a sampling here of the numerous simulation devices currently available or under development. The technology continues to advance at such a pace that future progress and applications seem limited only by the bounds of imagination.

Practical Suggestions for Use Now and Future Directions

The task of implementing simulation-based assessment methods, then, can be a daunting one for evaluation program planners: faced with choosing from among simulators that range so widely in terms of fidelity, cost, and features, how do we decide whether to use CEMs versus task trainers or VR simulators for a given assessment? Ultimately, the decision to use simulations for testing depends on local circumstances, the needs of the particular examination, and the competencies under evaluation. Wherever possible, we have tried to couch the foregoing discussion in terms that are broadly applicable, irrespective of particular health care disciplines or stage of

training. Clearly, however, many of the existing simulators pertain more to specific specialties and to education or evaluation at the postgraduate and continuing professional development levels. In this final portion of the chapter, we raise several important points for consideration by program directors wishing to implement simulation methods within their curricula now. In addition, we offer thoughts on what the future may hold for simulation-based assessments and suggest areas for ongoing research in this field.

First and foremost, in keeping with principles of curricular alignment, defined learning outcomes should drive the use of simulators for assessment, rather than the other way around. Any good curricular "blueprint" *begins* with the enumeration of competencies or learning objectives, which *then* determine the optimal instructional strategies to attain those goals and best assessment tools to document achieving the outcomes. Sometimes, however, programs acquire simulators without careful advance planning for their use—as stated earlier, high technology can be alluring—and then curriculum directors end up looking for ways to make them fit into their educational and evaluation schemes. Having a simulator that *can* be used to evaluate certain competencies does not mean that we *should* use it in this way, if these outcomes are beyond the scope of a particular course or inappropriate for our trainees' level.

Along similar lines, evaluators must match the features and fidelity of the simulator to the competencies under examination. For example, insertion of a bladder catheter is one skill that can be assessed on the Human Patient Simulator (HPS); if the *only* competency to evaluate is bladder catheterization, however, it makes little sense to purchase the very expensive HPS, if testing on a far less costly 3D anatomic (pelvic) model accomplishes the same goal. On the other hand, acquiring one full-featured device such as the HPS may be more economical than buying multiple single-task trainers to assess, say, endotracheal intubation, administration and pharmacology of intravenous medications, and induction of anesthesia, if all those are the outcomes to be assessed. Additional factors to balance include costs to maintain the equipment (HPS usually requires an annual service contract, whereas plastic models require little upkeep); value added in terms of higher face validity (realism) and presentation/assessment of a wider variety of clinical conditions or scenarios with multifeature simulators; and savings in rater time, if the simulator features built-in recording functions to capture assessment data.

Similar considerations of other feasibility issues, as discussed earlier, include the time and costs involved with training personnel and developing simulation scenarios. One way to surmount some of these challenges is to avoid "reinventing the wheel." Simulation societies and other users groups publish guidelines, host online discussion rooms, and convene meetings for the sharing of ideas, "lessons learned," and actual resources, which can save considerable effort and expense. For example, members in the Society for Simulation in Healthcare[55] can access a list server where they share experiences using particular simulators, evaluation tools (such as checklists) to be used in simulation-based assessments, scenario scripts, etc. Its journal, *Simulation in Healthcare*,[141] publishes peer-reviewed research and commentaries on this area of health professions education, as well as best practice recommendations that can prove very useful to directors of new programs utilizing simulation modalities. International conferences[142] feature special tracks for those interested in establishing and operating simulation centers, dealing with issues ranging from construction and space planning to personnel recruitment and resource procurement.

Such "special interest" sessions arose because numerous institutions worldwide are now constructing dedicated clinical skills or simulation centers, but the notion that such facilities are required for a successful simulation program, whether for training or assessment, is sometimes intimidating to those with limited resources. We can make a persuasive argument, however, *against* conducting tests in such artificial or in vitro settings: more authentic and, therefore, perhaps more valid assessments of clinical competence may entail evaluation in the environments in which practitioners actually work (in vivo, if you will: in the operating room, emergency department, or clinic examination room). Assessments that combine simulation modalities (e.g., a part task trainer—skin suturing pad—strapped to the arm of a standardized patient) in such settings are probably our best approximations of real patient encounters, and these may become the clinical assessment method of choice in the near future.[38] Because these "testing centers" already exist (in the hospitals and clinics where trainees work) and some of the task trainers involved are relatively inexpensive, programs with limited resources may still enter the arena of simulation-based evaluations.

Other innovative ways of combining simulation modalities may be just around the corner. In addition to coupling task trainers with SPs, as above, we may see VR applications integrated with, say, mannequin simulators: this form of "augmented VR" will allow simulation designers to customize and alter the appearance of the plastic models on demand—they can change genders, appear older, display cyanosis, etc., depending on the particular scenario. The user's visual experience will be via special display headsets, while still manipulating the physical mannequin. By programming actual patient data (radiographic imaging, physiologic parameters, etc.) into the simulation, VR technology will also allow rehearsal and assessment of complex or rare procedures in advance of performing them on the real patient.

Future trends in the application of these technologies for assessment are also likely to include greater use for high-stakes testing (e.g., certification and recertification examinations). This is already occurring to a limited extent in some disciplines: for instance, the

Royal College of Physicians and Surgeons of Canada is utilizing computer-based and mannequin simulations in addition to SPs for their national internal medicine certification (oral) examinations.[23] The American Board of Internal Medicine employs similar simulations in the Clinical Skills Module that is part of their Maintenance of Certification Program.[143] Many sorts of ongoing evaluation processes, some including simulation modalities, are already figuring prominently in continuing professional development programs; these assessment methods, by helping to identify practitioners with sub-par skills and also by providing opportunities for remediation and re-examination through simulation, are receiving increasing support and, in some jurisdictions, legislative mandates.[144]

The inherent reproducibility of simulators makes them ideally suited to testing environments where these kinds of high-stakes decisions will be made and, consequently, where high reliability is essential; as more and more studies also demonstrate validity of these assessment methods (especially predictive validity), they will gain wider acceptance by certification boards and credentialing organizations. Procedure-based disciplines (surgery, cardiology, interventional radiology, etc.) are likely to lead this movement and, as with the case of carotid stenting described earlier,[65] actually require simulation-based evaluations in certifying proficiency for users of new medical devices and practitioners of high-risk procedures.

There is some discussion now of employing simulation-based evaluations even earlier in the process of specialty training: rather than just using formative evaluations throughout the residency program and summative assessments at the end of training for the determination of competence and eventual certification, program directors could use simulation-based testing during medical school itself to screen student candidates for aptitude in certain skills and to guide selection decisions for further training.[119]

Thus, spanning the continuum of educational levels and bridging multiple health care professions, simulations are increasingly finding a place among our tools for assessment. Technological advances have created a diverse range of simulators that can facilitate testing in numerous areas of health care education. In general, simulators are most appropriate for the evaluation of competence in performing clinical skills or procedures. Simulators provide standardization of the patient variable in clinical examinations and contribute to more reliable assessments of performance in these domains. Simulators complement other testing methods, such as the OSCE, and allow us to measure and judge the wide range of processes and outcomes encountered in clinical training.

CONFLICT OF INTEREST DISCLOSURE

Neither author (RJS, SBI) has significant financial relationships with any of the commercial manufacturers or products referenced in this chapter. Likewise, although both authors are on the faculty of the University of Miami School of

Medicine, which manufactures Harvey, the Cardiopulmonary Patient Simulator, they receive no compensation of any kind related to the distribution of Harvey. Mention in this chapter of specific simulation systems does not constitute endorsement by the authors, editors, or publisher. Particular companies or simulators are cited when, in the opinion of the authors, they have historical significance or represent common or exemplary models used in health care education today.

ANNOTATED BIBLIOGRAPHY

1. Dunn WF: Simulators in Critical Care and Beyond. Des Plaines, IL, Society of Critical Care Medicine, 2004.

   This book is based on a compilation of papers originally presented at the 2004 Society of Critical Care Medicine conference. It provides a comprehensive introduction to the role of simulators as educational tools for health care providers. Topics include tips on designing and setting up a simulation center, how to customize simulators based on one's needs, and strengths and weaknesses of screen-based simulations, part task trainers, and mannequin-based simulators. Several chapters provide case examples of successful simulation programs and courses from the authors' own institutions.

2. Gaba DM: The future vision of simulation in health care. Qual Saf Health Care 2004;13(Suppl 11):i2–i10.

   In this paper Gaba describes a comprehensive framework for future applications of simulations as the key enabling technique for a revolution in health care—one that optimizes safety, quality, and efficiency. Gaba proposes that simulators must be integrated into the fabric of health care delivery at all levels, an undertaking that is much more complex than just "piling it on top" of the existing system.

3. Gallagher C, Issenberg SB: Simulation in Anesthesia. Philadelphia, Saunders, 2007.

   This is a step-by-step "how-to" guide on conducting an anesthesia simulation. Topics include which equipment to use as well as suggestions for simulation scenarios that will help train staff with a theoretical basis for handling even the most unexpected complications. This simulation guide with video clips helps to close the gaps that may result when abnormal situations are not recognized quickly enough or the response to them is haphazard and slow. One chapter contains a very extensive and detailed annotated bibliography of the most significant peer-reviewed manuscripts in the anesthesia simulation literature over the past 35 years.

4. Issenberg SB, McGaghie WC, Petrusa ER, et al: Features and uses of high-fidelity medical simulations that lead to effective learning: A BEME systematic review. Med Teach 2005;27(1):10–28.

   This is the first published systematic review conducted under the auspices of the Best Evidence Medical Education (BEME) Collaboration. Its mandate was not to compare simulation to other educational methods but to distill those features of simulation-based training that the literature suggests lead to best learning outcomes. The comprehensive literature review spanned 34 years and encompassed nearly 700 publications. Among the 10 most frequently cited as important features of simulation-based education were the provision of feedback, opportunities for repetitive practice, controlled learning environment, and integration within a curriculum.

5. Lloyd GE, Lake CL, Greenberg RB: Practical Health Care Simulations. Philadelphia, Mosby, 2004.

   This textbook provides guidance needed to make an informed decision about whether to begin using patient simulators. It describes how to develop and operate a simulation center and discusses how to design educational and assessment simulations that reflect specific educational curricula. Chapters from multiple experts in the field explain the value of simulation for a variety of health care disciplines and discuss which types of simulations are most relevant for each field. It also evaluates the specific simulation products that are currently available; details the "nuts and bolts" of preparing relevant "patients" and scenarios; describes applications for assessment, certification, and re-certification; presents an overview of future trends in simulation (such as virtual reality simulations); and discusses issues related to planning for simulation center growth.

6. Tekian A, McGuire CH, McGaghie WC: Innovative Simulations for Assessing Professional Competence. Chicago, Dept. of Medical Education, University of Illinois at Chicago, 1999.

   This book is an introduction to simulations used for teaching, training, and assessing the competencies of students and professional practitioners in a wide array of educational disciplines. The scope includes coverage of simulations used worldwide in architecture, medicine, aviation, law, and military applications. This text is only an introduction to simulations and is not a manual of specific techniques.

REFERENCES

1. Abrahamson S, Denson JS, Wolf RM: Effectiveness of a simulator in training anesthesiology residents. J Med Educ 1969;44(6):515–519.
2. Issenberg SB, McGaghie WC, Hart IR, et al: Simulation technology for health care professional skills training and assessment. JAMA 1999;282(9):861–866.
3. Fincher R-ME, Lewis LA: Simulations used to teach clinical skills. In Norman GR, van der Vleuten CPM, Newble DI (eds): International Handbook of Research in Medical Education. Dordrecht, The Netherlands, Kluwer Academic, 2002, pp 499–535.
4. Collins JP, Harden RM: AMEE Medical Education Guide No. 13: Real patients, simulated patients and simulators in clinical examinations. Med Teach 1998;20:508–521.
5. Haluck RS, Marshall RL, Krummel TM, Melkonian MG: Are surgery training programs ready for virtual reality? A survey of program directors in general surgery. J Am Coll Surg 2001;193(6):660–665.
6. Institute of Medicine: To err is human: Building a safer health system. Washington, DC, National Academy Press, 2000.
7. Committee on Quality of Health Care in America/Institute of Medicine: Crossing the quality chasm: A new health system for the 21st century. Washington, DC, National Academy Press, 2001.
8. An organisation with a memory: Report of an expert group on learning from adverse events in the NHS chaired by the Chief Medical Officer. Accessed Sept. 23, 2007 at www.dh.gov.uk/en/PublicationsAndStatistics/Publications/PublicationsPolicyAndGuidance/Browsable/DH_4098184.
9. Building a safer NHS for patients—Implementing an organization with a memory. Accessed Sept. 23, 2007 at www.dh.gov.uk/PublicationsAndStatistics/Publications/PublicationsPolicyAndGuidance/DH_4006525.
10. Barach P: Delivering safe health care: Safety is a patient's right and the obligation of all health professionals. BMJ 2001;323:585–586.
11. Goodman W: The world of civil simulators. Flight Int Mag 1978;18:435.
12. Ressler EK, Armstrong JE, Forsythe GB: Military mission rehearsal: From sandtable to virtual reality. In Tekian A, McGuire CH, McGaghie WC (eds): Innovative Simulations for Assessing Professional Competence. Chicago, Department of Medical Education, University of Illinois at Chicago, 1999, pp 157–174.
13. Wachtel J, Walton DG: The future of nuclear power plant simulation in the United States. In Simulation for Nuclear Reactor Techonology. Cambridge, Cambridge University Press, 1985.
14. Kochevar DT: The critical role of outcomes assessment in veterinary medical accreditation. J Vet Med Educ 2004;31(2):116–119.
15. Scalese RJ, Issenberg SB: Effective use of simulations for the teaching and acquisition of veterinary professional and clinical skills. J Vet Med Educ 2005;32(4):461–467.
16. Langsley DG: Medical competence and performance assessment: A new era. JAMA 1991;266(7):977–980.
17. Norcini J: Computer-based testing will soon be a reality. Perspectives 1999;3:57.
18. Kassebaum DG, Eaglen RH: Shortcomings in the evaluation of students' clinical skills and behaviors in medical school. Acad Med 1999;74(7):842–849.
19. Edelstein RA, Reid HM, Usatine R, Wilkes MS: A comparative study of measures to evaluate medical students' performance. Acad Med 2000;75(8):825–833.
20. Swing SR: Assessing the ACGME general competencies: General considerations and assessment methods. Acad Emerg Med 2002;9(11):1278–1288.

21. Medical Council of Canada: Qualifying Examination Part II, Information Pamphlet. Ottawa, Ontario, Canada, Medical Council of Canada, 2002.
22. Ben David MF, Klass DJ, Boulet J, et al: The performance of foreign medical graduates on the National Board of Medical Examiners (NBME) standardized patient examination prototype: A collaborative study of the NBME and the Educational Commission for Foreign Medical Graduates (ECFMG). Med Educ 1999;33(6):439–446.
23. Hatala R, Kassen BO, Nishikawa J, et al: Incorporating simulation technology in a Canadian internal medicine specialty examination: A descriptive report. Acad Med 2005;80(6):554–556.
24. Issenberg SB, McGaghie WC, Petrusa ER, et al: Features and uses of high-fidelity medical simulations that lead to effective learning: A BEME systematic review. Med Teach 2005;27(1):10–28.
25. Boulet JR, Swanson DB: Psychometric challenges of using simulations for high-stakes testing. In Dunn WF (ed): Simulators in Critical Care and Beyond. Des Plaines, IL, Society of Critical Care Medicine, 2004, pp 119–130.
26. Carmines EG, Zeller RA: Reliability and Validity Assessment. Beverly Hills, CA, Sage Publications, 1979.
27. Crocker L, Algina J: Introduction to Classical and Modern Test Theory. New York, Holt, Rinehart, and Winston, 1986.
28. Brennan RL: Elements of Generalizability Theory, 2nd ed. Iowa City, IA, American College Testing Program, 1992.
29. Streiner DL, Norman GR: Health Measurement Scales: A Practical Guide to Their Development and Use, 2nd ed. Oxford, Oxford University Press, 1995.
30. Downing SM: Validity: On meaningful interpretation of assessment data. Med Educ 2003;37(9):830–837.
31. McGaghie WC: Simulation in professional competence assessment: Basic considerations. In Tekian A, McGuire CH, McGaghie WC (eds): Innovative Simulations for Assessing Professional Competence. Department of Medical Education, University of Illinois at Chicago, 1999, pp 7–22.
32. Maran NJ, Glavin RJ: Low- to high-fidelity simulation—A continuum of medical education? Med Educ 2003;37(Suppl 1):22–28.
33. Kalu PU, Atkins J, Baker D, et al: How do we assess microsurgical skill? Microsurgery 2005;25(1):25–29.
34. The ACGME Outcome Project: General Competencies. Accessed Sept. 23, 2007 at www.acgme.org/outcome/comp/compFull.asp.
35. Harden RM, Crosby JR, Davis MH, Friedman M: AMEE Guide No. 14: Outcome-based education: Part 5. From competency to meta-competency: A model for the specification of learning outcomes. Med Teach 1999;21(6):546–552.
36. Tomorrow's doctors: Recommendations on undergraduate medical education. Accessed Sept. 23, 2007 at www.gmc-uk.org/education/undergraduate/undergraduate_policy/tomorrows_doctors.asp.
37. The CanMEDS Roles Framework. Accessed Sept. 23, 2007 at http://rcpsc.medical.org/canmeds/index.php.
38. Kneebone RL, Kidd J, Nestel D, et al: Blurring the boundaries: Scenario-based simulation in a clinical setting. Med Educ 2005;39(6):580–587.
39. Miller GE: The assessment of clinical skills/competence/performance. Acad Med 1990;65(9 Suppl):S63–S67.
40. ACGME Outcome Project: Table of Toolbox Methods. Accessed Sept. 23, 2007 at www.acgme.org/outcome/assess/table.asp.
41. McGaghie WC, Issenberg SB, Petrusa ER, Scalese RJ: Effect of practice on standardised learning outcomes in simulation-based medical education. Med Educ 2006;40(8):792–797.
42. Swanson D: A measurement framework for performance-based tests. In Hart I, Harden R (eds): Further Developments in Assessing Clinical Competence. Montreal, Can-Heal Publications, 1987, pp 13–45.
43. Whelan GP, Boulet JR, McKinley DW, et al: Scoring standardized patient examinations: Lessons learned from the development and administration of the ECFMG clinical skills assessment (CSA). Med Teach 2005;27(3):200–206.
44. Seymour NE, Gallagher AG, Roman SA, et al: Virtual reality training improves operating room performance: Results of a randomized, double-blinded study. Ann Surg 2002;236(4):458–463; discussion 63–64.
45. Grantcharov TP, Kristiansen VB, Bendix J, et al: Randomized clinical trial of virtual reality simulation for laparoscopic skills training. Br J Surg 2004;91(2):146–150.
46. Reznek MA: Current status of simulation in education and research. In Lloyd GE, Lake CL, Greenberg RB (eds): Practical Health Care Simulations. Philadelphia, Mosby, 2004, pp 27–47.
47. Limbs & Things. Accessed Sept. 23, 2007 at www.golimbs.com/.
48. Resusci Anne Simulator [Laerdal Medical]. Accessed Sept. 23, 2007 at www.laerdal.info/document.asp?subnodeid=8282560.
49. Pelvic Exam SIM [METI]. Accessed Sept. 23, 2007 at www.meti.com/products_es_pelvic.htm.
50. Harvey, the Cardiopulmonary Patient Simulator. Accessed Sept. 23, 2007 at www.crme.miami.edu/harvey_changes.html.
51. Gordon MS: Cardiology patient simulator. Development of an animated manikin to teach cardiovascular disease. Am J Cardiol 1974;34(3):350–355.
52. Ewy GA, Felner JM, Juul D, et al: Test of a cardiology patient simulator with students in fourth-year electives. J Med Educ 1987;62(9):738–743.
53. Cooper JB, Taqueti VR: A brief history of the development of mannequin simulators for clinical education and training. Qual Saf Health Care 2004;13(Suppl 1):11–18.
54. Human Patient Simulator (HPS) (METI). Accessed Sept. 23, 2007 at www.meti.com/products_ps_hps.htm.
55. Society for Simulation in Healthcare. Accessed Sept. 23, 2007 at www.ssih.org.
56. Emergency Care Simulator (ECS) [METI]. Accessed Sept. 23, 2007 at www.meti.com/products_ps_ecs.htm.
57. PediaSIM and PediaSIM-ECS [METI]. Accessed Sept. 23, 2007 at www.meti.com/products_ps_pedia.htm.
58. SimMan [Laerdal Medical]. Accessed Sept. 23, 2007 at www.laerdal.info/document.asp?docID=1022609.
59. SimBaby [Laerdal Medical]. Accessed Sept. 23, 2007 at www.laerdal.info/document.asp?subnodeid=20232391.
60. AirMan [Laerdal Medical]. Accessed Sept. 23, 2007 at www.laerdal.info/document.asp?docid=1022661.
61. HAL [Gaumard]. Accessed Sept. 23, 2007 at www.gaumard.com/customer/product.php?productid=16345&cat=281&page=1.
62. Noelle [Gaumard]. Accessed Sept. 23, 2007 at www.gaumard.com/customer/product.php?productid=16352&cat=249&page=1.
63. Ursino M, Tasto JL, Nguyen BH, et al: CathSim: An intravascular catheterization simulator on a PC. Stud Health Tech Info 1999;62:360–366.
64. Tseng CS, Lee YY, Chan YP, et al: A PC-based surgical simulator for laparoscopic surgery. Stud Health Tech Info 1998;50:155–160.
65. Gallagher AG, Cates CU: Approval of virtual reality training for carotid stenting: What this means for procedural-based medicine. JAMA 2004;292(24):3024–3026.
66. Tuggy ML: Virtual reality flexible sigmoidoscopy simulator training: Impact on resident performance. J Am Board Fam Pract 1998;11(6):426–433.
67. Halvorsrud R, Hagen S, Fagernes S, et al: Trauma team training in a distributed virtual emergency room. Stud Health Tech Info 2003;94:100–102.
68. Korocsec D, Holobar A, Divjak M, Zazula D: Building interactive virtual environments for simulated training in medicine using VRML and Java/JavaScript. Comput Methods Prog Biomed 2005;80(Suppl 1):S61–S70.
69. Patel AD, Gallagher AG, Nicholson WJ, Cates CU: Learning curves and reliability measures for virtual reality simulation in the performance assessment of carotid angiography. J Am Coll Cardiol 2006;47(9):1796–1802.
70. PHANTOM Haptic Devices [SensAble Technologies]. Accessed Sept. 23, 2007 at www.sensable.com/products-haptic-devices.htm.
71. d'Aulignac D, Laugier C, Troccaz J, Vieira S: Towards a realistic echographic simulator. Med Image Anal 2006;10(1):71–81.
72. Reinig KD, Rush CG, Pelster HL, et al: Real-time visually and haptically accurate surgical simulation. Stud Health Tech Info 1996;29:542–545.
73. Burdea G, Patounakis G, Popescu V, Weiss RE: Virtual reality-based training for the diagnosis of prostate cancer. IEEE Trans Biomed Eng 1999;46(10):1253–1260.

74. Stalfors J, Kling-Petersen T, Rydmark M, Westin T: Haptic palpation of head and neck cancer patients—Implication for education and telemedicine. Stud Health Tech Info 2001;81: 471–474.

75. Mabrey JD, Gillogly SD, Kasser JR, et al: Virtual reality simulation of arthroscopy of the knee. Arthroscopy 2002;18(6):28.

76. Wang D, Zhang Y, Wang Y, et al: Cutting on triangle mesh: Local model-based haptic display for dental preparation surgery simulation. IEEE Trans Vis Comput Graph 2005;11(6): 671–683.

77. Crossan A, Brewster S, Reid S, Mellor D: Comparison of simulated ovary training over different skill levels. In Proceedings of Eurohaptics 2001. Birmingham, UK, 2001, p 17–21.

78. Baillie S, Crossan A, Brewster S, et al: Validation of a bovine rectal palpation simulator for training veterinary students. Stud Health Tech Info 2005;111:33–36.

79. CyberGlove. Accessed Sept. 23, 2007 at www.mindflux.com.au/products/vti/cyberglove.html.

80. Gallagher AG, Richie K, McClure N, McGuigan J: Objective psychomotor skills assessment of experienced, junior, and novice laparoscopists with virtual reality. World J Surg 2001;25(11): 1478–1483.

81. Grantcharov TP, Rosenberg J, Pahle E, Funch-Jensen P: Virtual reality computer simulation: An objective method for the evaluation of laparoscopic surgical skills. Surg Endosc 2001;15(3): 242–244.

82. Satava RM: Virtual reality surgical simulator. The first steps. Surg Endosc 1993;7(3):203–205.

83. Phillips NI, John NW: Web-based surgical simulation for ventricular catheterization. Neurosurgery 2000;46(4):933–936; discussion 6–7.

84. Larsen OV, Haase J, Ostergaard LR, et al: The Virtual Brain Project—Development of a neurosurgical simulator. Stud Health Tech Info 2001;81:256–262.

85. Goncharenko I, Emoto H, Matsumoto S, et al: Realistic virtual endoscopy of the ventricle system and haptic-based surgical simulator of hydrocephalus treatment. Stud Health Tech Info 2003;94:93–95.

86. Tanaka H, Nakamura H, Tamaki E, et al: Brain surgery simulation system using VR technique and improvement of presence. Stud Health Tech Info 1998;50:150–154.

87. Larsen O, Haase J, Hansen KV, et al: Training brain retraction in a virtual reality environment. Stud Health Tech Info 2003;94: 174–180.

88. Ai Z, Evenhouse R, Leigh J, et al: New tools for sculpting cranial implants in a shared haptic augmented reality environment. Stud Health Tech Info 2006;119:7–12.

89. Spicer MA, Apuzzo ML: Virtual reality surgery: Neurosurgery and the contemporary landscape. Neurosurgery 2003;52(3):489–497; discussion 96–97.

90. Wiet GJ, Bryan J, Dodson E, et al: Virtual temporal bone dissection simulation. Stud Health Tech Info 2000;70:378–384.

91. Weghorst S, Airola C, Oppenheimer P, et al: Validation of the Madigan ESS simulator. Stud Health Tech Info 1998;50:399–405.

92. Satava RM, Fried MP: A methodology for objective assessment of errors: An example using an endoscopic sinus surgery simulator. Otolaryngol Clin North Am 2002;35(6):1289–1301.

93. Grunwald T, Krummel T, Sherman R: Advanced technologies in plastic surgery: How new innovations can improve our training and practice. Plast Reconstr Surg 2004;114(6):1556–1567.

94. Smith DM, Aston SJ, Cutting CB, Oliker A: Applications of virtual reality in aesthetic surgery. Plast Reconstr Surg 2005; 116(3):898–904; discussion 5–6.

95. Montgomery K, Sorokin A, Lionetti G, Schendel S: A surgical simulator for cleft lip planning and repair. Stud Health Tech Info 2003;94:204–209.

96. Hsieh MS, Tsai MD, Chang WC: Virtual reality simulator for osteotomy and fusion involving the musculoskeletal system. Comput Med Imaging Graph 2002;26(2):91–101.

97. Sohmura T, Hojo H, Nakajima M, et al: Prototype of simulation of orthognathic surgery using a virtual reality haptic device. Int J Oral Maxillofac Surg 2004;33(8):740–750.

98. Procedicus Virtual Arthroscopy Simulator [Mentice]. Accessed Sept. 23, 2007 at www.mentice.com/.

99. Strom P, Kjellin A, Hedman L, et al: Training in tasks with different visual-spatial components does not improve virtual arthroscopy performance. Surg Endosc 2004;18(1):115–120.

100. Smith S, Wan A, Taffinder N, et al: Early experience and validation work with Procedicus VA—The Prosolvia virtual reality shoulder arthroscopy trainer. Stud Health Tech Info 1999;62: 337–343.

101. Heng PA, Cheng CY, Wong TT, et al: A virtual-reality training system for knee arthroscopic surgery. IEEE Trans Inf Technol Biomed 2004;8(2):217–227.

102. Cannon WD, Eckhoff DG, Garrett WE Jr, et al: Report of a group developing a virtual reality simulator for arthroscopic surgery of the knee joint. Clin Orthop Relat Res 2006;442:21–29.

103. Tsai MD, Hsieh MS, Jou SB: Virtual reality orthopedic surgery simulator. Comput Biol Med 2001;31(5):333–351.

104. Sinclair MJ, Peifer JW, Haleblian R, et al: Computer-simulated eye surgery. A novel teaching method for residents and practitioners. Ophthalmology 1995;102(3):517–521.

105. Kaufman DM, Bell W: Teaching and assessing clinical skills using virtual reality. Stud Health Tech Info 1997;39:467–472.

106. Dubois P, Rouland JF, Meseure P, et al: Simulator for laser photocoagulation in ophthalmology. IEEE Trans Biomed Eng 1995;42(7):688–693.

107. Hikichi T, Yoshida A, Igarashi S, et al: Vitreous surgery simulator. Arch Ophthalmol 2000;118(12):1679–1681.

108. Rossi JV, Verma D, Fujii GY, et al: Virtual vitreoretinal surgical simulator as a training tool. Retina 2004;24(2):231–236.

109. Laurell CG, Soderberg P, Nordh L, et al: Computer-simulated phacoemulsification. Ophthalmology 2004;111(4):693–698.

110. Webster R, Sassani J, Shenk R, Good N: A haptic surgical simulator for the continuous curvilinear capsulorhexis procedure during cataract surgery. Stud Health Tech Info 2004;98:404–406.

111. Webster R, Sassani J, Shenk R, et al: Simulating the continuous curvilinear capsulorhexis procedure during cataract surgery on the EYESI system. Stud Health Tech Info 2005;111:592–595.

112. EYESI [VRmagic]. Accessed Sept. 23, 2007 at www.vrmagic.com/eyesi/ausbildung_e.html.

113. Khalifa YM, Bogorad D, Gibson V, et al: Virtual reality in ophthalmology training. Surv Ophthalmol 2006;51(3):259–273.

114. Webster RW, Zimmerman DI, Mohler BJ, et al: A prototype haptic suturing simulator. Stud Health Tech Info 2001;81:567–569.

115. Liu A, Kaufmann C, Ritchie T: A computer-based simulator for diagnostic peritoneal lavage. Stud Health Tech Info 2001;81: 279–285.

116. Kaufmann C, Liu A: Trauma training: Virtual reality applications. Stud Health Tech Info 2001;81:236–241.

117. Bro-Nielsen M, Helfrick D, Glass B, et al: VR simulation of abdominal trauma surgery. Stud Health Tech Info 1998;50:117–123.

118. Hassan I, Sitter H, Schlosser K, et al: [A virtual reality simulator for objective assessment of surgeons' laparoscopic skill]. Chirurgia 2005;76(2):151–156.

119. Rosenthal R, Gantert WA, Scheidegger D, Oertli D: Can skills assessment on a virtual reality trainer predict a surgical trainee's talent in laparoscopic surgery. Surg Endosc 2006;20(8):1286–1290.

120. McDougall EM, Corica FA, Boker JR, et al: Construct validity testing of a laparoscopic surgical simulator. J Am Coll Surg 2006;202(5):779–787.

121. Procedicus MIST [Mentice]. Accessed Sept. 23, 2007 at www.mentice.com/.

122. Gor M, McCloy R, Stone R, Smith A: Virtual reality laparoscopic simulator for assessment in gynaecology. Br J Obstet Gynaecol 2003;110(2):181–187.

123. Gallagher HJ, Allan JD, Tolley DA: Spatial awareness in urologists: Are they different? Br J Urol Int 2001;88(7):666–670.

124. Larsen CR, Grantcharov T, Aggarwal R, et al: Objective assessment of gynecologic laparoscopic skills using the LapSimGyn virtual reality simulator. Surg Endosc 2006;20(9):1460–1466.

125. Harders M, Bajka M, Spaelter U, et al: Highly realistic, immersive training environment for hysteroscopy. Stud Health Tech Info 2006;119:176–181.

126. Lim F, Brown I, McColl R, et al: A visual graphic/haptic rendering model for hysteroscopic procedures. Australas Phys Eng Sci Med 2006;29(1):57–61.

127. Hysteroscopy AccuTouch System [Immersion Medical]. Accessed Sept. 23, 2007 at www.immersion.com/medical/products/hysteroscopy/.
128. Shah J, Darzi A: Virtual reality flexible cystoscopy: A validation study. Br J Urol Int 2002;90(9):828–832.
129. Jacomides L, Ogan K, Cadeddu JA, Pearle MS: Use of a virtual reality simulator for ureteroscopy training. J Urol 2004; 171(1):320–323; discussion 3.
130. Matsumoto ED, Pace KT, D'A Honey RJ: Virtual reality ureteroscopy simulator as a valid tool for assessing endourological skills. Int J Urol 2006;13(7):896–901.
131. URO Mentor [Simbionix]. Accessed Sept. 23, 2007 at http://simbionix.com/URO_Mentot.html.
132. Michel MS, Knoll T, Kohrmann KU, Alken P: The URO Mentor: Development and evaluation of a new computer-based interactive training system for virtual life-like simulation of diagnostic and therapeutic endourological procedures. Br J Urol Int 2002; 89(3):174–177.
133. PERC Mentor [Simbionix]. Accessed Sept. 23, 2007 at http://simbionix.com/PERC_Mentor.html.
134. ANGIO Mentor [Simbionix]. Accessed Sept. 23, 2007 at http://simbionix.com/ANGIO_Mentor.html.
135. Procedicus VIST [Mentice]. Accessed Sept. 23, 2007 at www.mentice.com.
136. Winder J, Zheng H, Hughes S, et al: Increasing face validity of a vascular interventional training system. Stud Health Tech Info 2004;98:410–415.
137. Jensen U, Ahlberg G, Jensen J, Arvidsson D: There is a difference in performance level in diagnostic coronary angiography in the Procedicus VIST simulator between experienced PCI surgeons and cardiologists in training. In Proceedings of the 10th Annual Meeting of the Society in Europe for Simulation Applied to Medicine (SESAM). Sweden, Huddinge, 2004.
138. Hsu JH, Younan D, Pandalai S, et al: Use of computer simulation for determining endovascular skill levels in a carotid stenting model. J Vasc Surg 2004;40(6):1118–1125.
139. Rosenfield K, Babb JD, Cates CU, et al: Clinical competence statement on carotid stenting: Training and credentialing for carotid stenting—Multispecialty consensus recommendations. J Am Coll Cardiol 2005;45(1):165–174.
140. Endoscopy AccuTouch System [Immersion Medical]. Accessed Sept. 23, 2007 at www.immersion.com/medical/products/endoscopy/.
141. Simulation in Healthcare. Accessed Sept. 23, 2007 at www.simulationinhealthcare.com.
142. International Meeting on Simulation in Healthcare. Accessed Sept. 23, 2007 at www.ssih.org/.
143. ABIM Maintenance of Certification Program. Accessed Sept. 23, 2007 at www.abim.org/moc/semmed.shtm#5.
144. Cregan P, Watterson L: High stakes assessment using simulation—An Australian experience. Stud Health Tech Info 2005;111:99–104.

APPENDIX 12-1
List of Simulators and Their Characteristics

Simulator	Features	Specialty	Cost*	Comments
Human Patient Simulator (HPS) www.meti.com	Full-sized, high-fidelity mannequin that functionally simulates all organ systems and responds physiologically to procedures and IV medications	Anesthesia Critical care Emergency medicine Neurology Internal/family medicine	$$$$	Numerous studies demonstrate validity of simulator as assessment tool. Best used when assessing multiple competencies and used in a "theater" setting.
Emergency Care Simulator (ESC) www.meti.com	Full-sized, high-fidelity mannequin that is more portable than the HPS and is programmed for more emergency scenarios; less sophisticated physiologic response to interventions	Critical care Emergency medicine	$$	Newer simulator that uses much of the same technology as HPS, but is designed to be more portable so that it can be used in numerous environments.
PediaSIM PediaSIM-ECS www.meti.com	Small child-sized, high-fidelity mannequin that functionally simulates the anatomy and physiology of a child and responds appropriately to interventions	Pediatrics Emergency medicine	$$	Newer simulator that uses much of the same technology as HPS, but is designed to function and react differently than an "adult." The ECS version has less sophisticated physiologic responses to interventions.
Pelvic Exam SIM www.meti.com	Female adult-sized, high-fidelity pelvic simulator that functionally simulates a variety of gynecologic findings and automatically and objectively tracks user examination technique	GYN Internal/family medicine	$$	Several studies have demonstrated its validity as an assessment tool. Currently being evaluated by NBME for potential use in high-stakes examination settings.
BabySIM www.meti.com	Infant-sized, high-fidelity mannequin that functionally simulates the anatomy and physiology of a 3- to 6-month-old infant and responds appropriately to interventions	Pediatrics	$$	Newer simulator that uses much of the same technology as HPS.
AirSIM www.limbsandthings.com	Adult-sized, high-fidelity head and neck mannequin that functionally simulates a variety of airway emergencies and responds appropriately to interventions	Anesthesia Critical care Emergency medicine	$$	Several studies demonstrate validity of airway mannequin as assessment tool. Best used when assessing complex airway scenarios.
SimMan www.laerdal.com	Full-sized, high-fidelity mannequin that is portable and provides functionally realistic anatomy for multiple clinical tasks and procedures	Anesthesia Critical care Emergency medicine Internal/family medicine Surgery	$$$	Several studies demonstrate validity and feasibility of simulator as assessment tool. One of the most widely used high-fidelity simulators for a broad range of learner populations and levels.

Name	Description	Specialties	Cost	Comments
AirMan www.laerdal.com	Adult-sized upper torso, head and neck that provides functional anatomy and physiologic signs of normal and difficult airway conditions	Anesthesia Critical care Emergency medicine Internal medicine	$$	Uses much of the same hardware and software as SimMan, but focuses on airway management skills.
Resusci Anne www.laerdal.com	Adult-sized, medium-fidelity, portable task trainer that provides functional anatomy for critical lifesaving skills; optional built-in assessment system that evaluates adequacy of chest compressions and ventilations	Critical care Emergency medicine Internal/family medicine	$$	Numerous studies demonstrate reliability, validity, and feasibility of device as assessment tool.
CathSim www.immersion.com/medical	High-fidelity task trainer that provides haptic feedback for intravenous access skills; contains built-in assessment system that evaluates IV access performance	Critical care Emergency medicine Internal medicine Pediatrics OB/GYN	$$	Several studies demonstrate validity of simulator as assessment tool. Advantage is built-in objective assessment system.
Noelle Maternal and Neonatal Birthing Simulator www.gaumard.com	Adult- and neonate-sized simulators that provide functional anatomic and medium-fidelity physiologic signs to perform complete delivery and postnatal care	OB/GYN Pediatrics	$$	New simulator that also offers interactive features for more complicated pregnancies and deliveries.
HAL Mobile Team Trainer www.gaumard.com	Full-sized, high-fidelity mannequin that is very portable and programmed for emergency scenarios; has monitoring and programming components that come in the form of a wireless tablet computer	Emergency medicine Critical care Internal medicine	$$$	Very portable and durable high-fidelity simulator that is suited for a wide range of emergency scenarios for pre-hospital providers.
Harvey, the Cardiopulmonary Patient Simulator www.crme.med.miami.edu	Adult-sized high-fidelity mannequin that provides comprehensive cardiac and pulmonary physical findings	Internal/family medicine Pediatrics Critical care Emergency medicine Surgery	$$$	Longest continuous high-fidelity simulator with numerous studies demonstrating validity as assessment tool.
Suture Simulator www.limbsandthings.com	Adult-sized arm that provides anatomic functional wound for suturing skills	Surgery Emergency medicine OB/GYN Family medicine	$	Inexpensive task trainer that provides hundreds of assessment opportunities.
Clinical Female Pelvic Trainer www.limbsandthings.com	Partial adult-sized task trainer that provides functional anatomy of lower abdomen and pelvis, vaginal and rectal findings	OB/GYN Internal/family medicine	$	Inexpensive task trainer for assessing recognition of appropriate landmarks, vaginal and bimanual exam, cervical smear, dry catheterization, and digital rectal exam.
Breast Examination Simulator www.limbsandthings.com	Partial adult-sized task trainer that provides functional anatomy of female upper chest and breast with normal and abnormal findings	OB/GYN Internal/family medicine	$	Inexpensive task trainer that provides opportunity to assess breast exam technique (including lower neck, clavicle and both axillae), identification of anatomic landmarks, and pathologic diagnosis.

*Estimates (as of 12/2006): $, < $1,000; $$, $1,000 – $10,000; $$$, $10,000 – $50,000; $$$$, > $50,000.

Continued

APPENDIX 12-1
List of Simulators and Their Characteristics (Continued)

Simulator	Features	Specialty	Cost*	Comments
Episiotomy Suture Simulator www.limbsandthings.com	Partial adult-sized task trainer that provides functional anatomy of vagina and perineum with varying degree lacerations	OB/GYN	$	Inexpensive task trainer that provides opportunity to assess episiotomy technique (superficial, subcuticular, deep musculature) and identification of tissue layer.
Central Line Simulator www.kyotokagaku.com	Partial adult-sized task trainer that provides functional anatomy of neck and upper chest including all landmarks for subclavian and internal jugular vein catheterization	Surgery Internal medicine Critical care medicine	$	Newer task trainer that allows assessment of central venous catheter insertion technique (and incorrect technique—pneumothorax, arterial puncture), identification of local anatomy.
Diagnostic Prostate Simulator www.limbsandthings.com	Partial adult-sized task trainer that provides functional anatomy of male rectum, perineum, and prostate	Surgery Internal/family medicine	$	Inexpensive task trainer that provides opportunity to assess prostate exam technique and identification of normal, bilateral BPH, unilateral nodule, uni-/bilateral carcinoma
Eye Exam Simulator www.kyotokagaku.com	Partial adult-sized task trainer that provides functional anatomy of external and internal eye with normal and abnormal retinal findings	Internal/family medicine Ophthalmology	$	Inexpensive task trainer that provides opportunity to assess ophthalmologic exam technique and identification of normal and common abnormal retinal findings.
Ear Exam Simulator www.kyotokagaku.com	Partial adult-sized task trainer that provides functional anatomy of external and middle ear with normal and abnormal findings	Internal/family medicine Otolaryngology	$	Inexpensive task trainer that provides opportunity to assess otoscopic exam technique and identification of normal and abnormal middle ear findings.
Spinal Injection Simulator www.adam-rouilly.co.uk	Partial adult-sized task trainer that provides functional anatomy and landmarks for lumbar puncture and various spinal injections.	Neurology Internal medicine Anesthesiology	$	Relatively inexpensive task trainer that provides opportunity to assess technique of lumbar puncture and identification of critical anatomic landmarks. Fluid can be added to provide feedback regarding correct placement of needle.
Infant Lumbar Puncture Simulator www.laerdal.com	Partial infant-sized task trainer that provides functional anatomy and landmarks for lumbar puncture technique	Pediatrics Neurology	$	Inexpensive task trainer that provides opportunity to assess technique of lumbar puncture and identification of critical anatomic landmarks. Fluid can be added to provide feedback regarding correct placement of needle.

Product	Description	Specialty	Cost*	Features
Procedicus Virtual Arthroscopy Simulator www.mentice.com	A combination virtual reality (VR) trainer and task trainer that comprises a base platform and modules for various joints and procedures including the shoulder and knee	Orthopedic surgery	$$$	Users can train to overcome orientation and instrument handling problems as well as hand-eye coordination difficulties. This system tracks data for performance assessment including time to locate structures, efficiency of scope movement, and errors.
EYESI Ophthalmologic surgery simulator www.vrmagic.com	A mannequin head with cut-outs where the virtual eyes would be located, realistic foot pedals for equipment control, a position-tracking stylus to simulate instruments, and a surgical microscope that receives virtual images	Ophthalmology	$$$	There are options for objective assessment and several different procedure modules that permit evaluation of a range of intraocular surgical skills.
Procedicus Minimally Invasive Surgical Trainer (MIST) www.mentice.com	VR-based simulator that consists of a structural frame supporting 2 mechanical arms that hold standard laparoscopic instruments linked to a computer monitor; provides training and assessment of fundamental laparoscopic skills	General surgery Trauma surgery GYN Urology	$$$	One of the most extensively studied simulators. The system records data that enable evaluation of performance. Several studies have demonstrated transfer of skills from simulator to real patients.
Hysteroscopy Accutouch System www.immersion.com/ medical	VR-based trainer that uses force feedback haptics to simulate the appropriate resistance as the user navigates through the cervical canal and uterus; contains digital simulations of real-life procedures, complications, and tool/tissue interactions	OB/GYN	$$$	The system tracks time and precision in completing psychomotor tasks and generates metrics that can aid in performance evaluations.
URO Mentor www.simbionix.com	Combined VR and task trainer that supports the use of flexible and rigid endoscopes with working channels for tool insertion; the user can control instruments with actual tools that function realistically with virtual computer display	Urology	$$$	A versatile simulator that provides a range of diagnostic and therapeutic endourologic procedures. The system tracks multiple parameters to aid in performance assessment, including time to complete task and number of errors.
PERC Mentor www.simbionix.com	Combined VR and task trainer that can be used as a stand-alone device or combined with the URO Mentor; consists of a mannequin simulating a patient's back and flanks that enables practice for performing percutaneous renal access procedures	Nephrology Interventional radiology	$$$	The simulator has a built-in capability to record data for use in assessment exercises, including time to perform tasks and number of errors.

*Estimates (as of 12/2006): $, < $1,000; $$, $1,000 – $10,000; $$$, $10,000 – $50,000; $$$$, > $50,000.

Continued

APPENDIX 12-1
List of Simulators and Their Characteristics (Continued)

Simulator	Features	Specialty	Cost*	Comments
ANGIO Mentor www.simbionix.com	A VR trainer that uses haptic devices to mimic the use of guidewires, balloons, stents, and other devices; includes dynamic indicators of patient status that change with drug administration and procedural maneuvers	Cardiology Interventional radiology Vascular surgery	$$$$	Embedded tracking system allows assessment of user's medical decision-making and management skills. The system tracks a set of parameters and generates statistical reports on individual or group performance.
Procedicus Vascular Intervention System Trainer (VIST) www.mentice.com	Virtual and mannequin trainer that enables the user to manipulate real tools and devices that are passed through an introducer; haptic mechanisms reproduce tactile feedback with simulated fluoroscopic images on a monitor	Cardiology Interventional radiology Vascular surgery Neurosurgery	$$$$	In addition to renal, iliac, and carotid artery endovascular techniques, the system also simulates a range of interventional cardiology procedures—angiography, angioplasty/stenting and pacemaker placement. It has become the primary simulator for clinicians to become trained to use the only FDA-approved carotid stent. It contains a sophisticated tracking system that measures time to complete task, efficiency of movement and errors.

*Estimates (as of 12/2006): $, <$1,000; $$, $1,000 – $10,000; $$$, $10,000 – $50,000; $$$$, >$50,000.

Working with Problem Residents: A Systematic Approach

Catherine R. Lucey, MD, FACP, and Robert McL. Boote, JD

Most program directors choose to enter the field of medical education because of their love of teaching and desire to foster the careers of young physicians. Once in the position, they realize the importance of their role as arbiter of professional competency. The program director is responsible for using teaching and evaluation to ensure that the graduates of their residency program are fully competent to provide safe and effective medical care. We are indeed fortunate that the talented residents with whom we work generally make it easy to reconcile the dual program director roles of resident coach and competency judge. Unfortunately, we periodically encounter residents who demonstrate career-threatening deficiencies in knowledge, attitudes, or skills. When faced with such a resident, program directors may feel that their roles as resident advocate and patient advocate are at odds.

A problem resident is a resident who is unable to meet the standards of performance in one or more of the competency domains delineated by the Accreditation Council on Graduate Medical Education (Box 13-1).

There is a severity spectrum of competency deficiencies. As leaders of educational programs, residency directors are accustomed to providing the opportunities for young physicians to enhance their skills and move from novice to expert. Minor competency deficiencies, often considered "areas for improvement" that disappear with usual training, do not constitute problems. At the other end of the spectrum are residents who, despite participation in opportunities that allow their peers to become proficient in the field, fail to demonstrate progress toward competence. These are problem residents. Figure 13-1 schematically represents the learning curves of normal and problem residents. Curve A depicts the normal progression of competency. Curve B represents a resident whose knowledge and skills at baseline are similar to his peers but whose growth during residency is slow. Curve C represents a resident whose skills at entry are far below expected and who has difficulty catching up with his peers.

The limited literature on problem residents suggests that virtually all program directors have been

BOX 13-1   ACGME Core Competencies

Medical knowledge
Patient care
Interpersonal skills and communication
Professionalism
Practice-based learning and improvement
Systems-based practice

confronted with a problem resident. Statistics from the field of internal medicine suggest a prevalence of problem residents between 7% and 15%.[1] This literature also suggests that program directors often feel uncertain about how to identify and remediate problem residents. Concerns about possible legal action may exacerbate this difficulty.

This chapter will outline a systematic approach to dealing with the problem resident. Program directors and faculty must build an evaluation infrastructure, recognize the clues that a problem may exist, appropriately investigate the extent and possible causes of the problem, determine a suitable educational corrective action plan in an appropriate administrative setting, evaluate the outcome of the intervention, and deal with issues of legal due process. Resident threats of legal action need never alter a training program's considered professional judgment. Though dealing with a problem resident is never easy, adhering to the process outlined in this chapter will give program directors the best chance of successfully reconciling a difficult situation. Although the concepts and framework introduced here are applicable to students as well as residents, we have chosen to focus this chapter on residents

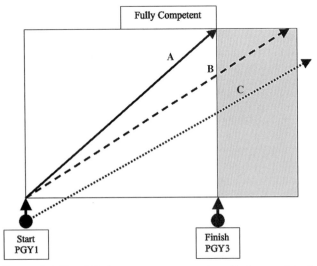

Figure 13-1 The clinical competency curve schematic for a prototypic 3-year residency. Curve A represents normal academic progress; curve B represents a resident who enters with the usual skills but learns at a rate incompatible with finishing during the normal residency duration but who may be successful with a short extension of training time; curve C represents a resident who enters with deficiencies and learns at a rate that is incompatible with finishing a program even after a short extension of training time.

with problems for several reasons. First, most medical schools have explicit policies and processes for dealing with the underperforming preclinical students. Second, residency lacks the testing framework and culture (i.e., course finals and USMLE step I and II) that exist in undergraduate medical education and that often make early identification of a problem student easier. Third, the domains of competency for students in the clinical years are identical to residents, and thus, it is logical to generalize from the resident with problems to the clinical student with problems. Finally, program directors dealing with problem residents must deal with both educational law as well as employment law.

Establishing the Necessary Evaluation Infrastructure

Program directors should build evaluation systems that can deal with the inevitability of a problem resident. The necessary evaluation infrastructure will help the program director avoid charges that their decisions about problem residents were either arbitrary (not based on defined standards) or capricious (made on a whim). The best way to avoid the appearance of arbitrary and capricious decision making is through the use of a clinical competency committee. The charge of this committee is to ensure that all residents meet the appropriate performance standards prior to promotion within or graduation from the program. In consultation with the program director, this committee should:

1. Establish program performance standards
2. Conduct ongoing reviews of the evaluation files of all residents to determine whether their records reflect acceptable academic progress or the possibility of a problem
3. Investigate and manage the remediation of any resident who is not meeting the program standards

Optimal functioning of the committee requires members who have skills in and a commitment to accurate evaluation of residents. These committee members should receive training in evaluation biases (discussed later in this chapter) as well as in effective strategies and institutional policies for dealing with problem residents. In small residency programs that are subspecialties of larger residency programs (e.g., plastic surgery as a subspecialty of general surgery) and fellowship programs, the clinical competency committee that establishes formal performance standards and reviews resident evaluations may be composed of the entire teaching faculty. When this is the case it may be helpful to use competency committee of the parent residency program to assist in the investigation and remediation of trainees with problems.

Program directors should also take steps to develop a relationship with the institutional attorney responsible for handling academic and disciplinary actions before a problem resident crisis emerges. It is as beneficial for her to understand your approach to competency assessment as it is for you to understand her approach to protecting the institution and its faculty from legal issues resulting from the management of problem residents. Together, the institutional attorney and the program director should document the policies and procedures that will be followed in the evaluation and management of residents who fail to meet program standards.

Systematic Approach to Evaluating and Remediating Problem Residents

Recognizing Clues That a Problem Might Exist

Concern about a resident's performance may surface in many ways. More than three quarters of program directors responding to Yao's survey on problem residents stated that the majority of problems are identified because of substandard performance in the clinical setting. Sixty percent of program directors identified problem residents because of critical incidents, such as a patient complaint about unprofessional behavior or a witnessed temper lapse in a clinical environment. Poor performance in conferences, particularly morning report, was another common way in which program directors recognized the presence of a problem. The observation that a resident is always too busy to attend conference or can never complete work on time to meet work hours restrictions should also raise concerns about a possible problem.

The way in which program directors become aware of these performance deficiencies is interesting. Although 74% of program directors commonly identified problem residents because of verbal complaints from faculty, only 31% of the same group identified problem residents using written evaluations from faculty. Problem residents rarely volunteer that they are not meeting performance standards, although they may admit to life stressors that are significant enough to cause difficulty with work.[1]

It can be surprisingly difficult to identify the presence of a problem. Although evaluation and feedback are essential functions of an educator, inter-rater reliability for faculty evaluations of residents can be extremely poor. Many faculty physicians take their responsibility as evaluators very seriously and are careful to provide and document thoughtful feedback to all residents. These faculty members recognize that early identification of a performance deficiency may allow corrective action that protects the resident from failure and patients from harm. Other faculty members are less skilled in, confident about, or committed to accurate observation and feedback and thus fall prey to common evaluation errors: range restriction and halo effect. Range restriction describes the tendency for faculty to only use a limited portion of the evaluation scale. When the faculty restrict their rating to the higher end of the scale (often the highest three

numbers on a 9-point Likert scale) while completing evaluations, this leads to the "Lake Wobegon effect"—all residents are above average. Faculty who are less attentive in their evaluation role may exhibit the halo effect, rating a resident's competency in all domains as equally strong (or weak) as their dominant performance behavior. For example, a faculty member who accurately assesses a resident's professionalism and communication skills as superior is operating under the halo effect if he also rates the resident's knowledge as superior when it more truthfully would be described as marginal. Physician raters who are uncertain about the validity of their assessment, either because they are unsure about expectations or because they feel that their assigned time with the learner was too short to draw accurate conclusions, tend to err on the side of rating a resident as satisfactory or superior even if they believe their performance is lacking.

Other physicians avoid providing negative feedback because of concerns that the feedback may have adverse consequences on either the learner or themselves. Some may not know how to deliver negative or corrective feedback in a manner that doesn't harm their relationship with the resident. Concern about how negative feedback will be used by the program may lead some faculty physicians to verbally express reservations about a resident's performance to the program director and then turn in a satisfactory or superior evaluation of the same resident. Because of this common problem, program directors who receive any verbal complaints about residents from faculty should personally document these complaints in writing in a memo to the resident's file. These concern memos should be filed in a location easily accessible to the resident in question. Many electronic evaluation systems allow for spontaneous concern or praise cards to be filed; this may be an ideal location for these memos to be housed. A copy can also be provided to the involved faculty member for review and affirmation. Finally, faculty whose promotions or teaching awards depend on strong learner evaluations may fear that residents will retaliate if they are given less than superior ratings. Box 13-2 summarizes reasons why faculty physicians are often reluctant to document problems. Given these common evaluation problems, it is not surprising that problem residents may have

BOX 13-2	**Frequently Cited Reasons for Faculty Reluctance to Document Problems**

Lack of contact with residents ("I didn't see them enough to really get to know them.")

Lack of knowledge or disagreement with current program expectations ("I don't know what interns today are supposed to learn.")

Concern about loss of resident advocacy role ("I don't want to be viewed as the bad guy.")

Concern about how a negative evaluation will be used ("I don't want to get the resident fired.")

Fear of retaliation from the resident ("There goes my teaching award.")

an evaluation file that has a wide range of evaluations, from unsatisfactory to superior. Unfortunately, 60% of the program directors surveyed by Yao observed that the presence of this discrepancy in evaluations may make it difficult for the program director to convince a learner that a problem truly exists.[1]

Program directors should be aware of these evaluation biases and must take steps to ensure that the evaluation file accurately reflects the resident's true level of competency. The program director should periodically review all evaluations in a resident's file and write an analysis of each resident's performance, interpreting faculty evaluations according to program performance standards and with an understanding of individual faculty evaluation biases and trends. If the mean score for a resident in your program is an 8 (superior) on a 9-point Likert scale, then a resident who is receiving scores of 5 may be in trouble, despite the use of a scale which labels a score of 5 as satisfactory. Both the raw data and the program director's analysis of evaluations should be submitted to the clinical competency committee for their periodic review and assessment.

Given the tendency for rating inflation that exists in most programs, the program director and clinical competency committee should at least consider the possibility that a problem exists in any resident who receives even a single substandard evaluation. In assessing resident files, the committee and the hospital attorney must understand that competency is not a weighted balance of all submitted evaluations. Residents must meet a minimal threshold in all competency domains and in all care arenas to achieve a satisfactory rating. They cannot compensate for a serious deficiency in one or more domain(s) by performing particularly well in the others. A resident who excels in the intensive care unit but fails in the ambulatory environment cannot be considered satisfactory even if he never intends to practice in the outpatient setting. Similarly, one cannot overlook unprofessional behavior in a resident because she is brilliant. A resident who has received excellent ratings for the first 2 years of her residency and then turns in substandard performance during her third year cannot be considered satisfactory simply because the number of positive evaluations exceeds the number of negative evaluations.

Investigating the Extent and Possible Causes of a Problem

Once a program director suspects the existence of a problem, she/he should undertake an investigation to fully describe the nature and severity of the problem and to identify any secondary problems that may be contributing to suboptimal performance. Categorizing performance problems as cognitive (knowledge, judgment, clinical problem solving), noncognitive (interpersonal skills, attitudes, and professional behavior) and technical (psychomotor skills common to procedural specialties) can help program directors identify appropriate strategies for further investigation and remediation. When confronted with an apparent problem in a single arena,

it is prudent to initially consider that problems may exist in all categories. It is not unusual for a resident to use inappropriate behavior to mask knowledge deficits.

Investigation of a potential problem resident may necessitate the use of tools not usually employed in the day-to-day evaluation of the resident who is progressing in a satisfactory fashion. If concerns are raised about a resident's judgment or knowledge, a focused review of that resident's patient care records may provide more information. Chart-stimulated recall (CSR), whereby the resident is asked to elaborate on or justify decisions based on his or her chart documentation may help to confirm a cognitive deficiency and may simultaneously convince the resident that there is a problem. Alternatively, CSR may reveal that the resident's knowledge is sound but that documentation and communication practices are questionable. Concerns about professional behavior or interpersonal skills and communication might prompt the program to ask for feedback from more nursing professionals or even resident patients. Videotaped encounters with standardized patients may provide insight into communication or problem-solving difficulties. Arranging a rotation with the program's "gold standard faculty member" (a physician known to have excellent observation, evaluation, and feedback skills) can be useful. Other tools are listed in Table 13-1.

Table 13-1 Additional Evaluation Tools to Investigate the Resident with a Potential Problem

Concerns Raised About Competency in This Domain	Additional Tools to Further Investigate
Medical knowledge	Chart-stimulated recall Structured case-based discussions or other oral examinations Written tests
Patient care	Gold standard faculty evaluator Chart review Chart-stimulated recall Standardized patient encounters Performance on simulators
Interpersonal skills and communication	360° evaluations (multisource feedback from patients, peers, nursing personnel) Standardized patient encounters
Professionalism	360° evaluations (multisource feedback from patients, peers, nursing personnel) Standardized patient encounters
Systems-based practice	360° evaluations (multisource feedback from patients, peers, nursing personnel) Review of discharge planning activities Standardized patient encounters
Practice-based learning and improvement	Learning logs Mandatory literature searches Assigned conference presentations

BOX 13-3	Common Secondary Issues Complicating Resident Problems: The 7 Ds

Distraction: family concerns
Sleep **d**eprivation (sleep, relationship)
Depression and other affective disorders
Drugs and alcohol
Disease (acute or chronic medical illness)
Learning **d**isabilities (learning disorders and attention deficit/hyperactivity disorders)
Personality **d**isorders

Once a resident is identified as having a problem, it is essential to consider whether a secondary issue might be contributing to the situation. Common secondary issues impacting performance in residents are listed in Box 13-3 as the 7 Ds. The *distractions* of balancing work and life as a resident may cause problems in learning and meeting new professional responsibilities. The normal developmental challenges which occur at the end of formal education and the beginning of a career must be dealt with in the setting of a job with life and death responsibility. Young physicians who have moved to a new city may have a tenuous support structure. Some are managing their own finances for the first time. Others will have new spouses or children. Aging or ill parents may also become an issue during this phase of life. *Sleep deprivation* as a secondary cause of poor performance will hopefully decline in prevalence given the recent restrictions on workload and work hours. *Depression and other affective disorders* may manifest either for the first time or as a recurrent problem for as many as 30% of residents in training. Still others may begin or continue to *abuse drugs*. When surveyed, program directors estimate the prevalence of substance abuse among residents as 1%; however, simultaneous survey questionnaires of residents consistently indicate that 12% to 15% of residents either admit or meet criteria for probable or possible alcoholism.[2–6] According to

a 1991 survey of 3000 residents, the new prescriptive authority may tempt up to 10% of young physicians to self-medicate for stress with prescription opiates and benzodiazepines.[2] *Diseases*, such as diabetes or inflammatory bowel disease, may be more difficult to control with the erratic sleep and eating habits of busy residents. *Learning disabilities* (LD) or *attention deficit/hyperactivity disorder* (ADHD) may be suspected in residents who have longstanding difficulties with standardized tests or apparent problems with organizing or processing information. Table 13-2 lists common symptoms of learning disabilities and ADHD.[7,8] Approximately 5% of medical students have LD with or without ADHD; a small percentage of these students were diagnosed for the first time during medical school, generally because of difficulty with testing during the first 2 years.[9] No literature addresses the incidence or prognostic impact of newly diagnosed learning disabilities or ADHD in residents with problems. Finally, some residents truly are unsuited for the profession because of previously unrecognized major psychiatric illnesses such as *personality disorders*.

The presence of a secondary disorder does not excuse poor performance but does influence how the program addresses the performance problem. Residents with a significant secondary disorder are unlikely to benefit from remediation until the secondary disorder is brought under control. Not every resident with a performance problem requires a full evaluation for a secondary cause. Residents should be interviewed by the program director or a trusted faculty member and should be asked about distractions, acute or chronic illnesses, and signs and symptoms of depression. Program directors are cautioned that denial (the eighth D) is part of the disease of substance abuse. Thus, a resident with a sudden change in performance status or with overt signs of intoxication at work should undergo mandatory drug testing in alignment with the rules and regulations of their institution. The issue of possible learning disorders remains vexatious.

Table 13-2 Common Signs of Learning Disabilities in Physicians and Attention Deficit/Hyperactivity Disorder in Adults

Feature	Learning Disabilities*	Attention Deficit/Hyperactivity Disorder†
Working definition	Differences in the acquisition or use of information presented in oral or written format that lead to problems with reading, writing, listening, speaking, or reasoning	Symptoms of inattentiveness, restlessness, and impulsivity that affect performance and have existed since childhood
Common manifestations	Inefficient study skills
Reliance on study groups rather than reading
Poor performance on standardized tests
Strong verbal and interpersonal skills	Impaired auditory vigilance
Difficulty with executive functioning (sequencing and complex tasks)
Psychiatric comorbidity (anxiety, depression, substance abuse) is common
Less common manifestations	Difficulty with organization and sequencing activities	

*Data from Guyer BP, Guyer KE: Doctors with learning disabilities: Prescription for success. Learning Disabilities 2000;10(2):65–72.
†Data from Spencer T, Biederman J, Wilens TE, Faraone SV: Adults with attention-deficit/hyperactivity disorder: A controversial diagnosis. J Clin Psychiatry 1998;59(Supp 7):59–68.

Neuropsychologic testing can uncover learning disabilities and clues to the diagnosis of ADD/ADHD. Identifying such a disorder may help the resident identify alternate strategies for managing their learning and organization, allow them to seek accommodations on standardized tests, or investigate the benefits of pharmacotherapy. However, many learning disorders have caused years of problems with processing, storing, and accessing knowledge that are unlikely to be overturned quickly in the setting of a residency program.

If a secondary cause seems likely, the clinical competency committee should seek an independent evaluation of the resident's health from either another qualified physician or an institutional committee on physician health. If the resident is substantially performing her duties of patient care, learning, teaching, and supervising, the Americans with Disabilities Act states that the committee may only suggest and not mandate such an evaluation. The responsibility of the evaluating physician is fourfold:

1. To determine whether a secondary condition exists that impacts the resident's performance
2. To provide advice about whether the resident can reasonably be expected to perform his/her duties *and* continue to learn while this secondary problem is addressed or whether the resident should be placed on a leave of absence or light duty
3. To refer the resident for any needed treatment
4. To serve as a liaison between a treating physician and the program so that the program director's concerns can be relayed to the treating physician and decisions about the resident's ability to function in the usual environment can be transmitted from the treating physician to the program without interfering with the resident's confidential doctor-patient relationship

Neither the independent evaluating physician nor the treating physician should have academic evaluation responsibilities for the resident in question. Under no circumstances should program directors assume care for a resident under their authority, even if they are medically qualified to do so. If the evaluative or treating physician feels that the resident's condition is such that he cannot be expected to continue to work and learn, then the resident must be placed on either a leave of absence or offered restricted responsibilities until he is ready to assume the full responsibilities of the position. If a leave or accommodation is required, the program director should be aware that she is not entitled to know the specific diagnosis, proposed treatment, or the extent to which the resident is complying with treatment. Instead, the treating physician will provide information about the nature and duration of the accommodation (including a leave of absence) requested by the resident.

As suggested previously, the ADA provides that an employer may not mandate a medical evaluation when a disabling medical (including psychiatric) condition is suspected because to do so would be to discriminate against people with a perceived disability. This counterintuitive circumstance highlights the potential legal sensitivity in suggesting or requiring medical evaluations. A brief discussion with legal counsel should precede any action in which there is doubt about the correct course or the atmosphere has become contentious. As a practical matter, however, in most circumstances it is in the resident's best interest, as the resident recognizes, to identify a problem that, if diagnosed and treated, could result in better performance or could justify a request for accommodations. Residents who decline a suggested referral should be informed that academic evaluations will be made with the assumption that they are capable of adhering to the standards of the program without accommodation. (See the later discussion on the ADA.)

Determining the Administrative Setting of Action

If a problem requiring remediation is identified, the next step in working with a problem resident is to decide whether remediation can be accomplished while the resident remains on usual duty. To make this decision, the clinical competency committee must consider several constituencies—the resident, patients, students and junior colleagues, and the program. Box 13-4 outlines a series of questions for the committee to consider. If the answer to any of these questions is no, then the resident must be removed from usual duty and offered either restricted responsibilities or a leave of absence.

Patient safety must be paramount. The committee will need to decide whether this resident's deficiencies are serious enough to raise doubts about his ability to safely manage patients given the degree of autonomy usually afforded residents at his level. Even new interns are asked to function independently when called by a nurse about an ill patient. A resident with knowledge or judgment deficiencies who reliably calls for help may be able to remain in a monitored position. One who fails to appreciate his limitations may need to be removed from a clinical care rotation.

The integrity of the learning process must be maintained. Students and interns routinely depend on more senior colleagues for much of their clinical learning. A resident who is struggling may not be able to dedicate time to teaching or may convey false information.

The residents must be capable not only of work but of continued learning. Residency is a time-limited experience during which the resident must master a vast

BOX 13-4	Critical Questions to Decide on the Administrative Setting of Action

Will patients be safe with this resident?
Will students and junior colleagues learn from this resident?
Is the resident capable of continuing to learn while on this rotation?
Will the morale and standards of this program be maintained if this resident remains on duty?

amount of information and critical skills. When considering return to work issues for residents with medical illnesses, it is important to remember that the resident must have recovered sufficiently to tolerate a full work day along with the studying necessary to continue to make progress toward full competency. In addition, the feasibility of remediation while working in the clinical environment should be considered. A resident with significant cognitive deficits may be set up to fail at attempted remediation if he is assigned to busy ward rotations that do not allow time for studying.

Finally, occasionally the problems presented by residents are so egregious or public that the program directors must consider the morale and standards of their program when deciding on an administrative setting of action. Confidentiality between the program director and individual learners often precludes an open discussion of the resident's behavior with the program's other residents. If the presence of the problem resident is visibly disruptive to the program, a leave of absence may be required while the situation is further investigated.

If one of the above conditions cannot be met, the options for the program include a leave of absence or reduced duty. Leaves of absence can be useful to residents who need time to recover from a medical illness, resolve family stressors, reconsider a career choice, or undergo intensive remediation for a knowledge deficiency or learning disability. Leaves of absence should be time-limited and monitored. Conditions for return to duty should be explicitly identified at the start of the leave. Consequences of failure to meet those conditions should also be articulated at that time (e.g., if you are unable to meet the conditions for returning to duty by the end of your leave, you will be referred for dismissal). A mechanism for financial support during the leave of absence must be identified.

Reduced duty or assignment to a nonpatient care month is another option. Reduced duty may be helpful for residents who do not have a medical condition that would allow them to use sick leave or disability leave and therefore need to have a mechanism for maintaining their salary. Before initiating a reduced duty program, the committee should decide whether this reduced duty will count toward training time. It is important that residents not be rewarded for poor performance by being assigned less call! Strategies whereby required rotations are delayed until after remediation or whereby the resident continues to receive pay for reduced duty but is required to extend training time to make up the reduced duty are possibilities.

Developing an Appropriate Educational Corrective Action Plan

The clinical competency committee should be responsible for developing an educational corrective action plan (ECAP) for each problem resident. The ECAP is a professional development plan designed to help the resident correct his/her deficiencies. The goal of

such a plan is to move the resident to a spot on the clinical competency curve where usual training can be expected to be successful. *A good ECAP is time-limited, faculty mentored, targeted to the resident's specific deficiencies, and documented in writing.* The clinical competency committee should be charged not only with establishing the ECAP but also with monitoring the progress of the plan and deciding whether any noted improvement is sufficient for the resident to reenter normal training. It is crucially important that the ECAP describe the consequences if the resident fails to demonstrate sufficient improvement during the action plan. Although all residents assigned to an ECAP should have a faculty mentor, it should be explicitly stated that the role of the faculty is to assist the resident and that it is solely the resident's responsibility to improve.

In developing the ECAP, a hierarchy of issues is apparent for both efficiency and effectiveness. First, the committee should strive to make sure that any secondary issues are adequately resolved. Attempting to remediate cognitive difficulties in a resident with severe depression is not likely to be successful and thus is unfair to both the resident and their faculty mentor. Second, substantial professionalism issues should be addressed. If the resident is unable or unwilling to embrace the professional values and standards for behavior, it doesn't matter whether the remediation of cognitive skills is successful. Finally, once secondary and professionalism issues have been resolved or dealt with, then the program can focus on substantial cognitive and technical skill issues.

Two types of ECAP exist and differ in content and impact. We have chosen to use the nomenclature of remediation and probation to differentiate between these categories. *Remediation* is the term used for a program of intensive tutoring that is designed to help the resident improve knowledge and skills. *Probation* is the term chosen for ECAPs wherein the primary intervention is to clearly warn a resident that behavior is wrong and must be stopped. Table 13-3 summarizes the important differences between remediation and probationary ECAPs. Some programs use the term *remediation* to signify an administrative action that is less severe than probation, but in this chapter the two terms represent entirely different types of ECAPs of equal significance.

Faculty mentors are key elements in both types of corrective action plans. The ideal mentor will have strong skills in teaching and evaluation as well as time to meet regularly with the resident. The assigned mentor should be apprised of the nature of the resident's difficulties and the nature of the educational action plan. The mentor should prepare a report of the resident's performance during the intervention period for the clinical competency committee. If the ideal mentor is a member of the clinical competency committee, he should not vote on the final outcome of the resident's case.

Remediation is program mentoring designed to help the resident improve his/her skills. It is appropriate for

Table 13-3 Educational Corrective Action Plans: Remediation versus Probation

Consideration	Remediation	Probation
Definition	Program mentoring to help the resident improve	Program warning that the behavior is wrong
Appropriate deficiencies	Fund of knowledge, clinical judgment, technical skills, suboptimal but not inappropriate communication/behavior	Unmet professional responsibilities or inappropriate communication/behavior
Goal	Improvement in deficient areas	Cessation of inappropriate behavior
Faculty role	Tutors/mentors	Standard setters/mentors
Timing of improvement	Gradual and self-sustaining	Immediate and self-sustaining
Reportable to future authorities?*	Possibly	Probably
Next step if insufficient improvement	Extended remediation and training; dismissal/contract nonrenewal	Dismissal/contract nonrenewal

*Virtually all requests for verification ask about probationary periods; some more broadly inquire about any alteration in usual training.

deficiencies in fund of knowledge, judgment, clinical skills, technical skills, and behavior that could be classified as quirky or ineffective but not professionally inappropriate. Remediation programs help these residents gradually improve their skills. The role of the faculty member in such a program is that of a tutor. Remediation programs typically involve assigned readings and weekly case reviews with questioning by senior faculty. Programs may assign problem residents to co-manage a team with a resident with superior clinical and teaching skills or may ask chief residents to shadow them on rounds. The duration of a remediation program must be fixed—residents cannot expect to be tutored for the duration of a residency. At some point, they must demonstrate that they have internalized the necessary skills to be able to complete their training in a usual fashion without intense help.

Probation is a program warning that the behavior exhibited by the resident is wrong and must stop. It is appropriate for noncognitive issues such as unmet professional responsibility or inappropriate behavior, communication, or relationships. In contrast to a remediation program in which improvement in knowledge or skills must occur gradually, the goal of a probationary program is to have the resident cease the objectionable behavior immediately. In this setting, faculty function not as tutors but as professional standard setters, reminding the resident of his responsibilities and helping him to identify strategies to overcome disruptive impulses. Residents with noncognitive problems may benefit from referrals for anger management or self-control, tutorials in empathic listening, and instruction in conflict resolution or negotiation skills. The duration of a probationary period is more open ended than a remediation program. The resident on probation can expect to be under intense scrutiny for some period. However, continued surveillance after the probationary program is necessary to ensure that the resident truly internalized the necessary changes and can continue meeting standards after the period of intense surveillance has ended.

The labels of remediation and probation may have different implications for reporting to future employers and licensing or regulatory agencies. Requests for verification of training or letters of recommendation from these organizations almost always contain a question about whether a resident was on probation. Thus, a resident assigned to probation for an ECAP will need to answer affirmatively to that question on all future inquiries. Although residents who have undergone remediation will not have to answer yes to a question regarding probation, they would have to answer yes to a question about irregular training. This differential treatment of the individual with cognitive versus one with noncognitive deficiencies seems logical. It is relatively easy to assess whether a career-threatening knowledge deficiency has been corrected. Each specialty's certifying examination functions as the ultimate confirmation of adequate knowledge base. A physician who fully meets the profession's cognitive standards should not be branded for life as a problem physician simply because he required a period of tutoring early in his career. It is more difficult to confidently attest that a significant deficiency in professionalism has been corrected. Satisfactory behavior during a monitored probationary period does not mean that the individual will maintain professional behavior without that scrutiny. Because of this uncertainty, it may be more reasonable for residents with substantial professionalism problems during their residency to be subjected to more intense scrutiny by future employers and agencies. Indeed, recent literature documents those students with professionalism problems during medical school were statistically much more likely to be subject to subsequent disciplinary actions by state medical boards later in their careers.[10] Students whose academic records contained multiple faculty comments about irresponsibility were eight times as likely to be subject to state medical board discipline later in their careers as were matched peers. State board action was three times as likely to occur in students who were considered to demonstrate poor efforts toward self-improvement.

Evaluating the Outcome of the Educational Corrective Action Plan

An ECAP can be considered successful if the resident has demonstrated sufficient and *self-sustaining* improvement in the deficient areas. Residents on probation for noncognitive issues should demonstrate full correction of the behavioral or communications problems that led to probation. They should also understand that there will be a zero tolerance approach for future professionalism breaches. That is, any repeat of unprofessional behavior should result in the resident moving to the step beyond probation (typically dismissal), even if it occurs after the formal probationary period has ended. Figure 13-2 presents a graphic schematic for assessing the improvement of a resident on cognitive remediation. The ideal outcome of an ECAP is to move the resident from point X to point E on the competency curve—this indicates that the resident has corrected his deficiency and has caught up with his peers. Movement from X to D, although positive, still means that the resident is behind his peers. If the lag in competency is estimated to be less than 6 months, the resident on this type of trajectory may benefit from a short extension of training. Movement from X to F means that the resident has not been able to take steps toward correcting the deficiency and is likely to always remain below the expected level of competency.

For residents who demonstrate some but not sufficient improvement, two options exist. If the resident was unable to adequately correct the deficiencies despite a program's maximal educational efforts, the program should dismiss the resident from the program or refuse to renew his contract at the end of the year of training. Alternatively, the program could decide to offer the resident an extension in training to see whether continued or accelerated improvement is noted. The decision to extend an individual's training

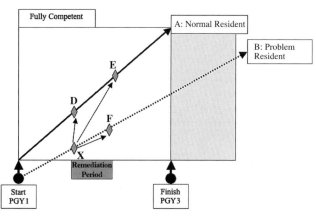

Figure 13-2 The clinical competency curve: necessary and sufficient improvement. Curve A represents the normal resident, curve C the problem resident. The ideal remediation outcome is a move from point X to point E: this resident has corrected any deficiencies and has caught up with his peers, who have continued to demonstrate growth during the period of the remediation. Movement from point X to point D shows improvement but the resident is behind his peers. Movement from point X to point F shows no change in the rate of growth in skills.

means added expense for the program and may require the program to apply for a temporary increase in resident complement from their residency review committee (RRC). If an extension of training is chosen, the duration of the extension should be clearly defined and the program should continue the resident on remediation or probation with the explicit understanding that if the resident does not improve sufficiently, he will then be dismissed or be subject to contract nonrenewal. One of the most common mistakes made by programs dealing with problem residents is failure to act decisively and discharge a resident who fails to demonstrate sufficient improvement after two remediation periods.

When remediation programs are unsuccessful and residents must be dismissed, there is a tendency for faculty members to view the unsuccessful remediation as a personal or program failure. In reality, they should realize that their obligations to the learner have been fulfilled through their attempts to help the resident overcome the performance deficiencies. It is possible that the resident who has not succeeded in their program may be more successful in another program, another discipline, or another career. More important, the program has also fulfilled their obligations to the profession and society by accurately identifying and removing a physician who was unable to meet program standards.

Attending to Legal and Due Process Issues

Legal Concepts in Academic Due Process

> . . . Courts are not supposed to be learned in medicine and are not qualified to pass opinions as to the attainments of a student in medicine.
> (*Connelly v. University of Vermont*, 244 F. Supp. 156, 161–62 (D. Vt. 1965)

Program directors and institutions often cite fear of legal repercussions as a reason for avoiding adverse actions in residents who are not performing well. Forty-nine percent of program directors surveyed by Yao and Wright received threats of legal action resulting from their dealings with problem residents; 15% of responding program directors were actually involved in lawsuits.[1] In actuality, academic due process has standards that are relatively easy for programs to meet. Courts have consistently shown their willingness to defer to the judgments of faculty who have made decisions about academic progress in a fair and understandable manner. Programs will prevail in courts of law if they:

- Have clear standards
- Notify residents of their deficiencies and the consequences of failure to correct these deficiencies
- Provide the resident with the opportunity to discuss and then correct their deficiencies
- Maintain clear written records

Routine consultation with your institutional attorney can help avert a crisis by ensuring that a program's evaluation process meets the standards of academic due process.

Courts, including the United States Supreme Court, have repeatedly applied the principle of judicial nonintervention when dealing with issues of grading, promotion, and the granting of academic degrees or professional titles. In *Board of Curators of the University of Missouri v. Horowitz*, 435 U.S. 78 (1978), the Supreme Court defined the essentials of due process for academic decisions. In *Regents of the University of Michigan v. Ewing*, 474 U.S. 214 (1985), the Court defined the narrow scope of review that due process requires of the substance of an academic decision. Scores of judicial decisions in federal and state courts throughout the United States apply and reaffirm the principles of *Horowitz* and *Ewing*. The Supreme Court cases involved medical students, but their principles apply with equal force to residents and fellows in training programs. A resident holds the dual status of *both* employee *and* student. Numerous judicial decisions hold that in the domain of academic evaluation a resident is a student and that a faculty has the right to make decisions such as contract nonrenewal, extension of training, or dismissal when a resident fails to meet program performance standards.

The courts will not reverse academic decisions if the following elements of academic due process defined by *Horowitz* and *Ewing* are met:

- The resident must be notified (preferably in writing) of the nature of the problem and its potential impact on his/her career.
- The resident must be given the opportunity to review the concerns and respond to those concerns. A meeting with the program director or with the clinical competency committee will satisfy this requirement.
- The decision to take adverse action must not be arbitrary or capricious. That is "such a substantial departure from accepted academic norms as to demonstrate that the person or committee responsible did not actually exercise professional judgment" *Ewing* at 214.

The specifics of the notification and the type of discussion necessary depend on whether the deficiency is an academic or disciplinary/misconduct issue. Table 13-4 compares the nature and the implications of

academic versus *disciplinary* issues with regards to due process rights. The definition of *academic* covers broad territory. Recognizing the need for a higher standard of decorum and appearance in professionals, the courts have supported the concept that not only cognitive issues but also behavioral/noncognitive issues (problems with personal hygiene, timeliness, abrasive behavior, and disrespect) can constitute academic deficiencies for the purposes of due process. (See, for example, *Horowitz* at 91, n.6; and *Stretton v. Wadsworth Veterans Hospital*, 537 F.2d 361, 368 [9th Cir. 1976]).

It is equally important to understand what elements are *not* required to satisfy *academic* due process standards. In essence, *residents are considered incompetent until judged by the profession to be competent*. Arguments about the resident's competence by individuals outside the medical field (i.e., lawyers) or by physicians who have not supervised the resident are not likely to overcome a program's conclusion that the resident does not meet professional standards. Thus, there is no requirement for a full adversarial hearing or inclusion of lawyers *unless required by your institution's contract*. There is no requirement to prove that patients would be harmed if the resident continues in the program. A reasonable concern that the resident might harm a patient is sufficient. There is also no requirement to prove that other residents have been subjected to similar actions. Programs must document only that the resident's record was reviewed in its entirety and that the resident did not meet performance standards. The burden of proof in disputed cases lies with the resident, who must prove that the program acted in an arbitrary or capricious manner in their assessment of his competency. As the Supreme Court stated in *Ewing*:

> When judges are asked to review the substance of a genuinely academic decision ... they should show great respect for the faculty's professional judgment. Plainly, they may not override it unless it is such a substantial departure from accepted academic norms as to demonstrate that the person or committee responsible did not actually exercise professional judgment.
> (*Ewing* at 223.)

Disciplinary due process standards apply if the resident exhibits behavior that breaks the rules of society as well as the profession. Examples include assault or

Table 13-4 Academic Versus Disciplinary Due Process Standards

Feature	Academic	Disciplinary
Application	Profession's standards for cognitive and noncognitive behavior	Society's standards for behavior of all citizens
Examples	Insufficient knowledge; poor interpersonal relationships; inappropriate professional demeanor	Stealing, assault
Judge	Only experts in the profession can judge whether someone meets the standards of the profession	Nonexperts could reasonably debate the facts of the situation
Burden of proof	On the resident, to show that the adverse decision was made in an arbitrary or capricious nature; the resident is assumed to be incompetent until the profession judges him to be competent	On the prosecutor to prove that the individual is guilty: "innocent until proven guilty"

theft. For disciplinary issues, a person outside the medical profession could reasonably dispute the facts of the matter; thus, in these circumstances, the resident is considered innocent until proved guilty. The burden rests with the institution to ensure that the alleged facts are true and that the punishment fits the crime. The requirements for due process in this case are much stricter. Involve institutional counsel immediately if a disciplinary issue has arisen. When resident conduct may justify both academic and disciplinary action, it may be appropriate to proceed on both pathways simultaneously. The outcome of the disciplinary proceeding should not govern the outcome of the academic evaluation. For example, a resident who is observed to strike a colleague while under the influence of alcohol may be successful in avoiding legal sanctions but could still be subject to academic sanctions.

Appeals of Adverse Actions

Though not required by law, many institutions provide residents who are subjected to adverse academic actions access to an appeal process. Program directors are advised to review the language in their institution's due process policy to make sure that it is not unduly burdensome. Residents should not be able to appeal the imposition of an educational corrective action plan that does not substantially impact the length of their training. A reasonable appeal process for a decision that a resident was academically deficient can be review of the matter by an academic officer outside the individual's training program such as a dean or the designated institutional official in an office of graduate medical education. The individual performing the review should have a clear understanding of evaluation processes, performance standards, and resident due process. An adversarial hearing is not required at an appeal stage. Residents who are afforded an appeal by a committee external to their discipline should be restricted to appealing the proposed action on the basis of due process issues only, because physicians outside a resident's discipline should not be able to dispute the program's judgment that a resident does not meet their performance standards.

Documentation to Prevent Legal Problems

Defense of academic adverse actions is easier when documentation of the process is complete. In addition to standard evaluations, the problem resident's file should include memos detailing any verbal complaints received from faculty, patients, or other involved parties about the resident; minutes from the clinical competency meetings at which the resident was discussed; and any evaluations received from outside experts.

A common concern when dealing with residents with problems is how to manage inconsistencies in the resident's performance record. The courts have upheld the authority of an individual charged with making the final academic decision to give a resident an overall failing grade when only a fraction of the resident's faculty evaluations were unsatisfactory (*Stoller v. College of Medicine*, 562 F. Supp. 403, 412–13 [M.D. Pa. 1983]). The program director and the clinical competency committee should document that the decision to initiate an educational corrective action plan was prompted *by a thorough review of the resident's evaluation file* and that the negative evaluations, though rare, represent a significant deviation from the program's standards.

Any resident subjected to an educational corrective action plan should receive a formal letter from the clinical competency committee including the following essential elements:

- A statement that the clinical competency committee has reviewed the resident's performance record in its entirety and has decided that he is failing to meet program standards in one or more of the ACGME domains
- A brief description of any critical incidents
- A brief description of the outcome of any evaluations for secondary problems
- A statement that the resident was given the opportunity to hear and offer his opinions regarding these concerns
- A description of the name, nature, and duration of the proposed educational corrective action plan, including the identified administrative setting of action
- The name of the faculty mentor
- The level of improvement that signifies successful completion of the corrective action plan
- A list of specific consequences for failing to demonstrate sufficient improvement, including extension of training, contract nonrenewal, or dismissal
- A statement affirming that the intent of this educational corrective action plan is to help the resident meet competency standards but that it is solely the responsibility of the resident to demonstrate sufficient improvement

Your institutional attorney may request that you provide her with a copy of the letter for review prior to giving the letter to the resident. Residents should sign and date the letter indicating receipt (though not necessarily agreement). Whether or not the resident signs the letter, a copy of the signed document should be placed in the resident's evaluation file.

Special Circumstances

The Americans with Disabilities Act

When dealing with residents with disorders such as learning disabilities, psychiatric or physical illness, questions about the impact of the Americans with Disabilities Act (ADA) on decisions to remediate or dismiss the resident are common. The ADA was designed to prevent discrimination against disabled individuals who are otherwise qualified for a position. "Otherwise qualified" means that they can perform the essential functions of the position with or without reasonable accommodation.

The ADA does not require programs to change their standards regarding the essential functions of a trainee. The essential functions of a trainee in most programs are to provide care to a panel of patients and to share in call during nights and weekends. Thus, requests to permanently remove a resident from required call rotations or assign him a reduced number of patients may be denied as not consistent with the essential function of the job. Similarly, programs may deny a proposed accommodation if it would lower academic standards, require an unreasonably large financial expenditure by the program, or alter the nature of training. Long-term changes in work hours that disrupt the schedules of other residents may not be considered reasonable. Reasonable accommodations include a leave of absence or a limited time of reduced duty. For learning disabled students and residents, extra time on multiple-choice tests is a reasonable accommodation. Finally, *residents seeking protection under the ADA must proactively request accommodations* and establish with reasonable medical documentation that they have a disability warranting accommodation. An accommodation may enable a resident to meet the performance standards of the program. But an accommodation should never lower program standards or excuse poor performance. The nature of the disability should be disclosed within the program only to the extent necessary to permit appropriate accommodation. Seek advice from your attorney if you are dealing with a resident for whom ADA protections may be invoked.

Alleged Sexual Harassment

Many institutions require all investigation of sexual harassment allegations to be referred to their human resource (HR) system. There are established protocols for these difficult investigations. Do not investigate such allegations yourself but contact your human resources attorney. A determination that sexual harassment has occurred may also have implications for core competencies such as professionalism. In that case it may be appropriate for the program to implement an educational corrective action plan in addition to whatever action the HR department imposes. For example, the residency program may recommend counseling and monitoring while the HR department invokes a warning or a suspension. If the action recommended by the HR department is more severe (e.g., termination) than that recommended by the training program, the decision of the HR department generally supersedes that of the residency program.

Adherence to Contracts

This chapter has summarized case law relevant to students, residents, and fellows failing to meet program expectations. As mentioned earlier, due process requirements for academic actions can be easily satisfied with nonadversarial meetings that do not include attorneys. However, many institutions have written resident contracts or personnel policies that fail to distinguish between a resident's status as a student and a resident's status as an employee. Academic judgments in medical training are not governed by labor law *unless* the institution so elects in its contracts either by inattention or by choice. Program directors should review their resident contract and any institutional policies on due process to make sure that they are not needlessly burdensome for academic evaluations. But if the institution's contract differs from the principles that this chapter outlines, the institution's contract controls, unless changed.

The Aftermath of Adverse Actions: Responding to Outside Requests for Verification of Training and Competency

Many states now mandate that program directors respond under penalty of perjury to inquiries from licensing boards and hospital credentialing committees about former residents. The program director should be in possession of a signed release from a resident prior to providing information to any requesting body. It is important to clearly identify the question they are asking and compare that to the action plan you used to deal with that resident. Answer the specific question honestly but succinctly. A question of whether the resident was ever on probation must be answered affirmatively if the resident was on probation but may be answered negatively if the resident was in a remediation program. The current practice of many regulatory bodies is to ask very broad questions such as, "Has this resident ever required anything other than usual training to complete his/her residency?" In these situations, it is important to honestly acknowledge the remediation or probation period and summarize its outcome, particularly noting any supportive data. Examples of honest and succinct responses include the following:

Dr. X required a 3-month remediation period for cognitive deficiencies during the second year of his residency program. Subsequent to that, he was able to successfully meet all program expectations and pass the ABIM certifying exam.

Dr. Y was placed on probation during his PGY-1 year for recurrent unexplained absences. This occurred during a family crisis. Since that time, his performance in all domains, including professionalism, has been exemplary and he was allowed to sit for the ABIM certifying exam.

Dr. Z was placed on probation during his PGY-2 year for unmet professional responsibilities. Despite counseling and remediation, he was unable to meet our program expectations and his contract was not renewed.

If a resident was successful in completing a remediation or probationary period, it is unlikely that acknowledgment of such a program on a licensing application will prevent him/her from being licensed or receiving hospital privileges. Problems arise when there is a discrepancy between information provided by the program (the resident was on probation) and information

Table 13-5 Comparative Educational Corrective Action Plans

Description	Cognitive		Noncognitive		
	Knowledge and Clinical Skills	Ineffective Interpersonal Relationships	Inappropriate Interpersonal Relationships	Unmet Professional Responsibility	Crimes
Examples	Deficiencies in Factual knowledge Clinical problem-solving skills History and physical examination skills	Tolerable but suboptimal communication or interpersonal interactions	Hostility, verbal abuse directed toward patients, colleagues or other health care professionals	Failure to accept feedback or work to improve Unexcused absences Leaving unstable patients Falsification of data	Stealing Assault Sexual harassment
Due process standards	Academic due process	Academic due process	Academic due process	Academic due process	Disciplinary
Initial educational corrective action plan	Remediation	Remediation	Probation	Probation	Investigation
Faculty role	Guidance/mentoring	Guidance/mentoring	Clarification of standards/surveillance	Clarification of standards/surveillance	Reporting only
Expected progress	Gradual but measurable and satisfactory	Gradual but measurable and satisfactory	Immediate improvement, zero tolerance for further misbehavior	Immediate improvement, zero tolerance for further misbehavior	Immediate improvement, zero tolerance for further misbehavior
Outcome if corrective action plan is unsuccessful	Extension of training Dismissal	Extension of training Dismissal	Dismissal	Dismissal	Dismissal

provided by the applicant ("I was never the recipient of adverse actions"). Prior to leaving a program, the resident should be informed of how the program will respond to inquiries and should be counseled on how he should respond to questions of this nature.

Candid, accurate evaluations are one of the fundamental purposes of a training program. Timely negative evaluations from faculty serve everyone's interest. Similarly, communication of the program's evaluations to third parties is also fundamental. The law provides incentives for providing accurate evaluations and sanctions for providing inaccurate ones. As of the end of 2005, 38 states had enacted statutes providing immunity or other protections for employers who provided accurate references. Under those statutes and the common law, someone who provides an inaccurate favorable evaluation can be liable to someone who relied on the evaluation and was damaged. See *Singer v. Beach Trading Co., Inc.*, 379 N.J. Super. Ct. 63, 876 A.2d 885 (2005); *Passmore v. Multi-Management Services, Inc.*, 810 N.E.2d 1022 (Ind. 2004).

Use of Attorneys

Following the advice outlined in this chapter and summarized in Box 13-5 will help the program avoid legal concerns. The program director should also establish a relationship with her institution's attorney before any crisis occurs. A well-timed phone call to ask for advice on handling a resident who may be the recipient of adverse action can save months of headache later.

Most lawyers want to be helpful and can be practical and constructive. A lawyer who truly *understands* your goals and standards will support them. This is true even for lawyers whose main focus is on "protecting" the hospital.

The attorney must understand that residency is an educational process, that residents are more than employees, and that the training program has clear and important goals and standards.

Abandoning standards is never in the fundamental interest of the training institution.

If the advice you receive from your attorney does not help you to support your program's standards, do not defer to their legal expertise. Instead, talk with your chief executive officer or upper management.

Conclusion

Table 13-5 summarizes the major concepts emphasized in this chapter. It is likely that all program directors will at some time work with problem residents. The willingness to identify and attempt to remediate a problem resident who needs extra help to succeed is the mark of a great resident advocate. The ability to recognize and remove a problem resident who is unable to meet the standards of our profession is a sign of a superior patient advocate and professional standard bearer. As program directors, we must embrace both roles. A systematic approach to working with residents in trouble will help all educators meet these critically important responsibilities.

ANNOTATED BIBLIOGRAPHY

1. Yao DC, Wright SM: National survey of internal medicine residency program directors regarding problem residents. JAMA 2000;284(9):1099–1104.
   This article describes the prevalence and presenting characteristics of problem residents and also examines attitudes and concerns of their program directors.
2. Papdakis MA, Teherani A, Banach MA, et al: Disciplinary action by medical boards and prior behavior in medical school. N Engl J Med 2005;353(25):2673–2682.
   This article correlates evidence of unprofessional behavior in medical school with subsequent adverse actions by state medical boards.
3. Kirk LM, Blank LL: Professional behavior: A learner's permit for licensure. N Engl J Med 2005;353(25):2709–2711.
   The editorial accompanying this article emphasizes the need for vigilance in identifying and remediating medical students whose professionalism is questioned.

Legal Issues in Dealing with Problem Residents

1. Irby DM, Milam S: The legal context for evaluating and dismissing medical students and residents. Acad Med 1989;64:639–643.
   This reference summarizes important case law that is relevant to the legal issues related to working with problem residents.
2. Losh DP, Church L: Provisions of the Americans with Disabilities Act and the development of essential job functions for family practice residents. Fam Med 1999;31(9):617–621.
   This reference describes the intent and application of the Americans with Disabilities Act for residency programs. The authors urge program directors to develop written documents outlining the essential functions of the job of residents.

Relevant Case Law Referenced in This Chapter

1. Board of Curators of the University of Missouri v. Horowitz, 435 U.S. 78 (1978). Accessed at http://caselaw.lp.findlaw.com/scripts/getcase.pl?court=us&vol=435&invol=78.
2. Connelly v. University of Vermont, 244 F. Supp. 156, 160–161 (D. Vt. 1965).
3. Regents of the University of Michigan v. Ewing, 474 U.S. 214 (1985). Accessed at http://caselaw.lp.findlaw.com/cgi-bin/getcase.pl?court=us&vol=474&invol=214.
4. Singer v. Beach Trading Co., Inc., 379 N.J. Super. Ct. 63, 876 A.2d 885 (2005). Accessed at www.peop7.com/peo/caselawDetail67086.htm.
5. Stoller v. College of Medicine, 562 F. Supp. 403, 412–13 (M.D. Pa. 1983). Accessed at www.paed.uscourts.gov/documents/opinions/98D1180P.pdf.
6. Stretton v. Wadsworth Veterans Hospital, 537 F.2d 361, 368 (9th Cir. 1976).

BOX 13-5	**Steps to Ensure Academic Due Process Standards Are Met**

Set and disseminate program standards for performance and essential functions of the resident's job

Use a committee to make decisions

Follow your institution's policies for due process

Review the record in its entirety

Notify the resident of his/her deficiencies as well as the career impact of that deficiency (extended training, dismissal, contract nonrenewal)

Allow the resident the opportunity to review the concerns and present her views about those concerns to the committee or present her views about the program director

Document everything in writing

Act decisively

7. Passmore v. Multi-Management Services, Inc., 810 N.E.2d 1022 (Ind. 2004); Accessed at www.in.gov/judiciary/opinions/archive/06290403.rts.html.

Learning Disabilities and Attention Deficit/Hyperactivity Disorder

1. Guyer BP, Guyer KE: Doctors with Learning Disabilities: Prescription for Success. Learn Disabil 2000;10(29):65–72.

   This interesting article describes the authors' work with learning disabled physicians. They describe the most common manifestations of learning disabled physicians and provide examples about useful accommodations.

2. Accardo P, Haake C, Whitman B: The learning-disabled medical student. J Dev Behav Pedatr 1989;10(5):253–258.

   This article describes the nature of learning disorders and explains why medical school may uncover learning disorders for which students had previously been able to compensate. They address counterproductive attitudes and comment on dealing with learning disabled students in medical school.

3. Spencer T, Biederman J, Wilens TE, Faraone SV: Adults with attention-deficit/hyperactivity disorder: A controversial diagnosis. J Clin Psychiatry 1998;59(Suppl 7):59–68.

   This review of the evidence of adult-onset ADHD from a behavioral and biologic perspective provides program directors with some insight into the types of behaviors that may signal the presence of ADHD.

Substance Abuse in Residents

1. Hughes PH, Conard SE, Baldin DC, et al: Resident substance use in the United States. JAMA 1991;265(16):2069–2973.

   This is the largest published survey of resident substance use. Compared with their lay peers residents are more likely to use alcohol and self-prescribed opiates and benzodiazepines but less likely to use illicit drugs. Though residents claim to be using the prescription drugs for therapeutic benefit, the authors point out that benzodiazepines and opiates are frequent causes of impairment.

2. McNamara RM, Margulies JL: Chemical dependency in emergency medicine residency programs: Perspective of program directors. Ann Emerg Med 1994;23(5):1072–1076.

3. Lewy R: Alcoholism in housestaff physicians: An occupational hazard. J Occup Med 1986;28:79–81.

4. Siegel BJ, Fitzgerald FT: A survey of the prevalence of alcoholism among the faculty and the housestaff of an academic teaching hospital. West J Med 1988;148:593–595.

5. Lutsky I, Abram SE, Jacobson GR, et al: Substance abuse by anesthesiology residents. Acad Med 1991;66:164–166.

   These four articles provide survey data on the prevalence of alcoholism and substance abuse in residents in different disciplines. Despite the different populations, a remarkably similar prevalence of self-reported substance abuse of 12% to 15% is seen. Program directors consistently underestimate the prevalence of substance abuse.

REFERENCES

1. Yao DC, Wright SM: National survey of internal medicine residency program directors regarding problem residents. JAMA 2000;284(9):1099–1104.
2. Hughes PH, Conard SE, Baldin DC, et al: Resident substance use in the United States. JAMA 1991;265(16):2069–2973.
3. McNamara RM, Margulies JL: Chemical dependency in emergency medicine residency programs: Perspective of program directors. Ann Emerg Med 1994;23(5):1072–1076.
4. Lewy R: Alcoholism in housestaff physicians: An occupational hazard. J Occup Med 1986;28:79–81.
5. Siegel BJ, Fitzgerald FT: A survey of the prevalence of alcoholism among the faculty and the housestaff of an academic teaching hospital. West J Med 1988;148:593–595.
6. Lutsky I, Abram SE, Jacobson GR, et al: Substance abuse by anesthesiology residents. Acad Med 1991;66:164–166.
7. Spencer T, Biederman J, Wilens TE, Faraone SV: Adults with attention-deficit/hyperactivity disorder: A controversial diagnosis. J Clin Psychiatry 1998;59(Suppl 7):59–68.
8. Guyer BP, Guyer KE: Doctors with learning disabilities: Prescription for success. Learn Disabil 2000;10(29):65–72.
9. Accardo P, Haake C, Whitman B: The learning-disabled medical student. J Dev Behav Pedatr 1989;10(5):253–258.
10. Papdakis MA, Teherani A, Banach MA, et al: Disciplinary action by medical boards and prior behavior in medical school. N Engl J Med 2005;353(25):2673–2682.

Constructing an Evaluation System for an Educational Program

Richard E. Hawkins, MD, and Eric S. Holmboe, MD

In Chapter 1, we began by discussing important changes in assessment in medical education and practice. A framework for implementing assessment programs, guidance for choosing individual assessment methods and tools, the importance of effective faculty development, and future challenges were described. Chapters 3 through 12 highlighted the strengths and weaknesses of a number of assessment methods with suggestions on how to implement such methods and related tools.* However, each assessment method must be integrated into an overall evaluation system embedded within an educational program and institution.†

This chapter will outline how educational leaders can facilitate and lead significant change in their programs and institutions through the creation of effective evaluation systems, both for the trainee and the program itself.

Challenges and Change

Introducing change in medical education programs and institutions can be a difficult process in which educational leaders confront a wide range of factors that

---

*A distinction is made between methods and tools used in assessment programs. A method is the generic process or means of gathering information about trainee competence or performance. A tool is the specific form, instrument, or device used in executing a particular method. For example, structured clinical observation is a method of observation whereby explicit direction or guidance is offered to facilitate, organize, or assure the completeness of observation. The mini-CEX is one tool that may be used to support structured clinical observation.

†Assessment and evaluation are often used interchangeably in the medical education literature. In this chapter assessment will refer to the process or means of measuring or gathering information about a trainee's (or program's) competence or performance. Evaluation will take this process a step further conceptually, representing the placement of assessment processes or outcomes in the context of educational objectives for the trainee's level. The process of evaluation involves making a judgment about the adequacy of competence or performance in comparison with educational objectives or defined competence or performance standards.

either support the need for or provide resistance to change. These factors include external trends and forces, institutional culture and values, and resource and logistical issues. External trends and forces arise from a variety of sources and may ultimately impact medical education through influencing accreditation processes. Growing demands for accountability in demonstrating educational and health outcomes as a primary measure of the quality of medical education and practice has stimulated change in many professional, clinical, and academic organizations and institutions. Increasingly, the focus of accreditation has been moving toward the demonstration of outcomes as the primary measure of education program quality. Although it is sensible to target educational and clinical outcomes as the primary measure of accountability, moving toward such an outcomes model can be difficult. In addition to methodological challenges and requirements for additional resources, any significant modification to an educational system or program is likely to confront challenges related to institutional inertia and logistical limitations. It is important for educational program leaders, as change agents, to recognize the wide range of variables involved that may facilitate or compromise their ability to be successful in introducing change in their programs.

Within educational programs, one of the elements most profoundly affected by evolving standards in accreditation is the approach to assessment of learning outcomes. That the quality of assessment processes and outcomes has become an important target for program accreditation should be no surprise to educators who understand the fundamental importance of assessment in medical education. Educators are well aware that "assessment drives learning" and understand that assessment practices have substantial influence on how trainees focus their learning priorities. Educators should recognize the potential for positive and negative effects of assessment when carefully planning or modifying their evaluation programs. They must avoid the temptation to rely simply on readily available methods, such as multiple-choice tests, which address primarily cognitive achievements. It is critically important that thoughtful development and integration of assessment approaches into our educational programs allow us to measure and reinforce not only the knowledge and skills, but also the values and behaviors, that foster achievement of the highest professional standards for performance in patient care.

The primary purpose of this chapter is to assist educational program leaders in responding to the forces influencing change in medical education, particularly in fulfilling their responsibility to the profession and the public to demonstrate the quality of their educational programs through the implementation of high-quality evaluation systems. To accomplish this purpose the chapter is divided into three parts. First the critical elements of an evaluation system are described. The second part focuses on developing and improving assessment of the individual trainee through an approach built around a structured portfolio, integrating all of the assessment methods discussed in the preceding chapters. The third part of this chapter focuses on programmatic assessment; a thorough discussion will be provided as this topic has not been specifically addressed in previous chapters.

Part 1: The Evaluation System

General Principles

An evaluation system includes a group of people who work together on a regular basis to provide evaluation and feedback to a population of trainees, from students to fellows. The human elements of an evaluation system can be considered analogous to a high functioning clinical microsystem.[1] In an effective evaluation system, members share common educational aims and outcomes, linked processes and information about trainee performance, and produce a student ready to enter residency, or a resident or fellow truly competent to enter independent medical practice at the end of training. The evaluation system has a structure (faculty, assessment methods, and resources) to carry out processes (teaching, clinical experiences, evaluation, and feedback) to produce an outcome (appropriate competence at the end of training).[2] This system must provide both summative and formative evaluation for trainees and, at a minimum, summative evaluation for the profession and public.

A systems approach provides the framework for effective evaluation (Box 14-1). The underlying assumption of the systems approach is that all components must be identified and integrated efficiently and effectively into the evaluation process. Attention must be directed toward the purpose of the evaluation, the competencies to be assessed, the evaluators, individuals to be evaluated, the settings of the evaluations, the quality of the learning environment, the timing of the evaluations, the methods used to collect and summarize the information about each trainee, and the management of information by the program.

This systems approach to evaluation optimizes the methods of collecting, acting on, and storing information

BOX 14-1	Elements of an Effective Evaluation System

Clear purpose of the evaluations
Clear definitions of the competencies to be assessed
Appropriate training and preparation of the evaluators
High-quality learning environment
Timeliness of evaluations
Reliable processes to collect, summarize, and disseminate assessment information
Transparency and trainee engagement
Efficient management of information

about trainees. A consistent, systematic process strengthens the ability of the educational leader to provide high-quality feedback and to respond to appeals by candidates over adverse judgments. In addition, this approach permits the eventual aggregation of data and feedback to clerkship and program directors about trainee problems, guides effective remediation for the problems identified, and facilitates delineation of the time frames in which improvements should occur.

Finally, a more structured evaluation system helps clerkship and program directors meet their responsibilities to the public and profession by encouraging recognition of early warning signals, facilitation of professional growth among trainees, clear decision making on the annual status of trainees, explicit documentation of problems and remedial attempts, and development of a final summary of the training and evaluation process.

Educational Leadership

Leadership in evaluation is essential. The leader of an effective evaluation system should possess several characteristics. First, the leader must be willing to do whatever he or she asks others to do (for example, take the time for direct observation and feedback of trainees). Research from the quality improvement world supports that "leading by doing" helps to promote change and give credibility to the process.[3–6] Second, leaders in an evaluation system must be knowledgeable about assessment and feedback methodologies. One of our main goals with this book is to provide practical information to educational leaders and faculty that can be used to implement an effective evaluation program. Third, the leader needs to interact collaboratively not only with other faculty and trainees but also with nurses, administrators, and other staff members responsible for comprehensive evaluations of the trainees' competence.[4] Educating all of these groups helps to promote a better assessment environment. Fourth, the leader needs to take negative evaluations seriously. Failure to do so can have substantial untoward consequences for the evaluator who had the courage to bring forth a negative evaluation and may squelch further negative evaluations from that individual as well as others in the program.

However, no single individual can manage all aspects of a successful evaluation system. Evaluation committees, often referred to as clinical competency committees in residency programs, can be effective and efficient mechanisms to detect deficiencies early, provide real-time faculty development, and promote positive changes in the evaluation culture. The collective wisdom and decision-making capacity of committees provide helpful support for educational leaders and faculty members, at times if only to provide encouragement to stand by one's convictions. In part, faculty can be insulated from making final decisions regarding trainee progress by referring ultimate decision-making authority to medical education, student promotion, or resident competency committees.

All committee members must be fully committed and not view this activity as simply another onerous task. The committee should not be a "rubber stamp" for the opinions of the department chair, clerkship director, or program director, but should collect and review meaningful evaluation information to help all trainees to progress and improve. A negative or disinterested climate on these committees, or breaches of trainee confidentiality regarding information shared at these meetings, can have a pernicious effect on the entire evaluation program.

Faculty Development

Many individuals with different qualifications and diverse roles participate in the evaluation of students and residents: clerkship and program directors, members of the evaluation committee, attending physicians who are full-time or voluntary clinical faculty, chief residents, other residents, fellows, peers, nurses, medical students, and potentially others in the education or health care environment. Evaluators should have sincere interest in their evaluative role; proper knowledge, skills, and attitudes for fulfilling the role effectively; and the time and opportunity to evaluate.

An assessment instrument or method is only as good as the individual using it. Evaluator training is absolutely essential in any effective evaluation system. Methods and tools do not magically produce an evaluation—they simply provide a means to guide, collect, and document the judgment of the evaluator about the trainee, whether it be a standardized patient (using a checklist) or a peer (completing a survey). We find it somewhat ironic that a standardized patient undergoes hours of training to provide a reliable and valid rating for a simulated patient encounter yet the faculty may receive no or little training for judging complex trainee interactions within unpredictable real patient encounters. Faculty development and support are essential to maintaining the health of the program. Faculty need to be trained to accurately appraise trainee performance and supported by program leaders when accurate evaluation leads to negative learner feedback or decisions. Accurate evaluation and feedback is, at its essence, a "willing and able" phenomenon. The ability to identify deficits must be accompanied by the willingness to report them. The techniques for helping individuals evaluate more effectively have been described throughout the book; readers are strongly encouraged to systematically incorporate faculty training in evaluation. Approaches to training faculty are described in Table 14-1.

Trainee Engagement

The evaluation system should be transparent to all of those involved in the assessment process, including the trainees. Transparency leads to an impression of fairness.[7] An explicit link with educational objectives and clear understanding of the evaluation goals and methods create an impression of fairness that is essential to acceptance of the results and incorporation of feedback. Students, residents, and fellows should clearly appreciate the dual nature of the evaluation process as it relates to the provision of feedback to encourage their continuous development as well as how it supports judgments about their progress and readiness to advance in their training. Trainees should

Table 14-1 **Methods to Train Faculty in the General Competencies**

Training Method	Rationale and Description	Example
Performance dimension training (PDT)	*Rationale*: Ratings can be improved if evaluators understand the dimensions and elements of a competency. *Description*: Familiarize faculty with appropriate performance dimensions or standards to be used in evaluation by reviewing the dimensions of a specific competency. Faculty members work in small groups to improve their understanding of these definitions with review of actual resident performance or clinical evaluation vignettes.	Faculty members discuss the elements of what constitutes an "effective utilization of resources" by a resident discharging a patient who needs physical therapy and follow-up (systems-based practice).
Frame-of-reference training (FORT)	*Rationale*: Get evaluators to share meaning and criteria of performance dimensions by teaching them how to use the evaluation tool. Specifically: What are dimensions of performance? (PDT) Does everyone agree on the dimensions? What is the meaning of different ratings? (e.g., low versus high) *Description*: After completing PDT, faculty members define what would constitute "satisfactory" performance, followed by the opportunity to practice evaluating residents performing at various levels of competence using the evaluation instrument of choice. The group then discusses reasons for the differences between faculty ratings.	Faculty members are given several vignettes along with examples of the medical record, regarding a discharge performed by this resident. For each vignette, the faculty members rate the level of performance (unsatisfactory, marginal, satisfactory, and superior). The vignettes provide examples of different levels of competence in systems-based practice. After each rating, the group discusses the ratings given. This exercise helps to "calibrate" faculty members to be able to discriminate between different levels of competence.
Rater error training (RET)	*Rationale*: By teaching evaluators about halo and distributional errors they will be more likely to recognize these errors in their own ratings. *Description*: Faculty members discuss the common errors (such as halo effect or compensation fallacy) in ratings. Each error is described and defined.	Examples of each error are provided for discussion and review. Actual examples from the program could be used.
Behavioral observation training (BOT)	*Rationale*: Improve observational accuracy and recall of behavioral events. *Description*: Provide tools to assist in guiding the observation and documentation of specific events related to competence.	Many tools can serve as observational diaries, such as the mini-CEX. Even simple aids such as a 3 × 5 card can be used to record events and observations.
Direct observation of competence training (DOC training)	*Rationale*: Improve the quality (validity and reliability) of the direct observation of clinical skills (patient-trainee interactions). *Description*: A systematic process that starts with a PDT exercise (define dimensions of a clinical skill such as counseling), followed by a frame of reference exercise to differentiate levels of performance. The focus is on observable behaviors. After the PDT and FORT, the participants practice observation skills with videotapes and if available, live standardized residents and patients.	Faculty members develop the criteria for an effective counseling session, followed by defining the minimum criteria for a satisfactory performance. Faculty members then apply this learning by observing and evaluating trainee-patient counseling sessions scripted at different levels of performance. Faculty members work in small groups to discuss differences in ratings and the reasons for those differences.

understand that clerkship and program directors are accountable to the public and to the profession to make important decisions about their attainment of professional standards and preparedness to deliver safe and effective care. The purpose of evaluation, and its relationship to the educational objectives and their educational experiences, should be explained at entry to the program, and reiterated on a regularly scheduled basis.

Because they are key stakeholders or "customers" of the educational process, a sound argument can be made for including trainees in decision making about the evaluation process and in providing feedback on its effectiveness. Indeed most residents feel that their participation in evaluation of the educational program and its faculty are important.[8] Even though published data suggest that residents could learn more about the assessment methods used in their programs, they are able to identify areas where assessment approaches to specific skills are inadequate.[9] Residents are aware that accurate evaluation of their clinical competence requires a multimodal approach and that different assessment methods capture different domains; they recognize that commonly used tools may not be ideal for measuring practice-based learning and improvement (PBLI) and systems-based practice (SBP) and are able to see the potential value of methods (multisource feedback, for example) for which they have no personal experience.[10]

Similarly, students are able to understand the need for multiple assessment tools in measuring their competence and are able to identify the relative value of individual methods for measuring specific aspects of competence.[11] In addition, students are able to recognize when assessment practices are driving learning approaches that may be maladaptive and not ideally suited to the particular educational content or conducive to durable acquisition of vocationally relevant knowledge.[12] The abilities of trainees to understand and meaningfully participate in development of the evaluation process should not be underestimated. Furthermore, opportunities to include them as evaluators should not be overlooked, particularly because ability to engage in peer assessment constitutes an important educational and professional achievement.

Part II: Developing or Improving the Evaluation System

General Principles

Constructing an effective evaluation system for an educational program is a difficult and challenging task, whether developed for an undergraduate course or clerkship or a postgraduate program. Yet, the return on investment in creating an effective evaluation system is substantial for the trainees, faculty, and institution. The individual methods used in any evaluation

system should meet the criteria discussed in Chapters 1 and 2 in order for users to be confident in their results. Assessment methods should yield results that are reliable and allow for valid interpretations regarding the individual domain or competency assessed. Although it may not be reasonable to expect program or clerkship directors to perform reliability and validity analyses for all of the tools they choose to employ, it is realistic to expect that educational leaders have sufficient understanding of the psychometric properties of the tools selected in order to apply them appropriately and accurately interpret their results. If they choose to develop new tools locally, directors should ensure those tools also possess sufficient reliability and validity.

The challenges to educational leaders, however, extend well beyond simply understanding the psychometric properties of the methods deployed in their evaluation systems. Such leaders function in an environment where resources are limited and support for educational programs is variable. Course and program directors must select or develop assessment tools that are both feasible to apply and credible to both faculty and trainees. They must consider the range of resources available to them and allocate them according to instructional and assessment priorities.

Understanding the core components of any educational program, and how they interrelate, is essential to the development of high-quality and cost-efficient evaluation systems. These core components include the educational objectives; the educational experiences (curriculum); and the evaluation system. The educational objectives and standards to be obtained during and at the conclusion of the training programs should be clearly communicated and understood by both teachers and trainees. The curriculum should be developed to ensure that trainees have the opportunity to participate in the educational activities that allow them to achieve expected performance standards in meeting program objectives. An optimally developed evaluation system should be closely aligned with educational goals and objectives and compatible with instructional methods and practices; it should provide accurate feedback to the individual trainees regarding their performance against clearly defined standards, and aggregate data from individual assessments should provide programmatic feedback regarding the adequacy of the educational experiences as a whole. Educational leaders should respect the important interrelationships between these core components and the need for their concomitant consideration in developing and modifying educational programs.

The implementation of new assessment modalities may be more difficult than the introduction of new instructional methods or educational activities. Changes in either component are likely to require modifications in the other to remain congruent. It is important to ensure that changes in assessment methods or educational activities remain consistent with relevant educational program objectives, and changes in both components should be introduced in close temporal proximity. Failure to do so may result in trainee dissatisfaction and demonstration of undesirable or unexpected learning behaviors compromising the acceptance and perceived value of program changes.[13] For example, an educational intervention focusing on improving communication skills in informed decision making is more likely to be successful if associated with an assessment of such skills via direct observation of real or standardized patient encounters.

The dual purpose of evaluation should be clearly understood and articulated to trainees and faculty alike. The formative nature of evaluation should be defined and evaluation leading to effective feedback should be exercised within the daily activities of trainees and their interactions with patients and faculty. The developmental nature of such evaluation requires thoughtful consideration regarding how the results of particular methods will be reported and feedback provided. For methods used in making summative judgments about trainees' readiness to move along the continuum of education and practice, more effort should be spent in ensuring that fair and equitable results are obtained. Reliability and validity properties of the tool take primacy over amenability to providing feedback. Realistically speaking, however, particularly at the residency and fellowship program level where the assessment infrastructure is often less well developed, many assessment methods need to serve a dual purpose. Measures that are employed continuously to provide formative evaluation to facilitate learner growth and development may also be used to inform interval judgments about the adequacy of learner progress. Thus, ensuring that our measurement tools meet reasonable quality standards is important, whether they be used for formative or summative intent. Furthermore, it is reasonable to expect that tools used for feedback in shaping trainee skills and behaviors and patient care practices, even if not used for summative purposes, meet appropriate psychometric standards.

Approaches to Constructing the Evaluation System

A variety of approaches may be used for planning and introducing change in evaluation systems. We will suggest a few possible tactics here that provide a mechanism, either through defining a framework for thinking about change or conceptualizing change within a model or simulation as a means of clarifying or organizing the important factors and issues involved.

Program Blueprint

In planning for or implementing change in an evaluation system, it is useful to begin with a *blueprint* that conveys the relationship between educational program objectives, curriculum, and the related assessment approaches and modalities. The blueprint provides a matrix that links the competencies to the content areas that are deemed essential for a particular program. The blueprint should delineate a comprehensive approach to

evaluation that addresses all relevant learning objectives and outcomes through the deployment of multiple assessment modalities. Multiple methods are necessary to cover all of the competences and subcompetencies. Additionally, each of the competencies may be addressed by several different methods, with the overlap allowing for the assessment of different elements of, or providing unique perspectives regarding a particular competency. Ideally, a multimodal evaluation program will allow for an approach that is both efficient and thorough.

Performance Sampling

A fundamental requirement that must be addressed in evaluation systems is the need for an adequate "sample" of a student's or resident's performance. The breadth and number of observations of a trainee should be adequate to assess each relevant competency. The principle of content-specificity (may also be referred to as task-, case- or patient-specificity, depending upon the assessment context), describing the expected variation that occurs in performance depending upon the content or context of the patient or test material encountered, requires multiple observations for stable judgments about trainee proficiency. Here content may refer to the disease process, patient presentation, or organ system covered by the particular assessment. Context refers to the educational setting or clinical/learning situation. A reliable result for judgments regarding particular competencies requires a minimum number of observations that span broad content areas within that competency. This principle applies to the evaluation of a range of knowledge and skills that may be assessed using different methods, such as written examinations, observations using structured rating forms, multiple-station SP examinations, or chart-stimulated recall.

Preparing for Change

One relatively simplistic way to introduce change in assessment approaches involves creating an inventory of current assessment methods constructed within the framework of program objectives, as defined by the blueprint. Aligning current assessment tools with program objectives facilitates a judgment process regarding the adequacy of current methods and discussion regarding potential alternative approaches (Table 14-2). A process for considering the effectiveness of a given tool for a particular domain is depicted in Figure 14-1. One added value of this approach is that it defines the process as cyclical and endorses a continuous quality improvement perspective that is becoming an important component of the educational process.

A similar approach might begin with thinking about the various strengths and weaknesses of a given evaluation system, and then placing the discussion with the context of a particular institution or program by brainstorming about potential opportunities for change as

Table 14-2 **Inventory Form for Appraising the Adequacy of Individual Tools for Measuring the General Competencies**

Competency	Tool(s) Currently Used	Effective? (Yes/No)	Steps for Improvement*
Medical knowledge			
Patient care			
Interpersonal and communication skills			
Professionalism			
Practice-based learning and improvement			
Systems-based practice			

*Indicate how current tool may be improved or consider addition of new tool.

well as potential threats. This involves application of a form of SWOT analysis, with the four essential components being (1) identification of the *strengths* of the current program, (2) identification of the *weaknesses* of the current program, (3) consideration of potential *opportunities* for change, and (4) consideration of *threats* to change.[14] For example, a particular residency program may use peer and patient feedback very well to evaluate professionalism (*strength*), but is uncertain how best to assess practice-based learning and improvement (*weakness*). One approach to address this

weakness would be to affiliate with an institution in which resident participation in quality assurance (QA) and process improvement (PI) activities would contribute valuable personnel resources to that institution, and might provide an *opportunity* for both the institution and the residency program by providing QA projects for residents. A potential *threat* to the successful implementation of this change, inadequate baseline knowledge regarding process improvement concepts and practices, can be addressed through didactic or small group sessions for the residents or referral to appropriate online resources.

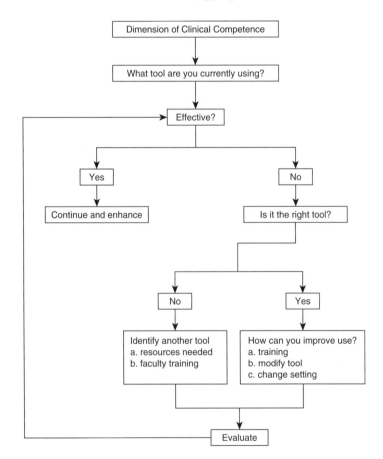

Figure 14-1 Approach to the evaluation of individual assessment methods and tools.

One of the most frequently encountered and serious threats to enhancing any evaluation system is limited resources. The enhancement of existing methods or addition of new methods often requires additional time, money, space, or personnel, or redistribution of such resources. Educational leaders may need to make difficult choices and sacrifices in deciding how to allocate limited resources within and across educational programs. It may be useful to delineate as thoroughly as possible the resources available for assessment in an educational program as a starting point for deliberation and decision making about allocation of such resources. Likewise, it is important to broadly consider the resource implications involved with introducing a new tool or enhancing an existing one. There are costs associated with developing, implementing, and monitoring various methods and tools; with preparing trainees and faculty to appropriately use the tools; and with the preparation of materials, instruments, and forms for providing scores, ratings, or feedback. The use of clinical faculty and space may result in lost revenues to the program or institution. Failure to consider all direct and indirect costs associated with selected methods may result in cutting corners that reduce their effectiveness or diversion of resources from other educational or assessment activities.

In the face of limited resources, educational leaders may apply more innovative approaches to stimulate creative thinking about how to develop or improve their evaluation systems. Mavis and colleagues described a simulation exercise in which curriculum deans from three medical schools were asked to decide upon what, when, and where various assessment methods were to be used across the 4-year curriculum, in the context of limited assessment resources.[15] The exercise, for which instructions for home use were provided in the article, was intended to provoke thoughtful consideration regarding the application of a comprehensive evaluation program that was consistent with institution goals. The simulation met its goals in forcing educational leaders to define their assessment priorities and make difficult choices in the context of limited resources. In addition, participants found the process useful in generating discussions about institutional values, expectations for standards of performance (excellence versus minimal competence level), and the purpose of assessment in different settings. The three participating schools developed programs that were quite different in light of differing institutional priorities, and it is likely that individual programs that initiate such a useful exercise will develop different evaluation systems based upon programmatic objectives and available resources.

Regardless of the approach taken to developing or modifying evaluation systems or individual methods, educator leaders should not be acting in isolation. Involvement of multiple participants is essential to successful implementation. Whether they are called project, program, or implementation teams, committees, or task forces, involvement of key, committed individuals is necessary if programmatic change is to be successful. Diverse membership with broad perspectives is ideal and should include academic and clinical leaders, administrative staff, faculty, students/residents/fellows as appropriate, and measurement expertise if available.[7]

The Assessment Framework

Consistent with current and evolving emphasis on the measurement of educational outcomes, the framework that we describe for constructing the evaluation system will comprise the six general competencies. As of July 2006, residency programs were expected to have fully integrated these competencies into their instructional and assessment practices; fellowship programs were required to begin the process (access at www.acgme.org). In preparing their graduates for entry into postgraduate training and future practice, medical schools have begun to introduce this model into undergraduate programs.[16]

The ACGME general competency model emphasizes the multidimensional nature of clinical competence and endorses a multimodal approach to its assessment. That clinical competence is defined as a multidimensional construct requiring the application of a variety of assessment approaches is not a new or novel concept.[17,18] However, the ACGME/ABMS model has proved somewhat difficult for educators to grasp conceptually, perhaps because it lacks a mnemonic such as KSA (knowledge, skills, attitude) or RIME (reporter, interpreter, manager, educator)[19] to facilitate recall and portability of the model, or maybe because it includes two relatively complex competencies, PBLI and SBP, that are not immediately amenable to assessment with commonly used tools. Indeed, residency program directors seem to struggle most with defining curriculum and assessment approaches to the PBLI and SBP competencies, and to a somewhat lesser extent, professionalism and interpersonal and communication skills.[20,21] One way of pursuing a more complete understanding of the ACGME competency model may be to view it as a KSA model at its core, supplemented with the addition of two competencies that are essential for providing high-quality patient care in our current health care environment. The competencies of PBLI and SBP each have their own knowledge base and skill set that can be approached with commonly used assessment methods. In addition, possession of the "attitudes" that the incorporation of evidence-based medicine and continuous monitoring and improvement of one's practice, as well as the ability to function effectively within multidisciplinary teams, are essential to quality patient care would seem to facilitate acquisition of the knowledge and skills underlying these competencies.

One question that frequently arises relates to the extent to which competence and performance should be measured. As highlighted in Chapter 1, competence refers to the capacity of a trainee to demonstrate the knowledge, skills, and behaviors relevant to a particular domain (or competence) in an assessment context. Performance is what the trainee actually does in practice, presumably when unobserved. In the context of medical education, it is reasonable to assume that some level of observation, whether direct or indirect, concurrent or retrospective, will be evident to trainees. The degree to which observation is evident, of course, influences the authenticity of trainee behavior and the extent to which competence versus performance is observed. Regardless, it is important to evaluate both, because each independently represents an important educational outcome and a measure of program quality.[22]

Selection of Assessment Methods and Tools

Most of the assessment methods that have traditionally been used in medical education programs focus primarily on measuring aspects of medical knowledge and patient care (using written examinations and global rating forms). The introduction of the general competencies has generated interest in development of new and better tools to assess communication skills, professionalism, and the more complex PBLI and SBP competencies. Additionally, there has been increased focus on the enhancement of existing methods, such as the facilitation of structured observation with behavioral checklists or rating scales to improve the quality of evaluation. Evaluation leaders need to decide upon and prioritize the incorporation of new or improved tools into their evaluation systems to better address the general competencies. Although some programs have been successful in developing a robust and comprehensive system for addressing the general competencies within a relatively short period,[23] it probably is more practical or achievable for the vast majority of programs to proceed at a more moderate pace. An incremental pace is more likely to gain buy-in from faculty and trainees and not overwhelm them.

It is not feasible for all tools to be developed by or within individual programs. In fact, as we've emphasized throughout this book, educators should try to adapt validated tools whenever possible. Many examples of validated tools can be found throughout the preceding chapters. Collaborative development of instruments across programs is a more efficient use of time and resources and has the additional advantage of allowing for the accumulation of comparison data to support program evaluation while supporting the measurement of the reliability and validity qualities of the tools.[23]

Regardless of the rate of introduction of new or modified assessment methods, educational program leaders should assume that additional time demands will result for administrative staff, faculty, and trainees.[7,23] For faculty and staff, more hours will be needed for performing or supporting assessment activities; for trainees the additional hours may be of value as they are likely to focus on activities intrinsic to their learner role rather than service responsibilities.[23]

One mistake that programs should avoid is the assumption that all of the general competencies could be covered by simple expansion of the monthly global rating scale. Simply stated, the monthly global rating form is not sufficient to assess the broad range of competencies necessary for the provision of quality patient care. Even with ideal training and form development the scale is not likely to be able to offer reliable and valid interpretation of the discrete attributes within the competencies (Chapter 3).[23]

The global rating forms themselves are not the primary problem; rather, difficulty arises due to the manner in which they are deployed (including the absence of appropriate faculty training and the frequency and timing of form completion). Rather than a single rating at the end of every month, a more appropriate application of global rating scales would involve capturing observed behaviors as they occur in actual clinical settings. Specific forms can be applied to assessment of more focused domains and completed in close temporal proximity so that they potentially reduce or eliminate two important threats to validity: halo effect and recall bias (see Chapter 3). Turnbull described the feasibility of such an approach using tailored rating forms, labeled "clinical work sampling," to provide more reliable and valid assessment of specific domains.[24] The approach is not without flaws and requires faculty development work, trainee orientation, ongoing communication, and increased administrative support.

However, the integration of more frequent, but targeted, assessment into the daily clinical activities of trainees is sensible and overall may not adversely affect efficiency. Such an approach changes the context of assessment, moving from a rotation-oriented to a more trainee- and patient-centered perspective. Indeed, it makes more sense to view the patient encounter or case, not the month or rotation, as the primary unit of assessment.[25] The end result of the deliberate selection over time of a range of patient encounters (see Performance Sampling above), spanning appropriate content areas and clinical tasks, provides a robust data source to be used in formative and summative assessment. Many opportunities for focused observation exist in the daily clinical lives of our trainees. Indeed, this general purpose underlies development of the mini-CEX approach for evaluating residents in internal medicine.[26]

A variety of methods and tools other than global rating forms may be used to assess competence and performance. Selection of the appropriate tools to create a comprehensive evaluation system is informed by knowledge regarding the appropriate application of each tool, awareness of their reliability and validity properties, and local program preferences, experience, and resources. The final battery of assessment tools will vary appropriately across individual programs. It is important to restate here that educational leaders should ensure faculty preparedness for effective use of each tool through faculty development and learner readiness and acceptance of the tool through careful orientation and ongoing transparency regarding its intended use.

Implementation of individual methods and tools should also involve careful deliberation about how they will be used for providing formative or summative evaluation (again with the realization that many tools will serve a dual function). With regard to formative and summative evaluation, one must strive to attain a balance between the professional and institutional requirement for reliability in making important decisions about trainee progress and the need for the learner to receive frequent and directive feedback in order to improve competence. Feedback can take a variety of forms and may be delivered in writing, often related to the scoring or rating of performance, or orally depending upon faculty preferences, nature of the performance, or goals of the feedback. Most important, to have the largest impact on trainee learning and development, it should be delivered immediately or as soon as possible.[27]

Assessment of the Individual Competencies (Table 14-3)

Medical Knowledge

Assessment should target the acquisition of a broad knowledge base within a particular field as well as the application of that knowledge base within a clinical context. Written examinations provide the most efficient and psychometrically sound approach to assessing a learner's fund of knowledge and basic cognitive skills. Educational leaders may use national standardized examinations or develop their own examinations. When using national standardized examinations it is important to ensure that the purpose and content of the test are consistent with the program's learning objectives and curriculum. For locally developed examinations, faculty should receive basic instruction in test development and item writing, in order to ensure that the content adequately represents program objectives and true knowledge competence is measured, rather that test-taking skills (Chapter 4).

The application of knowledge in clinical settings can be assessed using several different methods. Case-specific knowledge can be assessed during a structured direct observation exercise or a chart-stimulated recall exercise. Faculty development is important to enable faculty to ask the relevant questions in an appropriate manner and assess responses in an accurate and reliable manner (Chapters 5 and 9). Knowledge application can also be assessed during ward rounds, morning report, and other conferences. Here, construction of brief or focused rating forms to be completed during or after such conferences will facilitate the assessment process and provide documentation for the trainees' records or portfolios (also helpful in demonstrating a thorough assessment process for accreditation purposes).

Interpersonal and Communication Skills

Reliable and valid assessment of interpersonal and communication skills requires direct observation. This can be accomplished within the context of a structured patient encounter using a mini-CEX or structured clinical observation tool,[28] or a similar structured approach. Depending upon program or institutional resources, educational leaders may decide to supplement faculty observation with standardized patient (SP)–based assessment. SP-based approaches may be ideal for engaging in formative evaluation and instruction in sensitive or difficult situations in which risks to the safety or well-being of real patients might be expected, such as discussing end-of-life preferences or delivering bad news. Additionally, multiple station SP exercises might provide a reliable and efficient means of measuring the achievement of groups of trainees in important skill or content areas. Educational leaders should understand that the SP-based direct observation methods are a supplement to, but not a replacement for, direct observation and feedback by faculty (Chapter 8). It is important for faculty to observe the interaction of trainees with patients in real clinical settings in order for faculty to appreciate the ability of residents to respond to the spontaneity and idiosyncrasies intrinsic to real clinical situations and to fulfill their professional responsibility to mentor and facilitate the acquisition of clinical competence in future physicians.

Information regarding trainee communication and interpersonal skills can also be obtained via ratings by peers, patients, or other health care providers, either individually or as part of a multisource feedback (MSF) evaluation program (see Chapter 6). Using such ratings will allow for additional assessment of communication within the health care team, as well as provide supplemental data regarding patient-related communication and interpersonal skills.

Patient Care

The patient care competency is complex, consisting of several discrete domains that overlap to a variable extent with the other competencies. Effective communication, data gathering, patient counseling and education, elicitation of patient preferences in informed decision making, and caring and respectful behavior toward patients can be assessed using the observation and rating approaches listed under the interpersonal and communication skills competency. Further assessment regarding the use of information technology, clinical judgment, and the use of up-do-date scientific evidence can be accomplished via case discussion using structured observational approaches such as the mini-CEX, during review of the medical record using a deliberate interviewing technique such as chart-stimulated recall (CSR) (see Chapter 5), or by appraisal of trainees during conference presentation or participation. Other methods used in the assessment of PBLI also provide information on these overlapping dimensions. Similarly, methods used in evaluating SBP provide feedback on trainees' abilities to work on health care teams, an attribute found in both SBP and patient care domains. Medical record audits or review of other health care databases can be used to measure the provision of preventive health care.

Lastly, assessment of procedural and technical skills can be accomplished via direct observation of performance or through the application of appropriate simulation-based methods (see Chapter 12). Review of the medical record with CSR or focused discussion

Table 14-3 **Methods to Assess the General Competencies**

General Competency	Brief Definition	Preferred Evaluation Methods	Comments
Patient care	Trainees are expected to provide patient care that is compassionate, appropriate, and effective for the promotion of health, prevention of illness, treatment of disease, and at the end of life	Direct observation (with or without ratings or checklists) Standardized patients Multisource feedback Medical record audit with chart–stimulated recall	The best method for evaluating the patient encounter aspects of this competency is direct obser-vation. Direct observation is an area in which faculty development is important. Research suggests that without training faculty evaluations based on observation are often inaccurate.
Medical knowledge	Trainees are expected to demonstrate knowledge of established and evolving biomedical, clinical, and social sciences, and to apply their knowledge to patient care and the education of others	Standardized examinations (e.g., ITE) Chart-stimulated recall (for application of knowledge and clinical reasoning) Case- or vignette-based discussions	Different aspects of this competency should be emphasized. First, a certain amount of fundamental knowledge is required to function as a physician. Second, integration into the patient care context is required for assessment of application of knowledge (including clinical reasoning).
Professionalism	Trainees are expected to demonstrate behaviors that reflect a commitment to continual professional development, ethical practice, an understanding and sensitivity to diversity, and a responsible attitude toward their patients, their profession, and society	Multisource feedback Direct observation Standardized patients Portfolio (reflective narratives)	Obtaining a complete picture of a trainee's professionalism requires input from multiple sources: patients, family members, peers, and faculty and nonphysician medical staff.
Interpersonal skills and communication	Trainees are expected to demonstrate interpersonal and communication skills that enable them to establish and maintain professional relationships with patients, families, and other members of the health care team	Direct observation (with or without ratings or checklists) Standardized patients Multisource feedback Medical record audits (written communication)	Like professionalism, this competency requires input from different perspectives. Peer and nursing evaluations, patient surveys, or other medical surveys can be helpful.
Practice-based learning and improvement	Trainees are expected to be able to use scientific evidence and methods to investigate, evaluate, and improve patient care practices	Medical record audits with chart-stimulated recall Clinical vignettes Evidence-based medicine tools Clinical care audits Self–assessment Quality assurance/process improvement (QA/PI) projects Portfolios	This competency focuses primarily on the effective application of evidence-based medicine and quality improvement. The simplest approach is to use a clinical diary, in which trainees catalogue over time questions that arose during patient care activities along with copies of the data sources used to answer the specific question. Evaluation instruments have also been developed for evidence-based practice. A medical record audit can be an excellent method to assess quality improvement. More important, trainees can perform the audits themselves.

Table 14-3 **Methods to Assess the General Competencies** *(Continued)*

General Competency	Brief Definition	Preferred Evaluation Methods	Comments
Systems-based practice	Trainees are expected to demonstrate both an understanding of the contexts and systems in which health care is provided, and the ability to apply to improve and optimize health care	Clinical care audits Medical record audit with chart-stimulated recall Multisource feedback QA/PI projects Portfolios	Evaluation of systems-based practice depends heavily on the type of educational and care model in which the trainee is embedded. Evaluations from peers, nursing, patient care coordinators, social workers, and others can provide important information on how well the resident engages various care systems (such as discharge planning, social work, setting up referrals) and interacts with other health care providers to care for patients (teamwork). Medical record audits can show how the trainee facilitates care for specialty consultation, social services, and other services the trainee cannot provide.

in conferences or on rounds will provide information on the nontechnical aspects of procedural skills, such as the trainee's understanding of the indications and contraindications for the procedure and ability to interpret results and to deal with potential complications.

Professionalism

In that the overt behavioral manifestations of professionalism occur both episodically and continuously within the day-to-day experiences of physicians, it is important for assessment of professionalism to capture the many and varied interactions and behaviors demonstrated by trainees. It follows, then, that the ideal method for assessing professionalism would capture the wide range of behaviors exercised in various settings and would allow for inclusion of a broad array of observations and perspectives. Furthermore, it is essential that observations are provided in contexts and by individuals most likely to observe lapses in professional conduct, such as students, peers, administrative staff, and other health care providers. Although much is yet to be learned about the properties and value of MSF in medical education settings, it seems that this may be the ideal method for assessing professional behaviors. Of course, as discussed elsewhere in this volume, MSF should be thoughtfully implemented with appropriate orientation for raters and trainees (see Chapter 6).

Other approaches, such as direct observation with real or standardized patients, or performance on

rounds or during conferences, can yield important information about a given trainee's capacity to behave in a professional manner. Such methods may also be valuable in a diagnostic mode, should there be concerns about the degree or nature of unprofessional behaviors. However, it is important to be aware that such methods, to the extent that trainees are cognizant of being observed, measure to a variable extent the capacity to behave professionally, and do not necessarily predict professional behavior outside the assessment context.

PBLI and SBP

PBLI and SBP are complex competencies, each consisting of individual and overlapping knowledge, skills, and attitude domains. Measurement of such complex domains requires that assessment tools target the specific domains in a manner similar to that approached for each of the other four competencies. Additionally, thorough assessment of PBLI and SBP requires educational leaders to function within a paradigm that mirrors actual measurement of health care quality in a manner that reflects the continuum of education and practice with regard to physician performance. Accurate and thorough evaluation of PBLI requires *data* about a trainee's practice, through appraisal of specific clinical performance and review of other data sources regarding how the trainee pursues clinical questions and deals with uncertainty. The former can be accomplished through medical record and clinical care audits (measuring compliance with evidence-based health care processes and patient outcomes), the latter through learning logs and evidenced-based practice activities. SBP requires assessment from multiple other providers who work within the same clinical microsystem as the trainee. Evaluation of SBP requires gathering data regarding patient management in the context of the larger health care environment and the human interactions that occur with other members of the team during the provision of care. Therefore, information on how trainees interact with other health care providers, through multisource assessments, is essential, but not always sufficient, to the evaluation of SBP.

Portfolios: A Method to Put It All Together

The tool that holds promise as an overarching method for encompassing and integrating the six general competencies, as well as providing a structure for data collection and analysis, is the portfolio (see Chapter 7). The portfolio may include a wide range of assessment data, evidence of learning achievement, and reflection as documentation of the internalization of formative assessment (Fig. 14-2). Furthermore, the portfolio is adaptable to supporting assessment across the continuum of education and practice in an efficient manner resulting from its learner-driven nature. The active and ongoing assimilation of evidence of learning and achievement and documentation of reflection into a

portfolio is consistent with the theoretical underpinnings of competency-based education and assessment. A critical role for the learner defines and underlies the utility of both.[29] The effectiveness of formative feedback, leading to improved competence, is exemplified in reflection. Unfortunately, meaningful and creative documentation of learning is not particularly amenable to reliable and valid interpretation regarding learning achievement—for this, structure is necessary. The power of the portfolio as an assessment tool depends upon the balance achieved between creativity and individualization and the need for structure and quantitative data[29] (see Chapter 7).

We view the portfolio both as a tool to illustrate learning and self-reflection and an instrument that provides a structure for collecting, analyzing, and demonstrating competence across the spectrum of education and practice. Most portfolios currently in use by medical educators possess more structure than the traditional learning portfolio.

The ''structured portfolio'' described in Chapter 7 includes contents that are determined by both the training program and trainee to maximize outcomes-based evaluation. Portfolios in medical education must be able to provide sufficient evidence that a trainee has attained the desired level of competence and performance. Therefore, medical educators will need to define many of the assessment tools used in the portfolio, contingent upon local needs and resources.

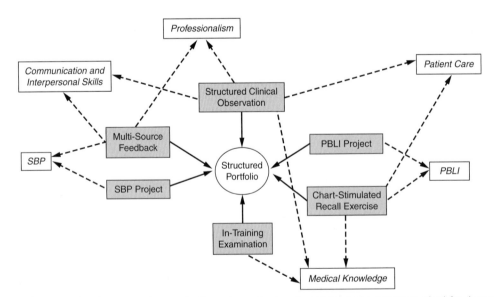

Figure 14-2 Example of a comprehensive approach to evaluation using a structured portfolio as the primary method for documenting evidence of learning and self-reflection. In this example, the six assessment methods in the gray boxes provide documentation of learning (either as evidence of learning or a stimulus for self-reflection). Self-reflection related to the documentation is contained in the portfolio. The six assessment methods provide coverage of the six general competencies (depicted in the other boxes). The frequency of assessment will vary depending upon the individual tool. For example, structured clinical observation or chart-stimulated recall may be scheduled four to six times per year, multisource feedback one or two times per year, in-training examinations once per year, and SBP or PBLI projects one or more times over the course of the training program. Information regarding the optimal frequency for each assessment method should be based upon their intended purpose (formative vs. summative) as well as knowledge regarding their reliability and validity properties.

Part III: Program Evaluation

In addition to the evaluation of individual trainees, educational leaders must also measure the success of the overall educational program in attaining curricular objectives. The LCME requires medical schools to include appropriate outcome measures in evaluating their students and graduates against national norms.[30] In July 2006, the ACGME accreditation process began to focus on the extent to which program directors and institutional authorities incorporate evidence from external sources in verifying impressions about resident performance and informing quality improvement efforts in their residency programs.[31]

In measuring the efficacy of educational programs, outcomes may be defined from the perspective of the learner, his/her patients, and the larger community. Learner outcomes include competence as reflected by incremental achievement in knowledge, skills, or behavioral domains; patient outcomes may include satisfaction or health care outcomes; and community outcomes may include the cost-effectiveness of medical education or changes in population health status.[32]

Program evaluation may focus on concurrent outcomes, those that occur within the training program or its sponsoring institution, or on the future performance of graduates. It may involve a wide variety of activities ranging from analysis of aggregated trainee assessment data (e.g., mean program in-training scores) to surveys of trainees, faculty, and future program directors and employers, to studies focusing on health care practices and outcomes of current trainees and graduates. The actual program assessment process may comprise inexpensive, broadly applied measures to support continuous monitoring of program performance (program director surveys, monitoring board certification rates or adverse licensure actions) or may involve the deployment of resource intensive assessment modalities for outcomes assessment of specific program initiatives (e.g., unannounced SPs to measure the success of an intervention to improve screening for domestic violence).

As in the evaluation of individual trainees, effective program evaluation depends upon the presence of clear educational objectives and the use of methods appropriately suited to those objectives. The evaluation process is continuous, involving stakeholders at multiple levels across the educational community and "measures learning as multidimensional, integrated and revealed over time."[33] Methods used to measure selected aspects of competence and performance at various stages and times during the training program will likely be different than those chosen to assess the performance of graduates.

Monitoring program processes and outcomes to inform ongoing development and improvement activities can be viewed as analogous to quality assurance/process improvement approaches used in the clinical care context. In educational program evaluation the quality assurance process intends to provide feedback regarding the success of such programs in achieving curricular goals and objectives. It comprises a systematic approach to gathering, analyzing, disseminating, and applying assessment data to continuous improvement in learning.[33] Broadly speaking, the elements essential to ensuring quality in medical education include qualified trainees, talented and motivated faculty, clear delineation and understanding of educational aims and objectives, a sound curriculum, and a good system of quality assurance.[34]

That the eventual product of educational programs depends on both the qualifications of entering trainees as well as the quality of the education process helps identify the important targets for program evaluation. Attention should be paid to program input (caliber of entering trainees and the selection process), internal processes and outcomes (program structure and quality of instruction and assessment), and program output (the competence and performance of program graduates).[35,36] The total quality management approach suggested by Suwanwela, including assessment of program input, educational processes, and program output, serves as a useful framework for program evaluation.[36]

Assessing Program Input

As the talent of the trainees entering an educational program is an important determinant of their subsequent performance it seems reasonable to consider the trainee selection process as well as trainees' initial abilities and characteristics in formulating judgments about the quality of the educational program and as a confounding variable when analyzing outcome measures.[37] What better way to document learning outcomes than to demonstrate improved knowledge, skills, and behaviors over time, related to educational program activities. A robust baseline assessment, such as that described by Lypson and colleagues, serves multiple purposes, including informing curricular priorities based upon demonstrated learner needs and enhancing patient safety by determining trainee's abilities to perform critical patient care activities without direct supervision. Their "Postgraduate Orientation Assessment" employs a variety of methods including SPs, computer-based formats, and paper and pencil exercises to reveal an intern's knowledge and skill levels, thereby identifying important learning needs. Structuring of the assessment exercise to align with the ABMS/ACGME core competencies also helps to meet accreditation standards for residency programs. As in this study, it is reasonable to predict that a wide range of competence and performance deficiencies will be uncovered by others introducing similar assessments, providing strong endorsement for such activities.[38]

Assessing Concurrent Processes and Outcomes

In terms of measuring relevant processes and outcomes within an educational program, it is important to plan carefully. Thoughtful consideration should focus on what is to be assessed, how it is to be measured, and how results will be used to inform program improvement. Although it will be challenging to design the perfect program evaluation scheme, efforts spent up front to balance the potential competing interests of stakeholder needs, methodological requirements, and resource constraints are likely to decrease the number of surprises and obstacles in moving forward. It is important to consider a range of issues in making decisions about how to proceed with program evaluation: the distribution of process and structure or outcome measures; the use of qualitative and quantitative methods; employment of internal and external methods and evaluators; measuring short- (current/intermediate) and long-term outcomes; and allocation of resources.[39]

While it is appropriate to emphasize educational and clinical outcome measures in evaluating the quality of the educational experience and informing program improvement, it is important to understand that quality is also measured by evaluating program structure and processes, including the elements of the curriculum, comprehensiveness and credibility of the instructional and assessment methods, number and involvement of faculty, etc.[36] Unless some understanding of a program's structure and processes exists, it may be difficult to explain or respond to outcomes data to effect program improvement. For example, a negative outcome result may be due to flaws in the design of a particular curricular innovation or may be due to problems in the way it was implemented (e.g., faculty or trainees were not properly oriented prior to introduction); one cannot interpret and properly act upon the outcome without some insights into the relevant processes.[39]

Both qualitative and quantitative methods are appropriately applied to program evaluation. Quantitative methods such as aggregated data from various written examinations, OSCEs, or medical record audits are generally considered superior in providing high-quality feedback to educational leaders. However, qualitative techniques such as focus groups, individual discussion and interviews, and faculty and trainee observation can play an equally useful role in selected aspects of program evaluation.[39] In particular, qualitative approaches to data collection and analysis may be important during periods of active program change and reform.[40] They may allow for more timely collection of data to identify unexpected problems or consequences to inform course correction before serious damage is done, and provide educational leaders a mechanism for continuous communication with learners, faculty, and other stakeholders, thus encouraging stakeholder buy-in and input into evolving program changes. The use of qualitative techniques is particularly useful when there is some uncertainty about what quantitative measures to select and when it is anticipated that new insights may shape continuing evolution in program development.[39] As above, qualitative assessment may complement quantitative outcomes by providing potential explanations for quantitative results.

Moving from qualitative to more quantitative approaches, surveys of key stakeholders can also provide an important source of information about program success. Multiple parties have a stake in undergraduate and graduate medical educational programs and therefore should have the opportunity to shape and participate in processes that measure the quality of such programs.[35] As previously stated, students and residents have expectations regarding the quality of their educational experience and are appropriately qualified to provide feedback on specific program performance elements. The faculty who devote time and effort to educational programs deserve to participate in and benefit from program performance assessment. Certainly, it is important to make sure that all stakeholders are provided with feedback from the program evaluation process, particularly those who have participated in providing information as well as those who are the subject of assessment data.[36] Those providing assessment data and opinions regarding program performance need to know that their efforts are appreciated and incorporated into program improvement activities.[40]

Surveys may be developed to focus on specific curricular interventions or may be designed with more broad intent to serve as an overall monitor of program performance. They should seek information on stakeholder perceptions regarding the adequacy of curriculum content as well as their perceived progress in mastery of essential skills or behaviors. Surveys of residents or graduates are a commonly used method for providing feedback on the ability of residency programs to prepare trainees for clinical practice. Such surveys may suggest that programs are doing a fairly good job of preparing graduates to provide high-quality care in a particular field; however, they also can be very helpful in detecting areas where graduates are not prepared to deal with some of the content, tasks, or nonclinical requirements of clinical practice. A recent paper describing the responses of senior residents in eight specialties to a survey regarding their preparedness for practice pointed to significant gaps across multiple programs and specialties in preparing residents to participate in and contribute to meaningful activities in clinical practice.[41] Residents about to graduate from their programs felt comfortable in caring for most of the common conditions seen in their specialty. However, occasional surprises were noted. Residents responded that they were not prepared to care for specific patient conditions or manage patients in certain contexts (e.g., 8% of psychiatry residents were unprepared for diagnosing and treating eating disorders; 29% of obstetrics and gynecology residents were unprepared to care for patients in nursing homes). Across all eight specialties surveyed, modest numbers of residents felt unprepared to choose cost-effective treatments, participate in quality assurance, care for populations of patients, collaborate with nonphysician caregivers, and practice in a managed care environment. These findings certainly suggest critical items for inclusion in most program surveys; however, the occasional unanticipated results for common specialty-based conditions and patient care contexts indicate that surveys should remain broad and unbiased by unfounded assumptions regarding program quality. Also, with regard to our and the ACGME/ABMS accountability to gather and examine the evidence regarding the utility of the current competency model, it would be interesting to track response rates over time and across programs for several of the above-mentioned domains, particularly those germane to practice-based learning and improvement and systems-based practice.

While assessment of internal structure and processes, the use of qualitative methods, and surveys of key constituents all play an important role in program evaluation, the ultimate product of the medical educational process is the learner's abilities in the context of patient care, and in the end the most valuable and revealing information will focus on the learner and learning outcomes.[33]

In deciding upon the methods for evaluating educational outcomes it is necessary to include more than written examinations and course grades or global ratings. In fact, well-designed performance-based assessments such as OSCEs are ideal tools for evaluating important skills and behaviors objectives, and may better predict future performance.[42] Aggregate data from other direct observation-based methods, medical record audits, or conference presentation/participation can also serve as a barometer for program performance in selected competence domains. It is also critically important to include measures of professional attitudes and behaviors beginning early in medical school as performance in this domain may have predictive value for identifying future problems in residency and practice.[43,44] Unfortunately, there is much work that needs to be done in order to fully understand, and develop appropriate instruments to measure, several of the important domains such as teamwork, lifelong learning, patient advocacy, and other aspects of professionalism.

Educational leaders should seek to attain a balance between the use of internal and external measures for assessing educational outcomes. Internal methods, such as the aggregate assessment data described here, or internal evaluators, such as faculty and residents, are likely to be somewhat biased by personal involvement with the program. However, internal measures can provide important information and feedback that is enriched by an understanding of program structure, history, goals and objectives, and the constraints under which educational managers operate.[39] External evaluators and methods provide for a more objective assessment of program processes and outcomes often with the additional advantage of providing norm-referenced comparison data, either across several programs or institutions or based on a national cohort of similar trainees and programs.[39]

Comparisons using external measures are more valid if the course or program objectives are matched with the appropriate assessment method; similarly, comparison between competence and performance at various levels is more appropriately performed through the use of the same or similar assessment

tools. Outcome measures that might be applied to assessing the quality of educational programs include both national and local methods. Standardized tests such as the NBME Subject Examinations, the USMLE, residency In-Training Examinations, and Board Certification examinations yield comparisons to national cohorts. Administration of clinical skills examinations through local or regional consortia may provide important information by comparing students and residents to local or regional peer groups. External evaluation processes, such as LCME or ACGME/RRC reviews, are often conducted by individuals with specific training and tend to have more credibility in influencing institutional change. Of course, despite the quality of the review process, most educational leaders do not wish to rely on such a high-stakes approach for valuable, yet critical program assessment information.

Although it is obviously essential to consider educational and clinical outcomes in evaluating the quality of individual trainees and the educational program, it is also helpful to think about the impact of an educational program on the educational and clinical environment in which it resides. From this perspective, evaluation of educational program outcomes extends beyond ensuring acquisition of competence among trainees to the larger impact of the educational program on infrastructural and cultural changes in the institutional environment.[45] To what extent does the program influence the teaching and learning experience of faculty and trainees, and to what extent do positive (or negative) effects spill over into the local clinical environment?

A measure of efficacy of the educational program can be obtained by assessing the impact on current health care outcomes within the home institution. For example, patient outcomes such as satisfaction, self-ratings of health status, or HbA_{1c} levels would be obtained during a resident PBLI project focusing on the quality of routine care provided to diabetics. Of course, in many cases it may be difficult to determine which came first, educational program initiatives or enhancements in institutional culture, or infrastructure. It is likely that some reciprocal relationship exists between the quality of educational programs and their environment. The quality of the clinical micro- and macrosystems of the institution undoubtedly influences the quality of local educational programs. In fact, the relationship between the quality of medical education and health care, in association with a culture supportive of innovation and scholarly pursuit within individual institutions, is an important underlying theme of the Educational Innovation Project sponsored by the Internal Medicine RRC. In return for demonstration of excellence and innovation in education and quality, participating residency programs are offered extended accreditation cycles.[46]

Institutional recognition of faculty contributions to educational programs also provides a measure of program success, endorsing professional values related to our responsibility to engage in the education and assessment of colleagues and professionals in training. As acknowledgment of grant support and research productivity in basic or clinical science results in faculty rewards such as promotion or other forms of recognition, so too should scholarly activity in medical education be rewarded. Do institutions embrace teaching as a valued community (professional) activity? There should be recognition of the diverse nature of scholarship in medical education, ranging from prospective research on teaching and assessment methodology to interpretation and application of existing knowledge into the development of educational programs and teaching approaches.[45]

One final element of the program evaluation process involves consideration of the evaluation system itself. Periodic review and critical analysis of assessment approaches are necessary to ensure that each assessment method is being used properly, in a manner that is congruent with the objectives and curriculum of the educational program and relevant to the total learning experience of the trainee.[27] At the very least, education program leaders should periodically ask themselves a series of questions about individual tools and the entire system (see Chapters 1 and 2). To begin with, they should question whether the assessment content is appropriate. Are the cases selected for a local OSCE targeting the important diagnoses and tasks? Is the distribution of real-patient encounters selected for observation sensible given overall programmatic goals? One must avoid uneven distribution of observations related to the location, preferences, or expertise of core faculty members. Are there an adequate number of faculty observers participating in trainee evaluation? Recently published data suggest that a larger number of raters observing fewer patient encounters each produces a more defensible result than fewer raters observing a larger number of encounters each.[47]

It is also helpful to compare the results of individual assessments within or across programs to make sure the results make sense. It is reasonable to expect that global ratings, OSCE results, and ITE scores may not correlate closely with each other as they are measuring different aspects of competence. However, if the results of local multiple-choice examinations are very different than ITE results, then one should question the purpose and assumptions underlying the local examination as well as its quality. Alternatively, program curriculum may not be aligned with national priorities, as reflected by ITE content.

Lastly, it is useful to consider the overall performance of a particular method related to constructs being assessed: Is it producing results that are consistent with beliefs about the competence being measured and knowledge about the trainees being evaluated? Recognizing significant variability may exist between trainees at a given level, it is reasonable, overall, to expect that most assessments will yield better results/higher scores for more advanced or experienced trainees. The failure of an assessment method to discriminate between trainees with expected different

levels of proficiency should trigger a review of that particular method (and/or reconsideration of assumptions about the trainees' level of competence). Beyond the internal assessment discussed here, additional information about the quality of a local assessment program can and should be obtained via periodic review by external parties, either through consultation or occurring as part of formal internal review and external accreditation processes. It is also important to consider future performance of graduates as another means of studying the validity of current assessment approaches.[27]

Assessing Program Output

Assessment of graduates' performance may target educational or professional outcomes or may focus on the clinical practices and patient health outcomes resulting from the care provided by graduates. Outcomes evaluation focusing on the competence and performance of graduates involves logistical and technical challenges. First are the difficulties in collecting information on graduates who may be spread across multiple institutions and geographic locations. Second, there remains uncertainty about the strength of connection between prior educational experiences and achievement and future abilities and practices of graduates.[30] Research has shown that it is difficult to demonstrate a consistent relationship between academic performance in medical school and residency, and the performance of residents and practicing physicians. There are several reasons for this inconsistent relationship; understanding the potential pitfalls in measuring the performance of graduates is critical in informing the development of sound program evaluation processes. Although most of the research on educational outcomes has focused on the relationship between learning in medical school and subsequent behaviors and performance in residency and practice, many of the limiting factors also pertain to measuring residency program outcomes in future practice. These limitations have been described by experts in medical education and assessment and include the following:[48-51]

1. *Dissimilarity in constructs between performances at different levels.* It is difficult to compare performances at different levels because expectations for the demonstration of competence and performance are different in medical school, residency, and practice. One should not assume that the performance of practicing physicians is an extension of that expected of residents, and the performance of residents represents an extension of that expected of medical students.[48] As one moves along the education-practice continuum the complexity of the practice environment and related situational effects (including clinical specialty) and constraints influence the practice behaviors and performance of physicians.[49-51] Achievement in medical school reflects more limited and relatively simple domains while performance in practice reflects a complex

relationship between knowledge and skills, personal and professional characteristics, and a wide array of patient- and system-related factors. Assessment in UME largely relates to educational process and outcomes; in practice, assessment should ideally focus on compliance with evidence-based processes of care and patient outcomes. The GME environment provides for the transition from educational to clinical outcomes measurement.

2. *Limitations in assessment methodology.* Performance at all levels is measured by instruments that are intrinsically flawed to a variable degree. In addition to the fact that predictor and criterion variables are likely to reflect different constructs, both are assessed by imprecise instruments that may be measuring different domains (or different aspects within the same domain), thus raising questions about the validity of interpretations.[49,50] For example, thorough analysis of scores from an OSCE for fourth-year students may find that they yield valid impressions about trainee communication skills, but history-taking scores (related to local case and checklist development practices) reflect assessment-related interviewing skills rather than their authentic clinical data-gathering practices (see Chapter 8). That predictor variable then may be compared to a sample of intern mini-CEX scores presumed to be measuring the same attributes, but the mini CEX actually measures some combination of cognitive and interpersonal skills (see Chapter 3). In this situation, one cannot assume that a difference in performance on the OSCE and the mini-CEX reflects changes in aptitude; the fact that the two tools are measuring different attributes may explain much of the difference.

3. *Intervening time.* The longer one waits between measuring the predictor and criterion variables, the more existing associations will diminish or disappear. This is due to a combination of factors including decay of original knowledge and skills and the introduction of a potential wide array of educational, professional, and personal events and activities during the intervening time.[49,50] Such limitations relate to the uncertain correlation between undergraduate education and subsequent practice behaviors and have resulted in a more focused assessment on the intermediate outcomes in graduate medical education, such as intern ratings. Concentration on intermediate outcomes in graduate medical education is appropriate though, as the goals and objectives of undergraduate medical education are to prepare graduates for the more limited patient care responsibilities in the supervised environment of GME.[39]

4. *Other measurement issues.* A variety of measurement constraints affect our ability to detect and accurately quantify relationships that exist across the education and practice continuum:

    a. Range restriction: Relatively speaking, the subjects (students and physicians) being assessed comprise a relatively homogeneous group. It may be difficult to detect significant differences using traditional correlation and regression-based analyses.[50]

    b. The skewed distributions typical of the global rating forms used in assessment obscure our ability to detect correlations.[50]

    c. Nonrepresentative nature of results related to response biases: The voluntary nature of participation in published studies influences their interpretation. Refusal of some students to participate and the failure of subsequent supervisors to return rating forms can be related to lower academic achievement of students as well as lower performance as residents.[52,53]

    d. See Gonnella[50] for a more detailed description of additional measurement constraints (nonlinear distribution of ratings, effects of variance of predictor and criterion variables, relationship between different predictor variables compared to criterion variables).

Despite the preceding limitations, studies have shown that a relationship can be demonstrated between performance in medical school and subsequent performance in residency and practice, although the strongest relationships exist for internship performances.[51,54] For example, students whose academic achievement is extremely low or extremely high are more likely to be classified in similar groups as interns.[51,55] In various studies, undergraduate measures such as individual and composite clerkship grades, licensure examination scores, faculty clinical ratings, class standing, and history of academic excellence or problems correlate to a variable extent with resident supervisor ratings, licensure and board certification scores, and subsequent academic affiliations.[50] When significant correlations have been observed, the magnitude of the relationship has not been particularly large, certainly not enough to endorse strong connections. As expected, stronger relationships exist for conceptually similar measures such as correlations between the separate licensure examination steps and between clerkship grades and residency supervisor ratings.[55]

These data suggest the potential value and limitations of assessing the performance of graduates as a program outcome measure. This information needs to be thoughtfully incorporated into an overall program evaluation plan. An important objective in designing program evaluation processes is to mitigate the effect of the limitations listed above when deciding upon attributes to be measured and the tools selected to assess them. To the extent possible, the instruments used to measure performance at various levels should be similar with reasonable expectations that they are measuring the same element of clinical competence or performance. One should understand what each tool is actually measuring, as well as its reliability, and apply that knowledge in interpreting results.[51,55]

Consider carefully the ultimate effects and potential end points of learning in selecting outcome variables. How will the knowledge and skills acquired at various

Table 14-4 Selected Methods for Assessing the ABMS/ACGME General Competencies Across the Continuum of Education and Practice

Competency	Assessment Method		
	Undergraduate Medical Education	Graduate Medical Education	Clinical Practice
Medical knowledge	Local examinations NBME subject examinations USMLE Step 1 and 2CK	Local examinations USMLE Step 3 Specialty in-training examinations Board certifying examinations	Recertification examinations Examinations linked to continuing medical education/CPD Clinical question logs
Interpersonal and communication skills	Direct observation SP examinations Global ratings Multisource feedback	Direct observation SP examinations Global ratings Multisource feedback	Multisource feedback or individual ratings by peers, patients, or supervisors Unannounced SPs
Professionalism	Direct observation SP examinations Multisource feedback	Direct observation SP examinations Multisource feedback	Multisource feedback Licensure/credentialing actions Maintenance of certification/ABMS board actions Unannounced SPs
Patient care	Direct observation SP examinations Global ratings Medical record audit +/− chart-stimulated recall	Direct observation SP examinations Global ratings Medical record audit +/− chart-stimulated recall	Clinical care audit Unannounced SPs Licensure/credentialing actions Recertification examinations and maintenance of certification components Multisource feedback or individual ratings by peers, patients, or supervisors
Practice-based learning and improvement	Medical record audits with chart-stimulated recall EBM exercises Portfolios	QA/PI projects EBM exercises Medical record audits with chart-stimulated recall Portfolios	QA/PI activities Clinical care audits Unannounced SPs Portfolios Web-based practice improvement modules Multisource feedback or individual ratings by peers, patients, or supervisors
Systems-based practice	SP examinations Medical record audit +/− chart-stimulated recall	QA/PI projects Multisource feedback Medical record audit +/− chart-stimulated recall	Multisource feedback Clinical care audits Unannounced SPs Multisource feedback or individual ratings by peers, patients, or supervisors Web-based practice improvement modules

CPD, continuing professional development; EBM, evidence-based medicine; PI, process improvement; QA, quality assurance; SP, standardized patient.

points in training be manifest in future practice contexts? What assessment methods are reasonably likely to be measuring the same or similar attributes across the continuum of education and practice? Table 14-4 provides some likely combinations of tests that might be considered as long as those performing the comparisons are cognizant of the potential limitations described above and are able to incorporate such understanding into the subsequent interpretation of results. Appropriate methods for comparison are somewhat obvious for the more "simple" domains of medical knowledge and interpersonal and communication skills, but more difficult to imagine for the more complex competencies. For example, how will you be able to distinguish a graduate who is performing well (or poorly) in applying the knowledge and principles of PBLI and SBP in their practices?

Educational leaders should address the participation of students and residents in program evaluation, not only as respondents providing input regarding program quality, but also as data sources for subsequent analysis. This requires that trainees participate in contributing current and future assessment and practice data that inform decisions about program quality and improvement. Informed consent for participation in longitudinal data collection should be obtained early in training so as not to obscure interpretation of future results with nonresponse bias.[52,53] It is also appropriate to minimize the time after graduation when selected variables are measured, primarily to reduce the effect of confounding variables such as additional educational interventions and evolution in practice context.[56]

Some experts suggest the use of statistical methods that are less affected by the measurement constraints described here. The use of nonparametric (distribution-free) statistics, focusing on more extreme levels of performance, including high, and in particular, low or marginal performance, is probably more effective in identifying important educational variables.[50] Such an approach would involve categorizing grades or ratings into arbitrary categories. For example, on a 9-point scale, ratings of 1 through 3 would place in the "low" category, 4 to 6 in an intermediate category, and 7 to 9 in the high category for comparison purposes. One would then compare the frequencies in which graduates fall into the specific categories in areas that constitute important program objectives. Alternatively, distribution into various categories using both predictor (current) and criterion (future) assessment measures would provide important validity information regarding the value of selected assessment methods. In general, it makes more sense for program directors to consider those factors that predict subsequent incompetence or poor performance (or, vice versa, high academic standing or clinical excellence) as constituting more critical and useful information than factors associated with relatively small correlation differences among graduates. Educational leaders should keep in mind that instruments such as global rating scales, even in the hands of program directors, may not be sensitive in detecting deficiencies and providing accurate feedback to medical school educational leaders.[54] As suggested earlier, failure of a residency program director or subsequent employer to respond to requests for information on graduates should be followed up as this may indicate cause for concern, and important information may not be communicated.

Clinical Outcome Measures

The final product of the medical education process is the quality of care delivered to patients, and to that end, it is appropriate to measure health care outcomes for the patients and populations treated by program graduates. However, the collection of clinical outcomes data to support programmatic assessment introduces even more significant logistical and measurement challenges than those involved in assessing educational and professional outcomes. As with the measurement of educational outcomes, the logistical challenges involved in collecting clinical performance data from graduates is especially daunting in that they are likely to be spread across multiple residency programs or practice sites. Beyond the logistical challenges, evaluators will confront the usual measurement concerns associated with health care outcomes assessment such as instrument flaws, case mix and selection bias, and attribution problems. Indeed, much work is still needed to address the limitations of health care processes and outcomes assessment as an indicator of physician competence before one can consider the routine use of such criteria in evaluating prior educational experiences.[57] Skepticism about the relationship between educational processes and clinical outcomes, particularly when there is a period of time separating the two, provides yet another obstacle to the use of

clinical data to inform program quality improvement.[58] Practicing physicians perceive little contribution of undergraduate medical education to their later practice performance, but do feel that graduate medical education has a more significant effect on their future medical practice.[59]

Nevertheless, there are studies demonstrating a relationship between health care–related outcomes and to prior educational experiences, and the impact is measurable.[58] For example, residency program characteristics have been found to correlate with board certifying examination scores, which have then been shown to correlate with peer ratings of professional competence.[37,60] More direct relationships have been identified in comparing specific medical education setting or performance parameters and practice variables such as medication prescribing and likelihood of adverse licensing actions.[61,62] However, the above mentioned studies involved significant resources, relatively complex designs and large numbers of participants. Most educational programs will not have the resources or expertise to enjoin such large projects. One potential way to address the need to obtain data on the performance of program graduates is to combine efforts and resources across multiple programs along the continuum of education and practice, perhaps in the form of research partnerships, networks, or consortia. It makes sense to focus on commonly encountered conditions for which appropriate (or inappropriate) treatment has important and measurable effects.[58] It is also more likely that one can actually obtain such data. Finally, as specialty certification boards continue to progress in incorporating the assessment of performance in practice into maintenance of certification programs, the data generated from these activities may become a useful source of assessment information in the future.

Educational program leaders should consider the development of broad and long-term collaborations spanning undergraduate and graduate medical education and engage communities of like-minded individuals addressing the similar challenges imposed by maintenance of licensure and certification activities. National efforts toward developing a coherent system of physician evaluation that simultaneously and continuously serves the needs of health regulators, credentials providers, and medical educators will promote the development of an infrastructure and methodology for monitoring acquisition of competence and performance across the education-practice continuum.[63]

Conclusion

This final chapter summarized and built upon the preceding chapters in suggesting approaches to developing a sound evaluation system within an educational program. The need for a comprehensive approach to competence and performance assessment through development of a multimodal program is emphasized.

Also highlighted in this chapter, and throughout the book, are the critical importance of faculty development and the essential role that assessment plays in relation to educational objectives and experiences. This chapter also outlines an approach to program assessment that embraces similar principles in providing means to continuously improve educational programs. We hope that this book has been helpful and wish our readers success in developing their evaluation systems.

ACKNOWLEDGMENT

The authors wish to thank Louis Pangaro, MD, for his thoughtful review and suggestions for improving this chapter.

REFERENCES

1. Nelson EC, Batalden PB, Huber TP, et al: Microsystems in health care: Part 1. Learning from high-performing front-line clinical units. Jt Comm J Qual Improv 2002;28:472–493.
2. Donabedian A: Explorations in Quality Assessment and Monitoring, Vol. 1. The Definition of Quality and Approaches to Its Assessment. Ann Arbor, MI Health Administration Press, 1980.
3. Hiss RG, MacDonald R, David WR: Identification of physician educational influentials in small community hospitals. Res Med Educ 1978;17:288.
4. Holmboe ES, Bradley EH, Mattera JA, et al: Characteristics of physician leaders working to improve the quality of care in acute myocardial infarction. Jt Comm J Qual Saf 2003;29:289–296.
5. Brennan TA: Physicians' professional responsibility to improve the quality of care. Acad Med 2002;77:973–980.
6. Gruen RL, Pearson SD, Brennan TA: Physician-citizens—Public roles and professional obligations. JAMA 2004;291:94–98.
7. Lee AG, Carter KD: Managing the new mandate in resident education: A blueprint for translating a national mandate into local compliance. Ophthalmology 2004;111:1807–1812.
8. Jones DR, Dupras D, Ruffin AL: Importance of the perspective of residents in defining and maintaining quality in GME. Acad Med 1996;71:820–822.
9. Day SC, Grosso LJ, Norcini JJ Jr, et al: Residents' perception of evaluation procedures used by their training program. J Gen Intern Med 1990;5:421–426.
10. Cogbill KK, O'Sullivan PS, Clardy J: Residents' perception of effectiveness of twelve evaluation methods for measuring competency. Acad Psychiatry 2005;29:76–81.
11. Usatine RP, Edelstein RA, Yajima A, et al: Medical student perceptions of the accuracy of various new clinical evaluation methods. In Scherpbier AJJA, van der Vleuten CPM, Rethans JJ, van der Steeg AFW (eds): Advances in Medical Education. Dordrecht, Kluwer Academic, 1997, pp 200–202.
12. Lindblom-Ylanne S, Lonka K: Students' perceptions of assessment practices in a traditional medical curriculum. Adv Health Sci Educ Theory Pract 2001;6:121–140.
13. Mennin SP, Kalishman S: Student assessment. Acad Med 1998;73:S46–S54.
14. SWOT analysis. Wikipedia, Accessed March 1, 2007 at http://en.wikipedia.org/wiki/Swot_analysis.
15. Mavis B, Henry R, Hoppe R, et al: $100,000 shopping spree: The home version. Teach Learn Med 1999;11:44–47.
16. Nierenberg DW, Eliassen MS, McAllister SB, et al: A web-based system for students to document their experiences within six core competency domains during all clinical clerkships. Acad Med 2007;82:51–73.
17. Miller GE: The assessment of clinical skills/competence/performance. Acad Med 1990;65:S63–S67.
18. Holmboe ES, Hawkins RE: Methods for evaluating the clinical competence of residents in internal medicine: A review. Ann Intern Med 1998;129:42–48.
19. Pangaro L: A new vocabulary and other innovations for improving descriptive in-training evaluations. Acad Med 1999;74:1203–1207.
20. Pasquina PF, Kelly S, Hawkins RE: Assessing clinical competence in physical medicine and rehabilitation residency programs. Am J Phys Med Rehabil 2003;82:473–478.
21. Heard JK, Allen RM, Clardy J: Assessing the needs of residency program directors to meet the ACGME general competencies. Acad Med 2002;77:750.
22. Anderson J: Commentary on ''A Vision of Quality in Medical Education'' by Charles Suwanwela. Acad Med 1995;70:S38–S40.
23. Dunnington GL, Williams RG: Addressing the new competencies for residents' surgical training. Acad Med 2003;78:14–21.
24. Turnbull J, MacFadyen J, Van BC, Norman G: Clinical work sampling: A new approach to the problem of in-training evaluation. J Gen Intern Med 2000;15:556–561.
25. Turnbull J, Gray J, MacFadyen J: Improving in-training evaluation programs. J Gen Intern Med 1998;13:317–323.
26. Norcini JJ, Blank LL, Duffy FD, Fortna GS: The mini-CEX: A method for assessing clinical skills. Ann Intern Med 2003;138:476–481.
27. Fowell SL, Southgate LJ, Bligh JG: Evaluating assessment: The missing link. Med Educ 1999;33:276–281.
28. Lane JL, Gottlieb RP: Structured clinical observations: A method to teach clinical skills with limited time and financial resources. Pediatrics 2000;105:973–977.
29. Carraccio C, Englander R: Evaluating competence using a portfolio: A literature review and web-based application to the ACGME competencies. Teach Learn Med 2004;16:381–387.
30. Kassebaum DG: The measurement of outcomes in the assessment of educational program effectiveness. Acad Med 1990;65:293–296.
31. ACGME Timeline. ACGME Web site. Accessed on March 1, 2007 at www.acgme.org/acWebsite/home/home.asp.
32. Bordage G, Burack JH, Irby DM, Stritter FT: Education in ambulatory settings: Developing valid measures of educational outcomes, and other research priorities. Acad Med 1998;73:743–750.
33. Stone SL, Qualters DM: Course-based assessment: Implementing outcome assessment in medical education. Acad Med 1998;73:397–401.
34. Gastel BA: Toward a global consensus on quality medical education: Serving the needs of populations and individuals. Acad Med 1995;70:S73–S75.
35. Vroeijenstijn AI: Quality assurance in medical education. Acad Med 1995;70:S59–S67.
36. Suwanwela C: A vision of quality in medical education. Acad Med 1995;70:S32–S37.
37. Norcini JJ, Grosso LJ, Shea JA, Webster GD: The relationship between features of residency training and ABIM certifying examination performance. J Gen Intern Med 1987;2:330–336.
38. Lypson ML, Frohna JG, Gruppen LD, Woolliscroft JO: Assessing residents' competencies at baseline: Identifying the gaps. Acad Med 2004;79:564–570.
39. Woodward CA: Program evaluation. In Norman GR, van der Vleuten CPM, Newble DI (eds): International Handbook of Research in Medical Education. Dordrecht, Kluwer Academic, 2002, pp 127–155.
40. Gerrity MS, Mahaffy J: Evaluating change in medical school curricula: How did we know where we were going? Acad Med 1998;73:S55–S59.
41. Blumenthal D, Gokhale M, Campbell EG, Weissman JS: Preparedness for clinical practice: Reports of graduating residents at academic health centers. JAMA 2001;286:1027–1034.
42. Smith SR: Correlations between graduates' performances as first-year residents and their performances as medical students. Acad Med 1993;68:633–634.
43. Brown E, Rosinski EF, Altman DF: Comparing medical school graduates who perform poorly in residency with graduates who perform well. Acad Med 1993;68:806–808.
44. Papadakis MA, Teherani A, Banach MA, et al: Disciplinary action by medical boards and prior behavior in medical school. N Engl J Med 2005;353:2673–2682.
45. Blumberg P: Multidimensional outcome considerations in assessing the efficacy of medical educational programs. Teach Learn Med 2003;15:210–214.

46. EIP Program Requirements. ACGME Web site. Accessed on March 1, 2007 at www.acgme.org/acWebsite/home/home.asp.

47. Margolis MJ, Clauser BE, Cuddy MM, et al: Use of the mini-clinical evaluation exercise to rate examinee performance on a multiple-station clinical skills examination: A validity study. Acad Med 2006;81:S56–S60.

48. Arnold L, Willoughby TL: The empirical association between student and resident physician performances. In Gonnella JS, Hojat M, Erdmann JB, Veloski JJ (eds): Assessment Measures in Medical School, Residency, and Practice: The Connections. New York Springer, 1993, pp 71–82.

49. McGuire C: Perspectives in assessment. In Gonnella JS, Hojat M, Erdmann JB, Veloski JJ (eds): Assessment Measures in Medical School, Residency, and Practice: The Connections. New York Springer, 1993, pp 3–16.

50. Gonnella JS, Hojat M, Erdmann JB, Veloski JJ: A case of mistaken identity: signal and noise in connecting performance assessments before and after graduation from medical school. In Gonnella JS, Hojat M, Erdmann JB, Veloski JJ (eds): Assessment Measures in Medical School, Residency, and Practice: The Connections. New York Springer, 1993, pp 17–34.

51. Hojat M, Gonnella JS, Veloski JJ, Erdmann JB: Is the glass half full or half empty? A reexamination of the associations between assessment measures during medical school and clinical competence after graduation. In Gonnella JS, Hojat M, Erdmann JB, Veloski JJ (eds): Assessment Measures in Medical School, Residency, and Practice: The Connections. New York Springer, 1993, pp 137–152.

52. Verhulst SJ, Distlehorst LH: Examination of nonresponse bias in a major residency follow-up study. In Gonnella JS, Hojat M, Erdmann JB, Veloski JJ (eds): Assessment Measures in Medical School, Residency, and Practice: The Connections. New York Springer, 1993, pp 121–127.

53. Vu NV, Distlehorst LH, Verhulst SJ, Colliver JA: Clinical performance-based test sensitivity and specificity in predicting first-year residency performance. In Gonnella JS, Hojat M, Erdmann JB, Veloski JJ (eds): Assessment Measures in Medical School, Residency, and Practice: The Connections. New York Springer, 1993, pp 83–92.

54. Lavin B, Pangaro L: Internship ratings as a validity outcome measure for an evaluation system to identify inadequate clerkship performance. Acad Med 1998;73:998–1002.

55. Markert RJ: The relationship of academic measures in medical scholl to performance after graduation. In Gonnella JS, Hojat M, Erdmann JB, Veloski JJ (eds): Assessment Measures in Medical School, Residency and Practice: The Connection. New York Springer, 1993, pp 63–70.

56. Gonnella JS, Hojat M, Erdmann JB, Veloski JJ: What have we learned, and where do we go from here. In Gonnella JS, Hojat M, Erdmann JB, Veloski JJ (eds): Assessment Measures in Medical School, Residency, and Practice: The Connections. New York Springer, 1993, pp 155–173.

57. Norcini JJ: Current perspectives in assessment: The assessment of performance at work. Med Educ 2005;39:880–889.

58. Tamblyn R: Outcomes in medical education: What is the standard and outcome of care delivered by our graduates. Adv Health Sci Educ Theory Pract 1999;4:9–25.

59. Renschler HE, Fuchs U: Lifelong learning of physicians: Contributions of different educational phases to practice performance. Acad Med 1993;68:S57–S59.

60. Ramsey PG, Carline JD, Inui TS: Predictive validity of certification by the American Board of Internal Medicine. Ann Intern Med 1989;110:719–726.

61. Monette J, Tamblyn RM, McLeod PJ, Gayton DC: Characteristics of physicians who:frequently prescribe long-acting benzodiazepines for the elderly. Eval Health Prof 1997;20:115–130.

62. Teherani A, Hodgson CS, Banach M, Papadakis MA: Domains of unprofessional behavior during medical school associated with future disciplinary action by a state medical board. Acad Med 2005;80:S17–S20.

63. Physician Accountability for Physician Competence Summit. Innovation Labs Web site. Accessed March 1, 2007 at www.innovationlabs.com/innovation-workshops.html.

Index

Note: Page numbers followed by the letter f refer to figures; those followed by the letter t refer to tables; those followed by the letter b refer to boxes.